Primary Care Cardiology

SECOND EDITION

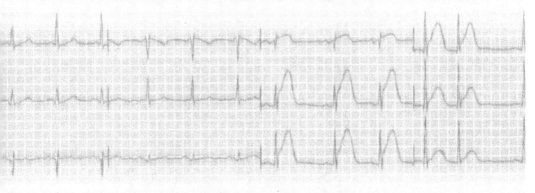

George J. Taylor

Primary Care Cardiology

SECOND EDITION

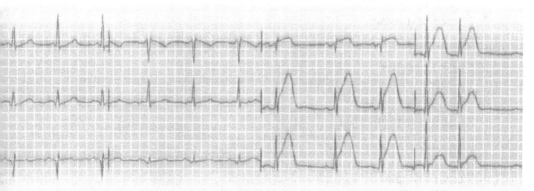

George J. Taylor

Professor of Medicine
The Medical University of South Carolina
Cardiology Clinics and Consult Service
The Ralph H. Johnson VA Medical Center
Charleston, South Carolina

Blackwell
Publishing

© 2005 by Blackwell Publishing

Blackwell Publishing, Inc., 350 Main Street, Malden, Massachusetts 02148-5018, USA
Blackwell Publishing Ltd, 9600 Garsington Road, Oxford OX4 2DQ, UK
Blackwell Publishing Asia Pty Ltd, 550 Swanston Street, Carlton, Victoria 3053, Australia

04 05 06 07 5 4 3 2 1

ISBN: 1-4051-0386-8

Library of Congress Cataloging-in-Publication Data

Taylor, George Jesse.
  Primary care cardiology: a complete guide for practitioners/George J. Taylor.—2nd ed.
    p. ; cm.
  Includes bibliographical references and index.
  ISBN 1-4051-0386-8 (pbk.)
  1. Heart—Diseases.   2. Cardiology.   3. Primary care (Medicine)
  [DNLM: 1. Cardiovascular Diseases—therapy.   2. Cardiovascular Diseases—diagnosis.
3. Primary Health Care. WG 166 T241pa 2004]   I. Title.
RC681.T39   2004
616.1'2—dc22

                                                                2004017775

A catalogue record for this title is available from the British Library

Acquisitions: Nancy Anastasi Duffy
Development: Kate Heinle
Production: Jennifer Kowalewski
Cover and Interior design: Leslie Haimes
Typesetter: International Typesetting and Composition in India

For further information on Blackwell Publishing, visit our website:
www.blackwellmedicine.com

Notice: The indications and dosages of all drugs in this book have been recommended
in the medical literature and conform to the practices of the general community. The medications described do not necessarily have specific approval by the Food and Drug Administration
for use in the diseases and dosages for which they are recommended. The package insert for each
drug should be consulted for use and dosage as approved by the FDA. Because standards for usage
change, it is advisable to keep abreast of revised recommendations, particularly those concerning
new drugs.

The publisher's policy is to use permanent paper from mills that operate a sustainable forestry
policy, and which has been manufactured from pulp processed using acid-free and elementary
chlorine-free practices. Furthermore, the publisher ensures that the text paper and cover board
used have met acceptable environmental accreditation standards.

To the memory of my father, George J. Taylor, III, MD

Table of Contents

Reviewers

Jason T. Bradley, MD
Cardiology Fellow
Texas Tech Medical Center
Lubbock, Texas

Andrea Charbonneau, MD, MSc
Assistant Professor of Medicine
Division of General and Geriatric Medicine
University of Kansas Medical Center
Kansas City, Kansas

Karen Fetzer, RN, FNP, PA-C
Physician Assistant, Transplant Surgery
Scripps Green Hospital
La Jolla, California

Laura L. Pickler MD, MPH
Instructor-Fellow, Family Medicine/Pediatrics
University of Colorado Health Sciences Center
Denver, Colorado

Preface

We spend about 60% of our time in adult medicine treating cardiovascular disease—hypertension, heart failure, dyslipidemia, cardiac arrhythmias, coronary and valvular heart disease. That is why the Internal Medicine and Family Medicine board exams tend to emphasize it. Our understanding and management of these illnesses have changed drastically over the decade following publication of the first edition of *Primary Care Cardiology*. There has been an explosion of clinical trials, and the treatment of heart disease is now evidence based.

The second edition of *Primary Care Cardiology* is a review of new management strategies that primary care physicians should incorporate into their practices. It also emphasizes basic principles critical to understanding and treating heart disease. For example, what is afterload? What is the difference between treating systolic and diastolic heart failure? What does surgical correction of mitral regurgitation do to left ventricular loading, and how does that affect the timing of surgery? What is the thallium scan, and how does pharmacologic stress testing work? How do statins, resins, and diet therapy lower cholesterol? What happens in the electrophysiology laboratory?

As a mixture of fundamentals and what is new, this is a curriculum for doctors who are studying for board examinations or recertification. It is also intended as a syllabus for students and house officers who are taking an elective cardiology rotation.

Primary Care Cardiology is not a comprehensive reference work. Rather, it provides a big picture, designed to be read through in a week. As a single author text, it describes the approach of a generalist in cardiovascular medicine. Academic appointment notwithstanding, I practice medicine full-time, and I write from the vantage point of having daily, hands-on experience with this material. My apologies if you find the tone of this book a bit casual. (I realize that this is a serious business!) Essentially, these are the conversations I have with students and house staff on the wards every day. When expressing opinion I try to make that clear. Most of the cited references are well-done review articles that summarize clinical trials, and I have avoided a literature review approach as much as possible.

My wife, Marilyn, is a patient woman, and I appreciate her forbearance during this writing adventure.

-*George J. Taylor*
Charleston, South Carolina
December 2004

CHAPTER 1

CONGESTIVE HEART FAILURE CAUSED BY SYSTOLIC DYSFUNCTION

Abbreviations

A_2	aortic second heart sound	ICD	implantable cardioverter-defibrillator
ACE	angiotensin converting enzyme		
AJT	abdominal-jugular test	JVP	jugular venous pressure (pulse)
ANP	atrial natriuretic peptide	LBBB	left bundle branch block
ARB	angiotensin receptor blocker	LV	left ventricle (ventricular)
AVP	arginine vasopressin	LVEF	LV ejection fraction
BiV	biventricular	MI	myocardial infarction
BNP	brain natriuretic peptide (or, type B natriuretic peptide)	MVO_2	myocardial oxygen demand
		P_2	pulmonic second heart sound
CBC	complete blood count	PMI	point of maximum impulse (LV apical impulse)
CHF	congestive heart failure		
ECG	electrocardiogram	RNA	radionuclide angiogram
EF	ejection fraction	RV	right ventricle

Epidemiology and Natural History

Congestive heart failure (CHF) is the clinical syndrome caused by insufficient cardiac output, leading to either pulmonary or systemic congestion. Extra-cardiac or valvular heart disease may limit cardiac output even though ventricular function is normal (see Chapters 2, 7, and 9), and there are rare cases of CHF with high cardiac output (Table 1.1). This is a review of CHF caused by ventricular dysfunction. Isolated failure of the right ventricle (RV) causes peripheral edema and splanchnic congestion. Left ventricular (LV) failure causes pulmonary congestion with symptoms progressing from exertional dyspnea to orthopnea, paroxysmal nocturnal dyspnea, and, eventually, pulmonary edema. Easy fatigue may be an early and subtle manifestation of both left and right heart failure.

There are 550,000 new cases of CHF diagnosed annually in the United States, and there has been an increase in the prevalence in the past decade.[1,2,3] It is the most common admitting diagnosis for elderly people, and the incidence of CHF more than doubles with each decade over age 45. This trend will progress, as reduced mortality in middle age from coronary artery disease leaves an older population at risk. Coronary artery disease is the most common cause of left ventricular systolic dysfunction and CHF (Table 1.1). Hypertension used to be a more

Table 1.1 Causes of Congestive Heart Failure (CHF)

Illnesses that inhibit ventricular filling, but do not effect ventricular function (result: low cardiac output)	Mitral stenosis (blocks LV filling) Pericardial tamponade or constriction (blocks RV filling)
Conditions influencing ventricular function, altering either preload or afterload (result: low cardiac output)	Aortic stenosis (high LV afterload) Aortic regurgitation (LV volume overload) Mitral regurgitation (LV volume overload) Pulmonic stenosis (high RV afterload) Tricuspid regurgitation (RV volume overload) Hypertensive heart disease (high LV afterload) Primary pulmonary hypertension (high RV afterload) Secondary pulmonary hypertension (high RV afterload caused by cor pulmonale, left heart failure, or Eisenmenger's syndrome)
Ilnesses causing LV systolic (contractile) dysfunction (result: low cardiac output)	Coronary artery disease (myocardial infarction) Idiopathic dilated cardiomyopathy Tachycardia induced cardiomyopathy (atrial fibrillation, incessant supraventricular tachycardia, or ventricular tachycardia) Viral myocarditis (Coxsackie A and B, echovirus, influenza A and B, polio virus, arbovirus, cytomegalovirus, mumps) Acute rheumatic fever (rheumatic myocarditis) Other bacterial and fungal infections Toxins (alcohol, cocaine, heroin, amphetamines, ethylene glycol, cobalt, lead, arsenic) Drugs (adriamycin, cyclophosphamides, sulfonamides, ipecac) Nutritional deficiencies (protein, thiamine, selenium, L-carnitine) Electrolyte disorders (low sodium, calcium, magnesium, or phosphate) Collagen vascular disease (lupus, rheumatoid arthritis, periarteritis nodosa, Reiter's syndrome, systemic sclerosis, Takaysau's syndrome, hypersensitivity vasculitis) Endocrine disorders (diabetes, hypo/hyperthyroidism, pheochromocytoma, hypoparathyroidism) Miscellaneous (peripartum cardiomyopathy, sleep apnea, hypereosinophillic syndrome, giant cell myocarditis)
Illnesses causing LV diastolic dysfunction (result: inadequate LV filling and low cardiac output, see Chapter 2)	Idiopathic diastolic dysfunction (usually elderly women) Hypertension Any cardiac condition that increases afterload and induces ventricular hypertrophy Hypertrophic cardiomyopathy (including idiopathic hypertrophic subaortic stenosis) Infiltrative cardiomyopathies or myocardial fibrosis (amyloidosis, sarcoidosis, hemochromatosis, other inflammatory conditions including collagen vascular disease)
High-output heart failure (in most cases high cardiac output alone does not lead to CHF, but precipitates it when there is underlying heart disease)	Anemia Thyrotoxicosis Arterio-venous fistulas (following trauma, A-V fistula for hemodialysis, Osler-Weber-Rendu disease, rupture of an aortic aneurysm into the inferior vena cava) Beriberi (thiamine deficiency may contribute to alcoholic heart disease; consider thiamine treatment when the cause of heart failure is obscure or there is an unusual dietary history) Paget's disease of bone

LV, left ventricular; RV, right ventricular; CHF, congestive heart failure common cause (it was in the initial Framingham study), but effective treatment of hypertension has changed this. Multiple other causes of LV dysfunction are surveyed in Table 1.1.

An interesting and recently discovered cause of LV dysfunction is persistent *tachycardia*; this is just now making it to board examinations.[4] Typically, a patient with a tachyarrhythmia—most commonly atrial fibrillation or flutter—is found to have a low LV ejection fraction (EF) on the echocardiogram. When the echocardiogram is repeated a few weeks after cardioversion or control of the ventricular rate, there is improvement in LVEF. Animal models using rapid atrial pacing show that LV function may decline within a couple days of the onset of tachycardia, and recovery begins soon after correcting it.[4]

Prognosis

Patient selection bias and differences in therapy have influenced assessment of prognosis with CHF in large clinical trials. For example, the Framingham study, conducted between 1949 and 1971, included a mix of patients with mild and severe CHF, and it reported a 40% 3-year mortality. However, in this pre-echocardiography era, the diagnosis of CHF was clinical; few patients had documentation of LV function, and many of them probably did not have CHF. Even with modern therapy, CHF remains a fatal illness with a 5-year mortality rate above 50% for those diagnosed currently.[2] The placebo arms of angiotensin-converting enzyme (ACE) inhibitor trials found a mortality rate of about one-third during 2–4 years of follow-up, and mortality paralleled the severity of symptoms. One-year mortality

Trial	n	Inclusion Criteria*	Therapy	Mean Follow-up	Treatment Mortality	Placebo Mortality
VHeFT-I	642	NYHA II-III EF < 45% CTR > 0.55	hydralazine/isordil vs. prazosin vs. placebo	30 mo	25% (hydralazine/ isordil)	34%
CONSENSUS	253	NYHA IV	enalapril vs. placebo	6 mo	25%	44%
VHeFT-II	804	NYHA II-III	hydralazine/isordil vs. enalapril	24 mo vs. enalapril	18% enalapril, 25% hydralazine/ isordil	NA
SOLVED	2561	NYHA II-III EF < 35%	enalapril vs. placebo	42 mo	35.2	39.7

Table 1.2 Effect of Afterload Reduction Therapy on Survival in CHF

* The New York Heart Association (NYHA) functional classes: I = no symptoms with physical activity but known disease, II = slight limitation of activity, symptoms with normal activity (but able to walk 3 blocks), III = symptoms with minimal activity and marked limitation of activity, IV = symptoms at rest and with any physical activity.

Table 1.3 Indicators of Poor Prognosis with Congestive Heart Failure

A. Functional Class

NYHA Class*	1-Year Mortality
I	5–10%
II–III	15–30%
IV	50–60%

B. Other Indicators of Poor Prognosis[†]

Clinical	Hemodynamic
Coronary artery disease etiology	Low LV ejection fraction
Resting tachycardia	Elevated LV end-diastolic pressure
Low blood pressure	Low cardiac output
Narrow pulse pressure	
S₃ gallop	
Cardiac cachexia	
Male gender	

Clinical laboratory	Cardiac rhythm
Low serum sodium	Sinus tachycardia
Elevated plasma renin activity and aldosterone	Atrial fibrillation
Elevated plasma norepinephrine	Frequent ventricular ectopic beats
Elevated BNP	Ventricular tachycardia
Low potassium, magnesium (increased arrhythmias)	
Increasing creatinine during hospitalization	

*New York Heart Association (NYHA) functional class: see footnote, Table 1.2.
[†] Thus, a patient with moderate symptoms (NYHA II–III) who also has resting tachycardia, low blood pressure, a gallop, and low serum sodium has an estimated 1-year mortality closer to 30%

for patients with class IV symptoms is 50–60%, and 15–30% for those with class II–III symptoms (Table 1.2).

There are a number of other clinical and laboratory markers of poor prognosis (Table 1.3). I teach students that LVEF is useful for determining survival in a general population, because it distinguishes normal from abnormal. However, when all patients in a population have low LVEF, the degree of depression of LVEF is not as predictive. For example, we encounter patients with LVEF below 20% who have good exercise tolerance and few CHF symptoms, and they tend to do well. By contrast, it is possible to have LVEF 30%, advanced CHF symptoms, and a poor prognosis.

The predictors of bad prognosis are usually found in combination. The patient with poor exercise tolerance, resting tachycardia (a particularly ominous finding), and an S₃ gallop often has low serum sodium and a high type B natriuretic peptide (BNP) level. When such a patient requires frequent hospitalization for control of congestion, or when diuresis is complicated by hypotension or worsening renal function, the prognosis is poor.[5]

Pathophysiology

Ventricular Anatomy and Function

The LV is thicker than the right. It works against a much higher pressure load, or *afterload*. Weight lifting builds muscle mass. What is true for the weight lifter's arms is true for heart muscle as well. Because aortic pressure is much higher than pulmonary artery pressure, the LV is more muscular than the RV. Increasing afterload increases the muscle mass of either of the ventricles, and lowering it allows a reduction in muscle mass. In the absence of infiltrative disease (i.e., amyloid or sarcoid), hypertrophy usually means high afterload.

The labels "right" and "left" ventricle do not accurately describe the position of the heart in the chest. Actually, the RV is positioned in front of (anterior to) the LV, and the plane of the interventricular septum is roughly parallel to the chest wall, positions that are readily apparent from the echocardiogram. The RV impulse, when palpable, is felt along the left parasternal border, and the RV is the first chamber punctured with an intracardiac injection.

Normally, the interventricular septum acts as a part of the LV. When you think about it, the septum has to choose sides, as it is anatomically a part of both ventricles. It chooses the side that is working hardest, normally the LV. On the echocardiogram (or with other imaging studies that show the heart in motion), the septum moves toward the posterior wall of the LV during systole, and away from the free wall of the RV. Conditions that produce RV overload or failure may lead to a reversal of this normal pattern, with the septum moving toward the RV and away from the LV during systole (this paradoxical septal motion is common with the volume overload of atrial septal defect, for example).

Cardiac Output and Ventricular Function

When all is said and done, what the body wants from the pump is blood flow. Output is the product of heart rate and the *stroke volume*, the volume ejected with each heartbeat. The units of measurement are fairly simple (Table 1.4). Increasing heart rate is an important early compensatory mechanism—the normal response to reduced cardiac output. In a normal young person, cardiac output goes up with increasing heart rate until the rate reaches 170–180 beats per minute, then it falls off, because there is not enough time between beats for ventricular filling. An elderly person with cardiac dysfunction may have cardiac output fall at rates above 150 beats per minute. Resting tachycardia, a rate above 100 beats per minute, is a commonly overlooked physical finding (perhaps because it is so easily measured); it indicates a bad prognosis in patients with CHF.

There are three things that influence ventricular stroke volume: preload, afterload, and contractility.

Preload—Precisely defined, preload is the length of each muscle fiber *before* contraction. When a strip of muscle is stimulated, it twitches and generates tension that can be measured. Within physiologic limits (meaning that the muscle is not

Table 1.4 Determinants of Cardiac Output and Stroke Volume
Cardiac Output (mL/min) = Heart rate (beats/min) × Stroke volume (mL/beat)
Stroke volume is augmented (+) or depressed (−) by 3 factors:
1 (+) Preload = the ventricular load or volume at the end of diastole. (Higher preload augments stroke volume.)
2 (−) Afterload = the load or resistance against which the ventricle empties during systole. (Higher afterload impedes the ventricle's ability to empty, lowering stroke volume.)
3 (+) Contractility = the basic state of ventricular muscle (its innate ability to contract independent of loading conditions—increased contractility, means greater ventricular emptying and greater stroke volume).

overstretched to the point of injury), increasing the resting length produces a stronger contraction (Figure 1.1). A century ago, Starling and others showed that this is as true for heart muscle as it is for skeletal muscle.

In the intact heart, muscle fiber length is proportional to ventricular diastolic volume. Thus, increased ventricular filling during diastole is the same as increased preload, and leads to more forceful contraction when the ventricle is stimulated. That is why volume expansion (salt and water retention) is a basic compensatory mechanism in heart failure. Increased vascular volume means increased venous return to both ventricles, an increase in ventricular diastolic volume, and higher stroke volume.

Ventricular diastolic volume may be measured using the echocardiogram, but continuous monitoring is not feasible. Instead, we take advantage of the fact that during diastole the ventricle works like a balloon, with volume proportional to pressure. Since LV diastolic pressure, or *filling pressure*, equals the pulmonary capillary

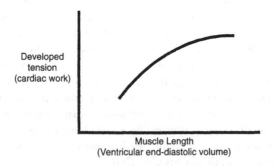

Figure 1.1 Ventricular function describing Starling's observation relating preload (muscle fiber length or ventricular volume just *before* ventricular contraction) and stroke volume (one measure of cardiac work) when the ventricle is then stimulated. With increased muscle fiber length, the strength of contraction increases. (Reprinted with permission from Taylor, GJ. The Cardiology Rotation. Malden, MA: Blackwell Science, 2001:6.)

bed pressure (there is no valve separating them during diastole), we use the pulmonary artery catheter to monitor ventricular preload (the *pulmonary capillary wedge pressure*). When a clinical trial reports that a drug produces a fall in the pulmonary wedge pressure, it is equivalent to saying that preload, vascular volume, and congestion are reduced.

A word about congestion: Because increasing preload increases stroke volume and cardiac output, it would seem that treatments to expand volume would be useful when ventricular function is depressed. But there is a limit to how much volume can be tolerated. When salt and water are retained and the pulmonary capillary hydrostatic pressure exceeds 25 mm Hg, the oncotic pressure that keeps fluid in the vascular space is overcome, and fluid is pushed into the interstitial space. The result is congestion, placing a limit on volume expansion and the Starling mechanism's capacity to compensate for low cardiac output.

Afterload—This is the load the ventricle works against when it contracts, during systole. Aortic or pulmonic valve stenosis impedes flow and raises afterload, and both induce ventricular hypertrophy. In the absence of ventricular outflow tract obstruction, vascular resistance and blood pressure provide rough approximations of afterload. Patients with hypertension have increased afterload, and LV hypertrophy is the first event in the development of hypertensive heart disease.

On the other hand, afterload may be reduced with no apparent change in blood pressure. The hydraulics equation (a.k.a. Ohm's law) states that *pressure = flow x resistance*. Thus, a vasodilator drug that lowers resistance by 20%, but that allows cardiac output (flow) to increase by 20%, causes no change in blood pressure. That is why vasodilator (afterload-reducing) therapy may be used in patients with CHF and low blood pressure.

On the ventricular function curve, a reduction in afterload produces a shift up and to the left (Figure 1.2). Reducing afterload with vasodilator therapy improves ventricular performance and cardiac output without increasing the myocardium's workload.

Hypertrophy, wall tension, and myocardial oxygen demand—The heart responds to increased afterload with an increase in contractility, and eventually, with hypertrophy. Myocardial oxygen demand (MVO_2) is proportional to wall tension, and tension is determined by the interplay of ventricular pressure and size described by Laplace's law (Box 1.1). A dilated ventricle thus has higher wall tension than a smaller one, and requires more oxygen. Interestingly, an increase in wall thickness tends to reduce tension and therefore MVO_2 (this may be the stimulus for hypertrophy). Conditions that lead to ventricular dilatation without hypertrophy, the usual case with dilated cardiomyopathy, may be considered maladaptive remodeling (Figure 1.3).

Laplace's law applies to many areas of medicine. A dilated aorta, loop of bowel, pulmonary bleb, or uterus all have increased wall tension, and are thus more prone to rupture.

Contractility—This third determinant of stroke volume is defined as an increase in the force of contraction when both preload and afterload are constant. Another

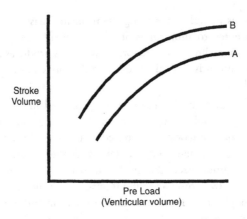

Figure 1.2 Manipulations that alter the ventricular function curve. Increasing *contractility* or reducing *afterload* shifts the curve up and to the left, from curve A to curve B. Thus, with either manipulation stroke volume is higher for a given preload. For this reason, drugs that augment contractility or reduce afterload are useful therapies for CHF. What about diuretics? They reduce vascular volume and thus reduce preload; the ventricular function curve does not shift, and the patient moves down and to the left on the same curve. Stroke volume falls, but this is a necessary intervention to reduce pulmonary congestion. (Reprinted with permission from Taylor, GJ. The Cardiology Rotation. Malden, MA: Blackwell Science, 2001:11.)

name for contractility is the *inotropic* state. In the muscle cell, the interaction of calcium ions with the contractile proteins initiates contraction. Increased calcium influx upon excitation leads to greater contractility (as with digitalis or catecholamines), and reduced calcium influx depresses contractility (as with the calcium channel blocker, verapamil, and beta adrenergic blockers).

Box 1.1 Chamber Size, Wall Tension, and Pressure: Laplace's Law

(A physical principle that applies to many areas of medicine.)

The law of Laplace describes the determinants of wall stress (or "tension"), and applies to any "container" of a fluid volume that has measurable intracavitary pressure. This would include chambers of the heart, blood vessels, airways, loops of bowel, the uterus, etc.

$$\text{Wall stress} = (\text{Pressure}) (\text{Radius}) / 2 (\text{Wall thickness})$$

Left ventricular wall stress is proportional to myocardial oxygen demand (MVO_2). A dilated LV or one with pressure overload requires more oxygen. Increased LV thickness, hypertrophy, tends to "normalize" wall stress, and therefore MVO_2, of the pressure overloaded or dilated LV.

This relationship is also important when gauging the possibility of rupture of an aneurysm, dilated loop of bowel, pulmonary bleb, etc. With higher wall stress there is an increased chance of rupture. The size of the chamber (radius) thus determines the "burst" pressure. Increased wall thickness reduces the chance of rupture. Thus, a thin-walled LV aneurysm is more likely to rupture than an equally dilated LV with normal wall thickness.

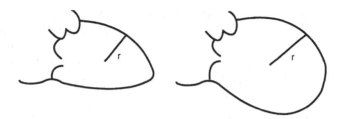

Figure 1.3 Ventricular "remodeling." The left ventricle is normally an ellipsoid (*left*). With the development of cardiomyopathy it enlarges and also changes shape, becoming more spherical (*right*). Both changes increase the radius of curvature (r), and this increases wall tension (see Box 1.1 for a description of Laplace's law). Wall tension is proportional to myocardial oxygen demand, so the remodeling process aggravates LV dysfunction. (Reprinted with permission from Taylor, GJ. The Cardiology Rotation. Malden, MA: Blackwell Science, 2001:13.)

An increase in contractility leads to a shift in the ventricular function curve to the left; there is an increase in stroke volume for a given preload (Figure 1.3).

Ejection fraction (EF)—A common measure of systolic function is ejection fraction, or that portion of blood ejected from the ventricle during systole. Thus, if the LV contains 150 mL at the end of diastole, and 50 mL at the end of systole, the LVEF equals 67%, and the stroke volume is 100 mL. It may be calculated by measuring the volume of the LV at end-diastole, and again at end-systole using either the LV angiogram or echocardiogram. It may also be measured with radionuclide techniques, measuring radioisotope counts at end-diastole and end-systole and doing the arithmetic.

EF is a measure of muscle shortening, and like stroke volume, it depends on both contractility and loading conditions. Increased contractility and reduced afterload both increase EF. However, stroke volume and EF cannot be equated. A dilated LV with a diastolic volume of 210 mL and an ejection fraction of 33% has a stroke volume of 70 mL. So does a normal ventricle of 140 mL and EF of 50%. This simple math indicates another way that ventricular dilatation compensates for LV dysfunction.

Neurohormonal Response to Low Cardiac Output

CHF due to systolic dysfunction is instigated by some insult to LV pump function, and the decrease in cardiac output provokes a neuroendocrine compensatory response. Best understood are the adrenergic nervous system and the renin-angiotensin-aldosterone systems. They are known to cross-regulate, with activation of one leading to activation of the other.

The immediate goal is maintenance of cardiac output and flow to vital organs, especially the kidneys, which function as a hemodynamic thermostat. Decreased renal blood flow turns on the renin-angiotensin-aldosterone system. Aldosterone promotes salt and water retention, boosting intravascular volume, ventricular preload, and cardiac output. Another immediate response to inadequate cardiac output is an increase in sympathetic tone with elevation of circulating catecholamines. This increases heart rate and contractility. Activation of both the adrenergic and renin-angiotensin systems causes vasoconstriction, which helps maintain blood pressure and flow to the kidneys and other vital organs. A byproduct of this increased vascular resistance is elevated LV afterload.

These responses to depressed flow help restore cardiac output over the short term. However, over the long run there may be adverse consequences. The increase in ventricular volume with fluid retention increases stroke volume, but this remodeling of the ventricle eventually is maladaptive because ventricular dilatation increases wall tension (the Laplace response, Box 1.1). High circulating catecholamines and angiotensin increase peripheral resistance, and therefore LV afterload, which provokes hypertrophy. More commonly, the patient with dilated cardiomyopathy is unable to mount a hypertrophic response, so LV wall tension and MVO_2 remain high.

The most important discovery about neurohormones is myocardial toxicity with sustained exposure. In addition to hemodynamic effects, norepinephrine and aldosterone function as growth hormones for myocytes and fibroblasts. At elevated levels, toxic effects may include accelerated cell death and/or fibrosis (increased myocyte apoptosis has been described).

History and Physical Examination

Left heart failure causes pulmonary congestion, right heart failure causes peripheral and splanchnic congestion. You hear that LV failure is the most common cause of RV failure, and that is true. Curiously, an occasional patient with biventricular failure has severe peripheral edema and ascites with minimal or no pulmonary congestion. Elderly patients with CHF may present with vague symptoms that do not point to heart failure, such as fatigue or a change in exercise tolerance. For all patients, history-taking should include a survey for conditions that may cause or aggravate CHF: myocardial infarction (MI) with few or subtle symptoms, viral illnesses, a family history of cardiomyopathy, alcohol use, and gastrointestinal symptoms that suggest blood loss and anemia.

General Examination

Frailty is not a nebulous physical finding, and its presence indicates a poor cardiac prognosis. An experienced surgeon often asked this question in cath conference, when discussing a high-risk surgical candidate: "How brightly does the fire of life burn in this patient?"

Cardiac cachexia is a diagnosis of exclusion. When weight loss develops in a patient with chronic heart failure, you must first exclude another etiology. Remember that occult bacterial endocarditis may cause weight loss in a patient with valvular disease. The pathophysiology of cachexia caused by heart failure is multifactorial. Anorexia is a common symptom of right heart failure because of splanchnic and hepatic congestion. Rarely, right heart failure may cause protein-losing enteropathy. Severe salt restriction may aggravate anorexia; food does not taste as good. Digitalis toxicity may contribute to anorexia, which may occur with a digoxin level in a therapeutic range. There may also be increased caloric needs. Both increased cardiac work (e.g., aortic stenosis or regurgitation) and the increased work of breathing with chronic pulmonary congestion increase caloric expenditure. More recently, patients with chronic heart failure have been found to have higher levels of the proinflammatory cytokine, *tumor necrosis factor*, and this may contribute to cachexia. Important physical findings include bitemporal and hypothenar wasting.

Vital signs—Resting tachycardia is a powerful sign of decompensation in a patient with chronic CHF, and it is a marker of poor prognosis. When present, it can be the most important physical finding. Systolic hypotension and narrow pulse pressure often accompany low stroke volume. Wide pulse pressure, on the other hand, is a finding of aortic regurgitation (or anemia or thyrotoxicosis—in all cases the mechanism is vasodilatation).

Jugular veins—There are three parts to this examination: estimation of venous pressure, testing for abdominojugular reflux, and assessment of the venous waveform. The sternal angle, or angle of Lewis, is 5 cm above the level of the right atrium. Thus, if the top of the distended vein is 3 cm above the sternal angle, right atrial pressure is 8 cm H_2O. Pressure greater than 7–8 cm water is abnormal (that is to say, a central venous column that is more than 2–3 cm above the angle). The patient may be examined in any position, and the optimal angle of inclination depends on the venous pressure. With high pressure, you may not see the top of the venous column unless the patient is sitting upright. With low pressure, it may be necessary to have the patient almost flat to see a distended vein.

In most cases, high venous pressure indicates high right atrial pressure. An exception is *superior vena cava obstruction*. In this case, there is no venous pulsation, because the veins are isolated from the heart. Furthermore, the vein fills from above and not from below.

Abdominal-jugular test (AJT)—I would guess that most doctors perform this test rarely, but I find it useful for making clinical decisions. It is also called *hepato-jugular reflux*. The maneuver is performed with the patient breathing normally (breath-holding may raise pressure). Push down in the periumbilical area for 10 seconds. When normal, there is a transient rise in venous pressure, less than 3 cm. A greater and more sustained rise occurs with *both right and left heart failure* as well as with tricuspid regurgitation. Although proposed as a test for *right heart* failure, most with a positive AJT have elevation of both pulmonary wedge and right atrial pressures (probably because right heart failure is usually caused by left heart failure).

The AJT is useful in determining the cause of peripheral edema when there is no jugular venous distention. If the AJT is negative, heart failure is less likely. The edema must be from some other cause (e.g., calcium channel blocker therapy, veno-occlusive disease, low albumen, lymphatic obstruction). It is useful for deciding whether there is early volume overload in a patient without edema or pulmonary congestion. When the AJT is negative, the patient probably is not volume overloaded, and current diuretic therapy is adequate (or perhaps excessive).

Jugular venous pulse waveform—Because there is no valve separating the right atrium from the superior vena cava and jugular veins, the pressure of atrial contraction is reflected back to the veins. Venous pressure waves are conveniently labeled: the A wave is generated by atrial contraction, and the V wave, by ventricular contraction.

To examine the pulse, have the patient breathe normally in a position where you can see venous pulsation through the sternocleidomastoid muscle (the internal jugular pulse) or pulsation of the more easily seen external jugular vein. Feel the brachial pulse while watching the vein to distinguish systole from diastole. *If the dominant venous pulse occurs before the brachial pulse (arterial systole), it is an A wave. If the dominant pulse occurs simultaneously with the arterial pulse, it is a V wave.* I state what I have observed on the chart: "JVP: A >V" (a normal examination), or "V > A" (an abnormal examination).

The V wave is created by RV systole, by either backward bulging of the tricuspid valve leaflets or slight backward movement of the valve ring during ventricular contraction. It is normally quite small. With an incompetent tricuspid valve the RV is no longer isolated from the atrium and veins during systole, and ventricular systolic pressure is transmitted back to the neck veins. A big V wave is not a subtle finding, and you have only to document that the dominant venous pulse wave is systolic (simultaneous with the arterial pulse). Look for a pulsatile liver, RV lift, and holosystolic murmur to confirm tricuspid regurgitation.

A giant A wave indicates high right ventricular diastolic pressures. This usually occurs with pulmonary hypertension (the Eisenmenger syndrome, primary pulmonary hypertension, or recurrent pulmonary emboli), or with pulmonic valve stenosis. Tricuspid valve stenosis or atresia is rare but potential cause. Right ventricular failure does not cause a giant A wave unless there is also pulmonary hypertension.

Be aware that the A wave in a normal person may be of such low amplitude that it is not visible. Instead, the most obvious event may be the collapse of the venous column after atrial contraction, at a time of rapid filling of the now-empty atrium. This prominent x descent occurs early during ventricular systole, and is a normal finding.

Examination of the chest—Inspection of the chest and the pattern of breathing shows little abnormality when CHF is mild or moderate. *Cheyne-Stokes respiration*, a cyclical breathing pattern with progressively deeper breaths followed by a brief period of apnea, may occur with advanced heart failure. It is caused, in part, by decreased sensitivity of the respiratory center of the brain to CO_2, and is more likely to develop in patients with cerebral pathology. It is aggravated by anything that further depresses the respiratory center including sleep, narcotics, and some sedatives (particularly barbiturates).

Advanced obstructive lung disease with a barrel-shaped deformity of the chest may point to cor pulmonale as the cause of right heart failure. Kyphoscoliosis may also cause cor pulmonale.

Increased respiratory rate and greater effort of breathing may accompany severe pulmonary congestion as well as obstructive lung disease. *Patients with emphysema and hyperexpansion may not have audible rales with congestion; a chest x-ray is needed to exclude congestion (this is always a board question).*

Pleural effusion may be a sign of either right heart or left heart congestion. Both the systemic and pulmonary circulations drain the pleural space. Physical findings include deviation of the trachea away from the effusion, absence of fremitus (palpable breath sounds), dullness to percussion, and softer or absent breath sounds. Heart failure is the most common cause of effusion; when it is unilateral, it usually occurs on the right side. An isolated left-sided effusion suggests a non-cardiac etiology.

Rales may be caused by heart or lung disease. I frequently hear inexperienced examiners describe rales as either "wet" (cardiac) or "dry" (pulmonary). However, when dealing with fine crackles, it is impossible to distinguish between the two based only on the quality of the sounds. More reliable is the *timing* of rales. With heart failure and early pulmonary congestion, fine crackles occur late in inspiration (end-inspiratory rales), and they are best heard at the bases of the lungs. Pulmonary fibrosis also causes fine crackles, but these rales are usually heard throughout inspiration (pan-inspiratory rales). The rales of pulmonary fibrosis may be isolated to the apices of the lungs or audible throughout the chest.

It helps to understand the mechanism of rales in heart failure and *interstitial* congestion. You are not hearing bubbles. Instead, the crackles are caused by the opening of collapsed airways. In the absence of congestion, there is little airway closure during expiration (Figure 1.4). However, lungs heavy with interstitial congestion have closure of small airways at a higher lung volume than is usual (it is the weight of the interstitium that is the problem). Thus, the airways close during normal expiration. To use the pulmonary physiology term, there is elevated *closing volume*. With subsequent inspiration, an even higher lung volume is needed to pop open the collapsed units, and the rales are thus end-inspiratory.

Wheezing is usually a sign of airway obstruction. It may develop in a patient with pulmonary congestion (cardiac asthma). Occasionally, an acutely ill older patient with wheezing and severe dyspnea may not have audible rales. The absence of a history of asthma points to the cardiac diagnosis, and the chest x-ray readily confirms pulmonary edema.

The Cardiac Examination

Apical impulse—The location of the point of maximum impulse (PMI) should be determined with the patient lying flat. Its normal location is the midclavicular line and fifth intercostal space. It is tapping in quality and occupies a space of no more than 2 cm. Left ventricular hypertrophy may not displace the PMI, but it becomes

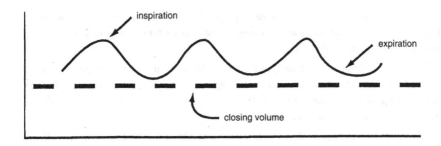

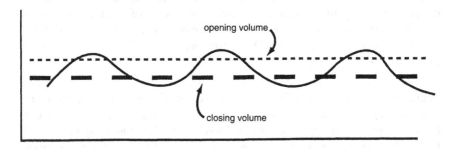

Figure 1.4 The pathophysiology of rales in congestive heart failure. In the normal state (*top*), the lung volume at which airways start to collapse, the "closing volume," is not reached during normal expiration. Pulmonary congestion changes this (*bottom*). The waterlogged lungs weigh heavily on the airways, and they collapse at a higher lung volume. Because the threshold for airway collapse has risen, the small airways close during normal expiration. Even greater volume is needed to pop the collapsed airways open, and that happens nearer to the end of the inspiration. For this reason, the inspiratory crackles of *interstitial* congestion occur at *end*-inspiration. The rales of pulmonary fibrosis (dry rales) are pain-inspiratory. (Reprinted with permission from Taylor, GJ. The Cardiology Rotation. Malden, MA: Blackwell Science, 2001:19.)

more forceful, like a fist hitting your hand. Systolic dysfunction and left ventricular volume overload and dilatation causes displacement of the PMI toward the anterior axillary line, and enlargement of the apex beat so that it may be felt in more than one interspace. The volume overload apical impulse is diffuse and rocking in quality.

A right ventricular impulse is not palpable in normal patients. RV pressure or volume overload produces a lift along the left parasternal border. When the lift is forceful and sustained, it suggests pressure overload. Volume overload causes a lift that is not sustained through systole.

The parasternal lift can be augmented by left atrial enlargement. The atrium is behind the right ventricle, and pushes it forward when enlarged. A rare patient with severe mitral regurgitation and left atrial enlargement may have a late-systolic parasternal lift in the absence of right ventricular enlargement.

Emphysema changes the position of the heart in the chest. There is clockwise rotation, and the left ventricle is more posterior. The heart seems to hang vertically on the chest x-ray. The PMI that is felt in the subxiphoid region comes from the RV, not the LV. A forceful and sustained apex beat in this position may reflect right ventricular hypertrophy secondary to pulmonary hypertension (*cor pulmonale*).

Heart sounds—CHF usually has no effect on S_1 and S_2. The intensity of both sounds may be diminished with advanced heart failure and severely depressed cardiac output. An especially loud S_1 may be an early finding of mitral valve stenosis, a potential cause of CHF. Similarly, an absent A_2 may indicate severe calcific aortic stenosis in an elderly patient. The rigid valve eventually stops moving, and A_2 disappears. To detect this, listen in both the pulmonic and aortic areas. P_2 is audible at the left sternal border but not to the right of the sternum. Thus, an absent S_2 at the right base indicates an immobile and probably stenotic aortic valve.

Gallops—These are low pitched sounds. The best way to hear a soft gallop is to concentrate on the segment of the cardiac cycle where it should be found. Thus, to hear S_3, listen to the space just after S_2, ignoring all other cardiac sounds. Ask yourself, "is there anything there?" If there is a soft thud, you are probably hearing a gallop. Occasionally the gallop is something you feel rather than hear. If you are convinced there is no sound in that space, there is no gallop.

Both of the left ventricular gallops are soft, and may be more audible with the patient rolled to the left side. The room must be quiet. As the sounds are low-pitched, use the bell of the stethoscope taking care not to press too firmly (which would, by tensing the underlying skin, make it work like the diaphragm). The S_3 may be localized, and you must carefully survey the apex and areas close to it. It may be hard to hear gallops in the patient with a thick chest wall. In such cases, the fourth heart sound (S_4) may be easier to hear over the sternum (bone conduction providing an aid). The timing of gallops is easier with a hand on the brachial pulse to identify systole. The S_4 is a presystolic sound, and the S_3, an early diastolic (protodiastolic) sound.

Think for a moment about the significance of gallops and the quality of the apical impulse. They are the physical findings that give you direct information about the state of the ventricle. Murmurs get a lot of attention, but they do not tell us much about the severity of disease. The gallops do just that: they tell us about ventricular size, function, and compliance.

- **S_3 gallop = big flabby ventricle (volume overload):** The low-pitched vibration in early diastole comes from rapid ventricular filling. The mechanism is related to both (1) high flow, and (2) the recipient ventricle being dilated and compliant. Any condition that causes ventricular dilatation and low cardiac output (with compensatory volume overload) may cause an S_3. It is the hallmark finding of dilated cardiomyopathy, regardless of the etiology, and it indicates poor prognosis.

- **S_4 gallop = stiff, noncompliant ventricle (pressure overload):** This gallop at the end of diastole corresponds to elevation of the ventricular end-diastolic pressure, and the A wave of the precordial impulse (Figure 1.5). It may be called the *atrial gallop*, because atrial contraction pushing the last increment of blood into a stiff

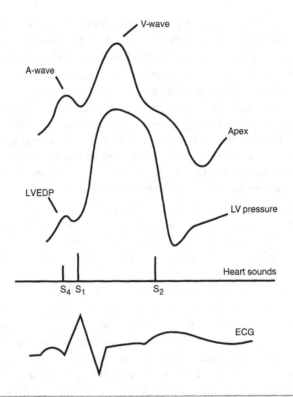

Figure 1.5 The contour of the LV apical impulse (*top tracing*) mirrors the LV pressure tracing. Just before ventricular systole, atrial contraction causes a small rise in LV pressure that is measured as the LV end-diastolic pressure (LVEDP). This is elevated in conditions that increase LV stiffness. It makes sense; the atrium is kicking into a ventricle that has higher pressure during diastole (it is stiff when it should be relaxed). When the apical A wave is greater than 15% of the total apical excursion, it is palpable as a shudder or glitch on the upstroke of the impulse. This is a reliable indicator of elevated LVEDP and is audible as the S_4 gallop. (Reprinted with permission from Taylor, GJ. The Cardiology Rotation. Malden, MA: Blackwell Science, 2001:23.)

ventricle generates the sound. The S_4 is absent when there is no atrial kick (e.g., atrial fibrillation, ventricular pacing, nodal or ventricular rhythms, or complete heart block). Any increase in ventricular stiffness may cause an S_4, including ventricular hypertrophy, infiltrative disease, and ischemia.

Note that I have referred to *ventricular* rather than *left ventricular* gallops. Right ventricular disease may produce gallop sounds, best heard over the left parasternal area. They may be subxiphoid in the patient with obstructive lung disease. RV gallops are augmented by inspiration (increased venous return and flow to the RV). I have had little luck hearing the right-side S_3 gallop; listen for it with tricuspid regurgitation and isolated right heart failure. The right-side S_4 that accompanies pulmonary hypertension is easier to hear (note the parallel with LV disease: volume overload causes the S_3; pressure overload, the S_4).

When the heart rate is fast, it may be impossible to determine whether the gallop occurs early or late in diastole. An occasional patient with ventricular dilatation may also have increased stiffness, and thus have both S_3 and S_4 gallops that are fused when the heart rate is elevated. In both cases, the patient is said to have a *summation* gallop. A "gallop rhythm" refers to this combination of sounds when the rate is high (it sounds like a galloping horse).

Heart murmurs—A loud murmur may indicate that the cause of heart failure is valvular disease. On the other hand, ventricular dilation tends to distort the orientation of the papillary muscles, and this may cause mild tricuspid or mitral regurgitation (MR). The resulting systolic murmur is usually soft. A mildly leaking valve does not aggravate ventricular dysfunction, but more severe mitral regurgitation may. Unfortunately, when severe MR is the result of a dilated, hypocontractile LV, mitral valve repair is not feasible (see Chapter 7).

Laboratory Examination

In addition to the comprehensive history and physical examination, all patients suspected of having CHF should routinely have the following studies: CBC and urinalysis, serum chemistries including electrolytes, renal function tests, liver function tests, albumin and thyroid function studies (especially over age 65 years or if in atrial fibrillation), chest x-ray, ECG, and echocardiogram with Doppler flow studies. These tests are used to: (1) confirm the diagnosis of CHF, (2) to rule out specific causes of heart failure such as occult valvular disease, and (3) to exclude conditions that may aggravate CHF (Tables 1.5 and 1.6).

Measurement of left ventricular ejection fraction—Demonstration of reduced LVEF is required for the diagnosis of CHF due to systolic dysfunction. While it is especially useful for determining prognosis in population studies, LVEF can be misleading when trying to predict outcome for the individual patient.

When there is an apparent disconnect between measured LVEF and symptoms, the clinical picture—especially functional class—tends to be a better predictor of outcome (Table 1.3). This is especially true when evaluating a patient with coronary artery disease who needs bypass surgery; a patient with good exercise tolerance and no clinical CHF can usually get through an operation, even when LVEF is low.

The echocardiogram is the most commonly used test to assess LV function. It also defines LV regional wall motion. A segmental or regional wall motion abnormality, a region that is akinetic, suggests prior infarction and therefore coronary artery disease, while global hypokinesis is more consistent with nonischemic cardiomyopathy.

Modern echo equipment includes image analysis programs that automatically measure LVEF, but more often the report describes the reader's estimate of LVEF. Studies have shown that an experienced reader's assessment is fairly reliable, but remember that it is still qualitative. When you are given an LVEF range, it is certainly the reader's estimate. The one time this may create a problem for the patient is in cases of cardiac disability. The Social Security Administration criterion for disability due to CHF is an LVEF of 30% or less. If your patient with clinically

Table 1.5 Diagnostic Studies Useful in the Initial Evaluation of Patients with Suspected Congestive Heart Failure

Laboratory Study	Clinical Issue(s)
CBC with differential	Anemia (may aggravate CHF; exclude high output failure)
Serum chemistry profile	Electrolyte disturbances Diabetes mellitus Renal insufficiency Hypoproteinemia
Thyroid function tests	Hyper/hypothyroidism
Urinalysis	Proteinuria (nephrotic syndrome, acute glomerulonephritis—both causes of edema)
ECG	Myocardial infarction Ventricular hypertrophy
Chest x-ray	Confirm congestion as the cause of dyspnea (especially important when there is obstructive lung disease) Pulmonary infiltrates/fibrosis Presence of pleural effusion
Echocardiogram	Differentiate systolic vs. diastolic dysfunction Document LV dysfunction and chamber size Wall motion abnormalities (CAD as an etiology) Valve abnormalities Pericardial effusion Intracardiac masses

CAD=coronary artery disease; CBC=complete blood count; CHF=congestive heart failure; ECG=electrocardiogram; LV=left ventricular.

significant CHF has an echo report with "LVEF 30–35%," you might ask the reader to review it with the clinical information in mind and, possibly, to redictate the report if the LVEF might just as easily be 28–30%. I believe that this is a fair request. The interpretation of laboratory and imaging data is always better when all clinical data are considered (a radiologist does a better job reading a chest x-ray knowing the patient has cough and fever).

A *radionuclide angiogram* (RNA), also called a MUGA scan, may be used to measure LVEF. Although more expensive, it may work when the echocardiogram is technically inadequate (often a problem with large patients or those with emphysema). Red blood cells from the patient are labeled with an isotope, and the cells are re-injected. This blood pool label allows scanning over the heart during peak systole and peak diastole. The math is simple: if there are 100,000 counts from the LV at end-diastole, and 50,000 counts at peak systole, the LVEF is 50%.

Coronary artery disease should be excluded, especially in younger patients with CHF and no apparent cause. A patient with ischemic cardiomyopathy usually has a

Table 1.6 Ancillary Diagnostic Testing for Congestive Heart Failure	
Diagnostic Study Laboratory Studies	Indication/Suspected Etiology
Serum iron/ferritin	Hemochromatosis
ACE level	Sarcoidosis
Toxicology screening	Heavy metal toxicity/other environmental toxins
Blood cultures	Bacterial and fungal infectious etiologies
Viral titers	Viral myocarditis
Sedimentation rate, ANA, rheumatoid factor	Collagen vascular disease
Radionuclide angiogram	Poor quality echocardiogram
Stress perfusion studies*	Patients with CHF without angina but with an intermediate risk of coronary artery disease as a possible etiology. Determination of myocardial viability in patients who may be candidates for revascularization.
Coronary angiography	All patients with CHF and a history consistent with angina or myocardial infarction (with or without recurrent angina). Patients with CHF and significant risk factors for coronary artery disease.
Hemodynamic monitoring (tailored therapy)**	Patients who respond poorly to initial empiric therapy (initiation of tailored therapy).
Endomyocardial biopsy	see text

*Non-ischemic cardiomyopathy may show patchy perfusion abnormalities.
**Tailoring therapy requires hemodynamic monitoring, then optimizing filling pressures and cardiac output with a combination of intravenous iotropes and vasodilators, then substituting oral medicines.
ACE, angiotensin-converting enzyme; ANA, anti-nuclear antibodies; CHF, congestive heart failure.

history of MI plus Q waves on the ECG, but not always. When the index of suspicion is low (e.g. no coronary risk factors, ECG findings, or suggestive symptoms), a perfusion scan may be adequate. When there is uncertainty, or when coronary disease seems likely, go directly to coronary angiography.

Brain natriuretic peptide—Brain natriuretic peptide (BNP) is synthesized and released from ventricular myocardium in response to myocyte stretch (it was first isolated from brain, hence the confusing name). Atrial natriuretic peptide (ANP) has similar properties but is less prominent in CHF.

BNP release is a counter-regulatory response to the actions of the sympathetic and renin-angiotensin-aldosterone systems. Short-term it does not boost cardiac output, but its long-term beneficial actions include natriuresis, sympathetic and renin-angiotensin system blockade, and direct venous and arterial dilatation (reducing both preload and afterload). When the LV fails, there is an increase in LV diastolic pressure and fiber length, and myocytes release BNP; a normal level excludes decompensated heart failure. This is true for heart failure caused by either systolic or diastolic dysfunction.

BNP measurement may thus prove useful when sorting out the cause of dyspnea for a patient with both heart and lung disease. A level above 100 pg/mL usually indicates CHF.[6] Furthermore, marked elevation of BNP (above 130 pg/mL) predicts poor prognosis and a higher risk for sudden death.[7] Elevated BNP at the time of hospital discharge is associated with a higher incidence of readmission or emergency department visits.[8] A caveat: remember that BNP increases with age, and it is higher in women. For a woman older than 65 years a BNP level over 100 pg/mL may be normal, and it can be as high as 155 pg/mL.[6] Like other laboratory tests, BNP must be evaluated in the clinical context.

Limitations notwithstanding, the use of *biomarkers*—and BNP appears the most useful—adds another dimension to the evaluation and management of CHF. The measurement of LVEF is essential when making a diagnosis of CHF, and it is closely related to prognosis in studies of large populations with disease. I indicated that there may be a disconnect between LVEF and clinical course, which limits its usefulness when dealing with the individual. Biomarkers like BNP may prove useful for tracking response to therapy and predicting outcome for a given patient. For example, a patient who has persistent elevation of BNP at the time of hospital discharge may need more aggressive therapy.[9,10]

Endomyocardial biopsy—The rationale for biopsy is detection of an illness that can be treated.[11] It is unusual for a biopsy to be abnormal; a histologic diagnosis was apparent in just 17% of a series of 673 patients referred with new-onset heart failure and low LVEF.[12] The most common abnormal finding was lymphocytic infiltration, suggesting previous or current viral infection.

Unfortunately, the results of immunosuppressive treatment for those with nonspecific inflammation have been disappointing. A study of patients with symptoms for 8 months showed no benefit with prednisone therapy, even for the subset with inflammation (positive biopsy or positive gallium scan or high sedimentation rate).[13] Other studies of patients with more acute illness and lymphocytes on biopsy also showed no benefits from immunosuppression using steroids with or without cyclosporine.[14] There is general agreement that the link between viral myocarditis and cardiomyopathy involves the host's immune response, and novel approaches to immunosuppression or modulation are currently being studied.[15]

Less common causes of cardiomyopathy may be diagnosed by biopsy (Table 1.7). Diagnosis of giant cell, hypersensitivity, or sarcoid myocarditis is the leading rationale for biopsy in the individual patient, because they may respond to steroid therapy. Wu and colleagues have suggested limiting biopsy to patients with the following characteristics:[11]

• Acute CHF refractory to medical therapy

• Rapidly deteriorating LVEF despite therapy and with no clear etiology

Table 1.7 Unusual Causes of Cardiomyopathy That May Be Diagnosed with Biopsy and That May Respond to Immunosuppressive Therapy[11]	
Giant cell myocarditis	Idiopathic, or with thymoma or drug hypersensitivity. Rapidly progressive (5-year survival = 10%). Improved clinical course with steroids plus azathioprine or cyclosporine.
Sarcoid myocarditis	Causes CHF in 5% of those with sarcoidosis; systemic disease is usually apparent. Ventricular arrhythmias and heart block more common than with idiopathic CM. Sensitivity of biopsy is 20–30%. If treated early, survival improves with steroid therapy.
Hypersensitivity myocarditis	Rapidly progressive heart failure, usually with eosinophilia and rash. Biopsy shows eosinophilic infiltrate, but little necrosis. Often a drug reaction (sulfonamides most common). Rx: stop the offending drug and give steroids.

- CHF plus ventricular tachycardia or heart block
- CHF plus rash or eosinophilia or fever
- Associated illness that can cause of CHF (i.e., collagen vascular disease, infiltrative diseases such as amyloid, sarcoid, or hemochromatosis)

Pharmacologic Treatment of Congestive Heart Failure

A summary of drug therapy is outlined in Table 1.8. The treatment of CHF has evolved over the past decade, and we now have therapies that are proven to lower mortality. The most potent is beta blockade (vide infra), with significant although less profound benefits from angiotensin and aldosterone blockade. If heart rate and blood pressure allow it, a patient with systolic heart failure should be on all the drugs that have been shown to prolong survival. If only one of the drugs can be tolerated, the first choice should be a beta-blocker.

Nonpharmacologic measures should be adopted in every case. Salt restriction is essential. Most patients benefit from modest fluid restriction, drinking only when thirsty. Our heart failure clinic advises fluid restriction (<2000 mL per day) for those requiring 80 mg or more of furosemide per day to control congestion, or for patients with serum sodium levels of 140 meq/dL or less. We recommend continued aerobic exercise even for those with moderate to severe symptoms. Abstinence from alcohol is critical for those with dilated cardiomyopathy, and thiamine should be given to alcoholics.

Beta Adrenergic Blockade

Patients with CHF have elevated circulating norepinephrine levels and a reduction in the number of myocardial beta receptors. This over-stimulation is toxic. On the other hand, some beta adrenergic support is needed by the failing heart, and overly aggressive blockade can have adverse effects. This may explain the small subset of

Table 1.8 Drug Therapy for Congestive Heart Failure Caused by Systolic Dysfunction		
Drug Class (Preferred agents)	**Action**	**Comment**
Beta adrenergic blockers*	Chronic beta stimulation has a direct toxic effect on the myocardium.	The most potent therapy for reducing mortality. Carvedilol or metoprolol. Must start with a tiny dose and slowly increase it. Temporary worsening of symptoms is common.
Angiotensin converting enzyme (ACE) inhibitors*	Blocks the formation of angiotensin II, a potent vaso-constrictor.	Improves symptoms and survival, and retards the progression of LV dysfunction. All drugs in this class are effective, with none shown to be superior. Most effective at high dose.
Angiotensin II (AII) blockers*	Action is similar to ACE inhibitors, but no cough.	ACE inhibitors plus AII blockers may be helpful (see text).
Diuretics	Relieve congestion, reduce preload	Monitor serum potassium and magnesium. If a loop diuretic is not enough, add a thiazide (see text). Consider spironolactone if there is low magnesium or potassium.
Digoxin	Increases contractility	No survival benefit, but improved symptoms and reduced hospitalization. Add if life-prolonging therapy does not control symptoms.
Calcium channel blockers**	Vasodilate, reducing afterload.	Studies of amlodipine showed improved symptoms, but no mortality benefit.
Intravenous dobutamine	Increases contractility and cardiac output.	Can be given at home. Intermittent therapy may be adequate (a 6-hour infusion two to three times each week). Palliative.
Anticoagulation (warfarin)	To prevent peripheral embolization	No clinical trial has supported routine anticoagulation for those in sinus rhythm with LV dysfunction. Definitely anticoagulate if there has been an embolic event, or for atrial fibrillation. Most start warfarin if the echo shows LV thrombus.

*Therapies shown to improve survival in patients with congestive heart failure.
**Avoid diltiazam and verapamil in those with CHF or low LVEF.

patients in clinical trials who get worse with beta blockade. The current treatment strategy aims at balancing stimulation and blockade.[16]

As noted, beta blockade is considered the most potent therapy for systolic CHF. There has been no study directly comparing beta blockade and ACE inhibition, but a review of available trials yields this estimate: the 1-year mortality rate in patients with class II–III CHF is about 16%. With ACE inhibition, the 1-year mortality rate decreases to 14%. Adding a beta blocker to the ACE inhibitor decreases the rate to 9–10%.[17] Because beta blockade was studied after the efficacy of ACE inhibition was established, all patients in beta blocker trials were on ACE inhibitors, making it impossible to estimate the effect of beta blockade alone.

Our experience in cardiology clinic supports the importance of beta blockade. For the first time we seem to be making patients with CHF "well," with dramatic improvement in clinical status. Most have a rise in LVEF, and a quarter of patients have LVEF increase by more than 15 percentage points. Those with the greatest rise in LVEF have the best prognosis.[18] The number of heart transplantation operations has declined in the United States in the past 5 years, and many attribute this to beta blockade therapy for CHF. One of our transplant specialists commented that "we are just buying CHF patients time," but that of course is what we do with transplantation. How much time is uncertain, as little is known about the natural history of CHF after beta blockade.

The earlier trials included patients with class II–III CHF. More recently, carvedilol has been found useful for those with class IV heart failure.[19] In this study, patients were excluded with systolic blood pressure below 85 mm Hg, or heart rate lower than 65 beats per minute.

Two beta-blockers are commonly used in the United States: carvedilol with a target dose of 25 mg twice daily, or long-acting metoprolol, 200 mg per day. At this time there is no clear-cut benefit of one versus the other when treating patients with class II–III CHF. Carvedilol may be preferable for the class IV patient. Clinical trials results have been comparable with bisoprolol, bucindolol, and nebivolol. Carvedilol and nebivolol are direct vasodilators and are both alpha and beta adrenergic blockers. Because of this combined action, it has been suggested that they may be more effective for African-American patients. However, large studies have shown that metoprolol is effective for all racial groups, and it is the least expensive drug available. Large drug comparison studies that are in progress will provide more information about drug selection for particular populations (perhaps indicating different strategies for racial, gender, heart failure etiology, or age subsets with CHF).

On the other hand, selection of a drug may be influenced by clinical status. Consider using carvedilol for the African-American patient with marked blood pressure elevation, because it is a more potent antihypertensive agent than a pure beta-blocker. Another special situation is the patient with bronchospasm. We generally avoid beta-blockers, but the cardioselective agent, metoprolol, may be tolerated at a lower dose by those with obstructive lung disease (the usual dose is ≤100 mg/day). Our heart failure clinic considers beta blockade important enough that they routinely try metoprolol for these patients with both CHF and advanced lung disease.

When initiating beta blockade, there is an initial period of myocardial depression (withdrawal of beta adrenergic support), followed by systolic improvement. For this reason, beta blockers are started at one-sixteenth to one-eighth of the target dose. The dose is then increased every 2 to 3 weeks. I tell patients they will experience fatigue when starting or increasing the dose of medicine: "you are used to elevated adrenaline levels, and when we dial that back, you will experience a temporary set-back until your system adjusts." I emphasize that over the long run, this therapy is their best chance to feel better and live longer, but that patience and perseverance will be needed while adjusting the dose. With frequent follow-up and coaching, 90% will reach the target dose.

When the patient's heart rate falls to 60 beats per minute, there is adequate beta blockade, and there is no need for further increase in the dose. Bradycardia is a contraindication to beta-blocker therapy, and special care is needed when the systolic blood pressure is under 100 mm Hg.

Afterload Reduction Therapy

Angiotensin converting inhibitors—ACE inhibitors block the conversion of angiotensin I to angiotensin II, which is a potent vasoconstrictor. Afterload reduction is an attractive strategy as cardiac output increases without an increase in cardiac work (the myocardium uses no more oxygen). It is one of those rare times in life that you get something for nothing.

ACE inhibitor therapy is indicated for CHF of all levels of severity, even for those with asymptomatic LV dysfunction (LVEF <40%). It has been shown to improve survival in patients with severe CHF as well as to retard the progression of heart failure in patients with less severe disease (Table 1.2). Note that patients with advanced aortic stenosis or LV outflow tract obstruction usually do not benefit from ACE inhibition, as their high afterload is structural, and lowering peripheral vascular resistance will not change it (an exception may be the patient with coexisting hypertension).

Although most of the earlier heart failure studies were performed using enalapril or captopril, the benefits of ACE inhibition are thought to be a class effect. Higher dose therapy yields the best results. Our heart failure clinic pushes the dose until the patient has postural dizziness, then backs off.

ACE inhibitors may also prevent CHF. The HOPE trial found a 23% reduction in the development of heart failure in a population with stable vascular disease. The benefit was greatest in—but not limited to—those with elevated blood pressure, and it was not the result of preventing MI.[20,21]

The most common adverse effect of ACE inhibitors is cough (in as many as 10–15%). It is caused by potentiation of bradykinin and does not resolve with cough suppressants. It is an intolerable side effect, but thankfully there is an equally effective alternative. Any suggestion of ACE inhibitor cough should prompt switching to an angiotensin receptor blocker (ARB). Less common is angioedema, which can be mild or severe; it requires discontinuation of ACE inhibitors with no rechallenge. ACE inhibitors are contraindicated in pregnancy due to fetal and neonatal morbidity and mortality.

Hyponatremia, renal dysfunction, and practical tips when starting ACE inhibitor therapy—Renal dysfunction may occur with ACE inhibition when there is renal artery stenosis. Maintaining adequate perfusion across the stenosed artery depends on high blood pressure, the result of elevated renin activity. Blocking the renin effect brings blood pressure down, leading to renal ischemia and an increase in creatinine. *Check electrolytes a couple days after starting ACE inhibitors (there is no need to wait longer); if creatinine increases by 0.3 mg/dL or more, stop the drug and evaluate for renal artery stenosis.*

Hyperkalemia is another side effect of ACE inhibition, which usually occurs when there is renal dysfunction. On the other hand, an elevated creatinine level is not a contraindication for use of ACE inhibitors or ARBs. In fact, most kidney diseases—with the exception of renal artery stenosis—respond favorably to ACE inhibition. Nevertheless, renal dysfunction indicates a need for careful monitoring when starting therapy.

Patients with CHF often have low serum sodium, and hyponatremia is a marker of poor prognosis. Serum sodium is inversely proportional to plasma renin activity (PRA). Those with high PRA are especially sensitive to ACE inhibitors. When there is hyponatremia, start with a lower than usual dose to avoid hypotension.

Hypotension may also occur with volume depletion. Remember that volume depletion increases the chance of symptomatic hypotension when starting any vasodilator. A "diuretic holiday"—holding furosemide for a couple days—before starting the ACE inhibitor may help the patient with borderline low blood pressure, or when you feel that the patient is dry. It is particularly useful when the serum sodium is below 140 mEq/dL. By the same token, if your patient becomes hypotensive after starting ACE inhibitors, you might try backing off diuretics, then restarting the drug at a lower dose.

Angiotensin II receptor blockers—Comparative trials have found that ARBs (irbesartan, candesartan, losartan, valsartan, etc.) are as effective as ACE inhibitors for CHF.[22] In fact, a recent trial found that adding valsartan to ACE inhibitor therapy reduced symptoms and a need for hospitalization.[23] Explanation: even with ACE inhibition, angiotensin II levels remain high, as angiotensin II can be generated through other pathways such as the chymase system (not dependent on ACE). Consider adding an ARB to ACE inhibition when blood pressure is not low.

A caveat: Val-HeFT found that triple therapy with ACE inhibition, ARB, and a beta blocker was not well tolerated, and suggested using just two of the three drugs in combination. Because beta blockade is so important, most patients will be taking that plus an ACE inhibitor or ARB. But for patients unable to take beta blockers, the ARB-ACE inhibitor combination is better than either of them alone.[23]

Why not just use an ARB (avoiding the possibility of ACE inhibitor cough and blocking all angiotensin II)? Some of the beneficial effect of ACE inhibitor therapy may come from the potentiation of bradykinin and increased production of nitric oxide. ARBs have no effect on this.

Afterload reduction with other vasodilators—Hydralazine works but is tough to use. A short half-life requires giving it four times a day. High doses are needed to achieve a demonstrable hemodynamic effect. The Veterans Administration trial that showed efficacy (V-HeFT I and II) treated patients with an average dose of 300 mg hydralazine per day and found little benefit in those who could not tolerate at least 200 mg.[24] Side effects are common at these high doses. Furthermore, these studies combined high-dose hydralazine with isosorbide 160 mg/day, and the beneficial effect probably requires this combination. Frankly, it is a difficult therapy to use, and large studies documented a high dropout rate. In the clinic, I commonly see a patient who is on hydralazine 50 mg twice a day for *afterload reduction*. At that dose, do not assume you are doing much good.[25]

Spironolactone

Aldosterone is another neurohormone that is apparently toxic when persistently elevated. The Randomized Aldactone Evaluation Study (RALES) found improved survival and symptoms with spironolactone 25 mg per day.[26] The patients had advanced CHF (class III–IV), and were treated with ACE inhibitors; a minority were taking beta blockers. Benefits could not be explained by hemodynamic changes or diuresis. Instead, reduced mortality and a 35% reduction in hospitalization for CHF were attributed to less myocardial and vascular fibrosis. The most common side effect was gynecomastia. Hyperkalemia was uncommon, but potassium should be monitored, especially with baseline creatinine greater than 1.5 mg/dL.

The role of aldosterone blockade with less severe CHF is uncertain.

Increasing Contractility (Inotropic Therapy)

Most patients with advanced symptoms benefit from digoxin therapy. One study stopped digoxin in patients who were also on ACE inhibitors, and found worsening of symptoms.[27]

There is concern about inotropic therapy as a strategy: that forcing an already sick heart to work harder can have deleterious effects. Indeed, the oral phosphodiesterase inhibitor, amrinone, had a favorable effect on symptoms but an increase in mortality when compared with placebo. The drug never made it to market. Based on this experience, many were concerned when digoxin was finally tested against placebo, anticipating an adverse effect on survival (the practice of cardiovascular medicine would not seem quite right without this old friend).

The DIG trial found no favorable effect of digoxin on survival, but at least it did not increase mortality.[28] It relieved symptoms and reduced hospitalization for CHF. Based on this experience, the current recommendation is to add digoxin for relief of symptoms when afterload reduction, beta blockade, and diuretics are not enough. Because of its narrow therapeutic window and renal excretion, it can be tricky to use, especially for those with advanced disease. Toxicity may develop with a change in renal function (e.g., with decreased cardiac output or excessive diuresis). Be sensitive to the noncardiac manifestations of toxicity such as visual changes, nausea, or anorexia, and check drug levels with any change in condition. Efficacy is slight at digoxin levels below 0.5 ng/mL, and the frequency of adverse effects and mortality increases at levels above 1.0 ng/mL, even though the laboratory usually indicates that the toxic level is 2.0 ng/mL.[28] The latest communication from the DIG trial suggests keeping the range between 0.5 and 0.8 ng/mL.

Catecholamine infusion is used for acutely decompensated heart failure, especially for the patient who is hypotensive or who has progressive renal dysfunction with diuretic therapy. This inotropic approach reverses the hemodynamic abnormalities of cardiac decompensation: cardiac output increases, and pulmonary wedge pressure falls. However, it does not shorten hospital stay, prevent readmission, or improve survival. Nevertheless, it may be crucial for the relief of symptoms for the patient with end-stage disease.

Intravenous *dobutamine* at 4–8 μg/kg/min stimulates beta 1 and 2 receptors, increasing cardiac output and lowering systemic and pulmonary vascular resistance, usually without raising heart rate.[29] The cardiac selective actions of this and other catecholamines are lost at higher doses. An alternative is *milrinone* (0.3–0.8 μg/kg/min), which may have less effect on heart rate and ventricular ectopy.[29] Home therapy is possible with either of these drugs with supervision by a visiting nurse—hospice nurses generally have experience with it. The dose is determined in hospital either (1) with pulmonary artery pressure monitoring, or (2) by observing heart rate, blood pressure, urine output, and symptoms. I do not think you are obligated to transfer a patient with end-stage heart failure to a tertiary center for hemodynamic monitoring to use this treatment. Start with a low dose and increase it until there is a slight rise in blood pressure, without an increase in heart rate. Back off if there is increased ventricular ectopy. You should then see improved urine output.

This minimal effective dose is used at home, with 6-hour infusions four times a week. Beneficial effects have been shown to persist for some time after the 6-hour infusion. With a reduction in congestion, many patients are able to reduce the frequency of treatments to once or twice a week. Note that intravenous catecholamine therapy is reserved for the patient with end-stage disease. While it clearly improves symptoms, there have been no large clinical trials that establish safety. Many who work in this area suspect there may be a negative effect on survival, but agree that it is justified for palliation.

Dopamine is an alternative to dobutamine, and tradition holds that it favorably affects renal blood flow. When tested, it had no specific renal benefits. Dobutamine is our first choice for chronic infusion therapy because it has less effect on heart rate.[30]

Preload Reduction: Diuretics

Congestion, either systemic or pulmonary, is the most problematic symptom with advanced CHF. Note that diuresis—a reduction in ventricular preload—does not improve ventricular function (on the contrary, it moves the patient down on the

Table 1.9 Diuretic Therapy				
			Elimination Half-life (hr)	
Drug (equivalent dose)	Oral Absorption (%)	Normal	Renal Insufficiency	Congestive Heart Failure
Furosemide (Lasix, 40 mg)	10–100%	1.5–2	2.8	2.7
Bumetanide (Bumex, 1 mg)	80–100%	1	1.6	1.3
Torsemide (Demadex, 20 mg)	80–100%	3–4*	4–5	6
Hydrochlorothiazide	65–75%	2.5	Increased	Uncertain

* The longer half-life is an advantage, facilitating diuresis. When multiple dosing is needed, the doses should be separated by 6 hours (more than with furosemide or bumetanide).

ventricular function curve; Figure 1.1). Nor does it improve survival—it is not on the list of treatments that will help the patient live longer. Instead, diuretics are used to control symptomatic congestion. While most patients with CHF need diuretics, an occasional patient does not require them once other therapy is working—because there is no effect on survival, diuretics are not "required" for heart failure. (It is obvious that the patient with severe pulmonary edema lives longer because of rescue by diuretics; the key is that prophylactic use of diuretics in the absence of congestion has no role.)

Loop diuretics are used initially because of their potency.[31] Furosemide (Lasix) is the cheapest, and we all have extensive experience with it. But bioavailability varies, and furosemide resistance is common. On average, about 50% of an oral dose is absorbed, but the range is 10% to 90%, making it difficult to know how much a particular patient is getting. We solve this by gradually increasing the dose until there is diuresis. The rate of absorption is slowed in heart failure, even more when there is splanchnic edema, so the effective dose may vary with the patient's condition.

The problem of variable absorption is compounded by reduced renal responsiveness to all loop diuretics in patients with advanced CHF, by as much as 70% compared with normals. Renal insufficiency further impairs delivery of furosemide to the site of action; there is reduced secretion of the drug into urine in the proximal tubule, so delivery to the distal tubule is reduced. The net effect is "diuretic resistance."

The maximum effect with furosemide is achieved with a daily intravenous dose of 160–200 mg. Above this there is little increase in natriuresis, and the risk of tinnitus increases. A hospitalized patient with severe pulmonary congestion may need this high intravenous dose several times a day. The maximum effective oral dose is about twice the intravenous dose when renal function is normal, but higher still with renal insufficiency.

When a patient is requiring high doses of oral furosemide, you may assume that there is poor absorption of the drug. That is the time to switch to one of the newer loop diuretics, bumetanide (Bumex) or torsemide (Demadex, Table 1.9).

They work like furosemide: they are secreted into the urine in the proximal tubule and act on the distal tubule. The difference is that bioavailability with oral dosing is much better, with 80% to 100% absorbed even in the presence of splanchnic congestion or renal insufficiency. Both are metabolized and excreted by the liver, and the elimination half-life is not affected by renal insufficiency. However, renal insufficiency does reduce the secretion of drug into the proximal tubule, so higher doses are needed.

If you are treating the patient with intravenous medicines, there is no advantage of bemetanide or torsemide over furosemide. However, with oral therapy, more reliable absorption makes the newer drugs almost as effective as intravenous furosemide. When comparing the newer drugs, the major difference is elimination half-life, which is longer for torsemide (Table 1.9). This may be advantageous, because there may be rebound sodium retention between diuretic doses. It is for this reason that continuous infusion furosemide has been suggested for congestion that is resistant to diuresis (a loading dose of 40 mg, then 10–40 mg/hr, with the higher dose for those with renal insufficiency). The costs of torsemide and bemetanide are similar, and equivalent doses are reviewed in Table 1.9.

Another issue is whether to give loop diuretics once or twice a day, especially as half-life is brief. Early in the course of CHF, when congestion is easily controlled, there is no reason for multiple doses. Active diuresis restricts the patient's activities. As congestion worsens, twice-daily dosing is usually needed. With furosemide or bemetanide, morning and noon dosing frees the evening for other activities. Because of its longer half-life, oral doses of torsemide should be separated by 6 hours.

Using multiple diuretics—There is synergy between the thiazide and loop diuretics, and adding an oral thiazide is the next step for the unresponsive patient. Thiazides work more distally in the nephron, blocking the absorption of sodium that escaped the loop of Henle (and thus, the action of the loop diuretic). Metolazone (Zaroxolyn) has been marketed for this purpose in the United States. However, hydrochlorothiazide (HCTZ) is more rapidly absorbed, has a shorter half-life (hours rather than 2 days), and is cheaper. For these reasons, HCTZ may be the preferable drug.[31] With severe CHF the dose of HCTZ is 100–200 mg/day, given in two doses. The dose may be increased with renal insufficiency.

An occasional patient resistant to loop and thiazide diuretics will respond to a potassium-sparing diuretic, such as spironolactone, that acts on the distal nephron. Although untested, there is a belief that it works well for peripheral (as opposed to pulmonary) congestion. Clinical responsiveness can be predicted by measuring urine electrolytes. Low urinary sodium and high potassium suggest that potassium is being exchanged for sodium in the distal nephron (the aldosterone mechanism), and spironolactone should work. If urinary potassium is low, spironolactone probably will not be effective. The half-life of spironolactone is sufficient for once-daily dosing (50–200 mg/day). It may take a couple of weeks before diuresis begins.

Another benefit of spironolactone is its effect on electrolytes. In addition to its potassium sparing effects, 50 mg spironolactone given daily has been shown to increase serum magnesium 13%.[32] With all diuretic therapy, electrolytes must be monitored.

Remember that sudden death accounts for more than half of CHF mortality; the mechanism is ventricular fibrillation. Either hypokalemia or hypomagnesemia may provoke ventricular arrhythmias in the failing heart. There is loss of potassium and magnesium with loop and thiazide diuretics. Because furosemide is a more potent diuretic, you would think that potassium wasting would be especially severe. However, in practice, I have encountered profound hypokalemia just as often with thiazide treatment.

An infrequently recognized complication of diuretic therapy is *thiamine deficiency*. Furosemide increases the urinary excretion of thiamine.[33] Thiamine replacement may lead to an increase in LVEF. Consider replacement therapy for the patient who has been taking furosemide long-term and has poor nutritional status. You may also consider it when a previously stable patient decompensates.

Nesiritide—Human recombinant brain natriuretic peptide (BNP, also called type B natriuretic peptide) is available for infusion therapy. When released by the stretched left ventricle, the peptide serves as a counter-regulatory response to increased sympathetic and renin-angiotensin-aldosterone activity in decompensated heart failure. Given intravenously, nesiritide blocks both systems and is a direct arterial vasodilator. Arterial and venous dilatation lowers both preload and afterload. There may be an increase in urine output, although this effect is variable. The VMAC trial comparing it with intravenous nitroglycerin found a greater fall in pulmonary wedge pressure with nesiritide.[29,33]

A curious finding in early trials has been persistence of dyspnea in almost half of those treated, despite a fall in pulmonary wedge pressure. This disconnect between symptoms and hemodynamics is unexplained.[29] If you are using the drug without pulmonary artery pressure monitoring, 25–50% will show no clinical response. On the plus side is a relative absence of side effects. Hypotension is possible and may prevent up-titration of the dose, but it is no worse than intravenous nitroglycerin in this regard. Nesiritide does not provoke ventricular or atrial tachyarrhythmias.

Currently nesiritide is used for acute pulmonary edema in place of intravenous nitroglycerin. We try it for the occasional patient with congestion that is resistant to diuretics, stopping it if there is no clinical improvement over 2 days.

Vasopressin receptor blockers—Arginine vasopressin (AVP) levels are elevated in CHF, contributing to fluid retention. AVP promotes water reabsorption by the kidneys (an antidiuretic effect), and it has a vasoconstrictor effect as well. AVP blockade leads to free-water diuresis (excretion of a large volume of dilute urine), and to elevation of serum sodium provided that water intake is unchanged.[17]

Oral AVP blockers are currently in clinical trials, and it appears they will be useful for both acute and chronic heart failure. When combined with standard diuretics they increase urine output and lower pulmonary wedge pressure (e.g., they relieve pulmonary congestion). Those with hyponatremia are particularly sensitive to AVP blockade, and experience an increase in serum sodium as well as relief of congestion.[17]

Other Therapies for Congestive Heart Failure

Biventricular Pacing: Resynchronization Therapy

The rationale for this new therapy is apparent from the pattern of LV shortening seen on the echocardiogram.[35] Normally, the interventricular septum and the posterior-lateral walls contract simultaneously, moving toward each other during systole. With left bundle branch block (LBBB) the septum is activated late, and therefore contracts after the lateral wall.

Late septal contraction persists beyond the completion of aortic ejection, and this phase of contraction therefore does not contribute to forward flow. Also, the late contraction continues into diastole, effectively shortening diastole and inhibiting diastolic filling of the LV. The net effect is lower LVEF and stroke volume.

Biventricular (BiV) pacing—that is, pacing the ventricle from two sites—resynchronizes the LV so that contraction of the septum and lateral walls is simultaneous. One pacing wire is positioned at the RV apex, capturing the septum. The second is threaded up the coronary sinus to the backside of the heart, where it stimulates the lateral wall. Current technology also calls for an atrial electrode, so that an optimal heart rate and PR interval can be programmed.

BiV pacing works best for the patient with LBBB and a wide QRS (>150 msec).[36] Efficacy is predicted by a narrow QRS with pacing, and the two ventricular leads are positioned so that the paced QRS is as narrow as possible.[37] The hemodynamic effects are impressive, with a reduction in the delay in septal activation and a 30% increase in LVEF.[38] This is accomplished with no increase in myocardial oxygen consumption, because the myocardium is not contracting more forcefully (just more efficiently). Mitral regurgitation, a frequent complication of dilated cardiomyopathy, tends to improve.[39]

Clinical trials have shown improved exercise tolerance and functional class, and a trend toward reduced hospitalization for CHF.[35,40] There have been no studies large enough to demonstrate an effect on survival, but the changes in LV geometry and function, an increase in maximum oxygen consumption, and a decrease in sympathetic tone suggest that large trials will show a benefit.[39–42]

Currently, there are no practice guidelines for this therapy. In practice, BiV pacing is being offered to those with class III–IV symptoms despite optimal medical therapy, and who have QRS duration greater than 130 msec.

Ultrafiltration—When other measures have failed, ultrafiltration relieves congestion. This approach affords greater hemodynamic stability than hemodialysis. Vascular volume is held constant and cardiac output remains stable, despite a decrease in total extracellular fluid volume. Electrolyte abnormalities can be corrected in the process.

Ultrafiltration removes plasma free water, usually at a rate of 1.5–2 L/hr, and the usual treatment schedule is 2 hours daily, or every other day, until a target dry weight is reached. The demonstrated benefits are relief of congestion, reduction in diuretic dose, and fewer hospitalizations.[34] Tradeoffs include a need for vascular access, adherence to a regular treatment schedule in the dialysis center, and possible aggravation of renal disfunction.

The frequency of treatment can usually be reduced when dry weight is reached, especially for patients who are able to restrict free water intake. Vasopressin receptor blockade—which also removes free water—will be preferable to ultrafiltration when treating the diuretic resistant patient (when it becomes available for clinical use).

Treatment of Anemia

Cardiac output is the product of heart rate and stroke volume, but oxygen-carrying capacity is also directly proportional to hematocrit. Lower it from 40% to 30%, and oxygen delivery is reduced by 25%, just as it would be with a 25% reduction in cardiac output. Low-grade anemia, usually the anemia of chronic disease, commonly accompanies heart failure.

A randomized Israeli study of patients with poor symptom control despite maximal therapy pushed hemoglobin from a baseline of 10.5 gm% to above 12.5 gm% with intravenous iron and subcutaneous erythropoietin.[43] Over 8 months of follow-up, the treatment group had improved functional class and LVEF, and a decrease in diuretic requirement.

With this result you may expect to see larger, multicenter trials to assess the role of mild anemia in the natural history of CHF. In the meantime, my threshold for treating anemia is lower.

Implantable Cardiac Defibrillators—MADIT II

Sudden death is common in patients with reduced LVEF, and the usual mechanism is ventricular fibrillation (VF). The MADIT II trial enrolled patients with prior MI and LVEF 30% or less to ICD or conventional medical therapy.[44] Electrophysiologic testing was not done before randomization.

During 20 months follow-up, there was a 31% reduction in mortality with defibrillator therapy. Patients in both treatment groups were on good medical therapy, with a high percentage of them on beta-blockers and ACE inhibitors. The rate of hospitalization for new or worsening CHF was slightly higher in the defibrillator group. This suggests that some patients who would have died suddenly lived long enough to develop clinical heart failure.

MADIT II substantially expands the indications for ICD therapy. Most who practice cardiology believe the result, although practice guidelines have not yet been changed to incorporate ICD therapy for all patients with ischemic cardiomyopathy. The economic impact is huge given the number of patients with chronic coronary disease and the cost of ICD therapy. Currently an ICD costs more than $40,000 over the life of the device, and the MADIT II indication potentially could add $40 billion per year to the US health-care budget. Stay tuned for a national debate that will determine the role of this effective, although perhaps too expensive, therapy.

Table 1.10 Heart Transplantation	

Indications	End-stage congestive heart failure (CHF)
	   Cardiogenic shock requiring mechanical assistance
	   Low output state requiring continuous intravenous inotropic support
	   NYHA class III or IV CHF and poor 12-month survival (see Table 1.1)
	Refractory angina pectoris, unsuitable for revascularization
	   Symptoms prevent normal daily activities
	   Objective evidence for ischemia
	   Recurrent hospitalization for unstable angina
	   Life-threatening coronary anatomy
	Hypertrophic cardiomyopathy and NYHA class IV symptoms (see Table 1.1)
	Life-threatening ventricular arrhythmia that cannot be controlled

Contraindications	Advanced age (varies, but some programs transplant into the 60s) Irreversible lung, kidney, or liver disease Diabetes mellitus with end-organ disease Active infection Cancer Poor medical compliance Pulmonary hypertension (severe) Systemic disease limiting survival or rehabilitation Inadequate social support*

* A nebulous category. Programs are reluctant to transplant a patient who does not have adequate family support. A team is needed to get a person through this complicated and difficult treatment, and equally difficult follow-up. Support includes financial resources. Although partially funded by the state, transplantation and follow-up are expensive, and no program can afford to give it away.

(There may have to be a practical answer to the question, "how can you put a price on a human life?")

The first study of ICD prophylaxis for *nonischemic cardiomyopathy* found a 35% reduction in all cause mortality ($p = 0.08$ with 458 patients), and an 80% reduction in suddent death ($p = 0.006$).[45]

Surgical Therapy

Indications for revascularization or valve surgery are reviewed elsewhere. Surgery to reduce ventricular volume has been shown to improve symptoms for those with dilated cardiomyopathy, but has not been widely adopted or subjected to randomized trials. It is considered experimental at this time.

Heart transplantation both relieves symptoms and prolongs survival for the end-stage patient. Indications and contraindications are summarized in Table 1.10.

Palliative Care

All of our therapies for CHF may be considered palliative, as they relieve symptoms as well as prolong survival. None of the standard medical treatments for CHF is withdrawn from the patient with end-stage disease.

When all else fails to control severe pulmonary congestion, morphine usually provides relief. It is a venodilator, reducing blood return to the heart. Pulmonary capillary pressure and symptoms of congestion are quickly reduced. In addition, it blunts the anxiety that comes with severe dyspnea.

Morphine is safe for patients with pulmonary congestion or the dyspnea of advanced lung disease. Despite widespread concern, respiratory depression is rare, short of extremely high doses. Regular oral dosing is useful (Roxanol starting at 2.5–5 mg at 2- to 4-hour intervals). It may be preferable to use the medicine as needed rather than throughout the day, especially if attacks of dyspnea are intermittent. Within reason, there is no maximum allowable dose, and the dose may be increased at 4- to 12-hour intervals as needed to control symptoms.

I encourage hospice care for those with end-stage CHF. The hospice nurse monitors salt and water intake, and regulates diuretics and other drugs. Patients often improve dramatically. There is no doubt that physicians are qualified to man patients taking opioids. But there are practical advantages to having hospice involvement. The first is that narcotics may not appear to be usual treatment for CHF; hospice care avoids any suggestion of abuse. Another is that hospice nurses are expert at regulating the morphine dose and at managing possible complications.

Extreme Symptoms in the Terminally Ill Patient

There is often uncertainty when treating a patient with terminal symptoms. Many with CHF have ventricular fibrillation and die suddenly. Others die from heart failure and may come to the emergency department with pulmonary edema that is refractory to intravenous diuretics.

Many of our patients with advanced disease make the decision to avoid interventional, heroic therapies at the end-of-life. It is unfortunate when the doctor tells the patient and family that intubation and mechanical ventilation is the only hope for relieving symptoms. Despite a previous decision to avoid ventilator therapy, a desperate patient and family may have a change of mind, especially when this seems the only chance for relief.

An effective alternative that should be considered is higher dose morphine, titrated to relieve dyspnea. There may be depression of respiration with a dose sufficient to relieve symptoms. In this case the moral imperative is to provide relief of suffering for the dying patient, even if high-dose morphine contributes to more rapid death. There is no culpability. This is not considered assisted suicide or euthanasia, but rather, necessary therapy for extreme symptoms.[46]

References

1   2002 Heart and stroke statistical update. Dallas: American Heart Association, 2001.

2   Levy D, Kenchaiah S, Larson MG, et al. Long-term trends in the incidence of and survival with heart failure. N Engl J Med 2002;347:1397–1402.

3 McCullough PA, Philbin EF, Spertus JA, et al. Confirmation of a heart failure epidemic: findings from the Resource Utilization Among Congestive Heart Failure (REACH) study. J Am Coll Cardiol 2002;39:60–69.

4 Shinbane JS, Wood MA, Jensen DN, et al. Tachycardia-induced cardiomyopathy: a review of animal models and clinical studies. J Am Coll Cardiol 1997;29:709–715.

5 Forman DE, Butler J, Wang Y, et al. Incidence, predictors at admission, and impact of worsening renal function among patients hospitalized with heart failure. J Am Coll Cardiol 2004;43:61–67.

6 Shapiro BP, Chen HH, Burnett JC, Redfield MM. Use of plasma brain natriuretic peptide concentration to aid in the diagnosis of heart failure. Mayo Clin Proc 2003;78:481–486. Also note, Mueller C, Scholer A, Laule-Kilian K, et al. Use of B-type natriuretic peptide in the evaluation and management of acute dyspnea. N Engl J Med 2004;350:647–654. (*Rapid measurement of BNP in the ER allowed identification of those without CHF—with a normal BNP—reducing the need for hospitalization, and allowing more rapid diagnosis.*) And, Mark DB, Felker GM. B-type natriuretic peptide—a biomarker for all seasons? N Engl J Med 2004;350:718–720.

7 Berger R, Huelsman M, Strecker K, et al. B-type natriuretic peptide predicts sudden death in patients with chronic heart failure. Circulation 2002;105: 2392–2397.

8 Harrison A, Morrison LK, Krishnaswamy P, et al. B-type natriuretic peptide predicts future cardiac events in patients presenting to the emergency department with dyspnea. Ann Emerg Med 2002;39:131–138.

9 Bozkurt B, Mann DL. Use of biomarkers in the management of heart failure: are we there yet. Circulation 2003;107:1231–1233.

10. Anand IS, Fisher LD, Chiang Y-T, et al. Changes in brain natriuretic peptide and norepinephrine over time and mortality and morbidity in the Valsartan Heart Failure Trial (Val-HeFT). Circulation 2003;107:1278–1283.

11. Wu LA, Lapeyre AC, Cooper LT. Current role of endomyocardial biopsy in the management of dilated cardiomyopathy and myocarditis. Mayo Clin Proc 2001;76:1030–1038.

12. Kasper EK, Agema WR, Hutchins GM, et al. The causes of dilated cardiomyopathy: a clinicopathologic review of 673 consecutive patients. J Am Coll Cardiol 1994;23:586–590.

13. Parrillo JE, Cunnion RE, Epstein SE, et al. A prospective, randomized, controlled trial of prednisone for dilated cardiomyopathy. N Engl J Med 1989;321:1061–1068.

14. Mason JW, O'Connell JB, Herskowitz A, et al. A clinical trial of immunosuppressive therapy for myocarditis. The Myocarditis Treatment Trial Investigators. N Engl J Med 1995;333:269–275.

15. Feldman AM, McNamara D. Myocarditis. N Engl J Med 2000;343:1388–1398.

16. Bristow M. Antiadrenergic therapy of chronic heart failure: surprises and new opportunities. Circulation 2003;107:1100–1102. Also, Gheorghiade M, Colucci WS, Swedberg K. Beta-blockers in chronic heart failure. Circulation 2003;107:1570–1575.

17. Jessup M, Brozena S. Heart failure. N Engl J Med 2003;348:2007–2018. Also, Mehra MR, Uber PA, Francis GS. Heart failure therapy at a crossroad: are there limits to the neurohormonal model? J Am Coll Cardiol 2003;41:1606–1610.

18. Metra M. Marked improvement in left ventricular ejection fraction during long-term beta-blockade in patients with chronic heart failure: clinical correlates and prognostic significance. Am Heart J 2003;145:292–299.

19. Packer M, Coats AJ, Fowler MB, et al. Effect of carvedilol on survival in severe chronic heart failure. N Engl J Med 2001;344:1651–1658.

20. Arnold JM, Yusuf S, Young J, et al. Prevention of heart failure in patients without known left ventricular dysfunction in the Heart Outcomes Prevention Evaluation (HOPE) study. Circulation 2003;107:1284–1290.

21. Linseman JV, Bristow MR. Drug therapy and heart failure prevention. Circulation 2003;107:1234–1236.

22. Manohar P, Pina IL. Therapeutic role of angiotensin II receptor blocker in the treatment of heart failure. Mayo Clin Proc 2003:78:334–338.

23. Cohn JN, Tognoni G. A randomized trial of the angiotensin-receptor blocker valsartan in chronic heart failure. N Engl J Med 2001;345:1667–1675.

24. Cohn JN, Archibald DG, Ziesche S, et al. Effect of vasodilator therapy on mortality in chronic congestive heart failure. Results of a Veterans Administration Cooperative Study. N Engl J Med 1986; 314:1547–1552.

25. Cohn JN, Johnson G, Ziesche S, et al. A comparison of enalapril with hydralazine-isosorbide dinitrate in the treatment of chronic congestive heart failure. N Engl J Med 1991;325:303–310.

26. Pitt B, Zannad F, Remme WJ, et al. The effect of spironolactone on morbidity and mortality in patients with severe heart failure. Randomized Aldactone Evaluation Study Investigators. N Engl J Med 1999;341:709–717.

27. Packer M, Gheorghiade M, Young JB, et al. Withdrawal of digoxin from patients with chronic heart failure treated with angiotensin-converting-enzyme inhibitors. RADIANCE Study. N Engl J Med 1993;329:1–7.

28. The effect of digoxin on mortality and morbidity in patients with heart failure. The Digitalis Investigators Group. N Engl J Med 1997;336:525–533. Also, Rathore SS, Curtis JP, Wang Y et al. Association of serum digoxin concentration and outcomes in patients with heart failure. JAMA 2003;289:871–878. (*This update from the DIG trial showed increasing mortality with digoxin level >0.9 ng/mL. At 0.8 ng/mL the mortality was lower than it was with placebo. Bottom line: it is a tricky drug to use.*)

29. Jain P, Massie BM, Gattis WA, et al. Current medical treatment for the exacerbation of chronic heart failure resulting in hospitalization. Am Heart J 2003;145(suppl):3–17. Also, Forman DE, Butler J, Wang Y, et al. Incidence, predictors at admission, and impact of worsening renal function among patients hospitalized with heart failure. J Am Coll Cardiol 2004;43:61–67. (*When creatinine rose during the first three days in hospital, there was a 7-fold increase in hospital mortality. Diabetes and hypertension predisposed to worsened renal function.*)

30. Vargo DL, Brater DC, Rudy DW, Swan SK. Dopamine does not enhance furosemide-induced natriuresis in patients with congestive heart failure. J Am Soc Nephrol 1996;7:1032–1037.

31. Brater DC. Diuretic therapy. N Engl J Med 1998;339:387–395. (*Best available review—pull this article!*)

32. Barr CS, Lang CC, Hanson J, et al. Effects of adding spironolactone to an angiotensin-converting enzyme inhibitor in chronic congestive heart failure secondary to coronary artery disease. Am J Cardiol 1995;76:1259–1265.

33. Shimon I, Almog S, Vered Z, et al. Improved left ventricular function after thiamine supplementation in patients with congestive heart failure receiving long-term furosemide therapy. Am J Med 1995;98:485–490.

34. Publication Committee for the VMAC Investigators (Vasodilation in the Management of Acute CHF). Intravenous nesiritide vs nitroglycerin for treatment of decompensated congestive heart failure: a randomized controlled trial. JAMA 2002;287:1531–1540. Also, Fonarow GC, Stevenson LW, Walden JA, et al. Impact of a comprehensive heart failure management program on hospital readmission and functional status of patients with advanced heart failure. J Am Coll Cardiol 1997;30:725–732.

35. Pavia SV, Wilkoff BL. Biventricular pacing for heart failure. Cardiol Clin 2001;19: 637–651.

36. Kay GN, Bourge RC. Biventricular pacing for congestive heart failure: questions of who, what, where, why, how and how much. Am Heart J 2000;140:821–823. Also, Mehra MR, Greenberg BH. Cardiac resynchronization therapy: caveat medicus. J Am Coll Cardiol 2004;43:1145–1148.

37. Bax JJ, Molhoek SG, van Erven L, et al. Usefulness of myocardial tissue Doppler echocardiography to evaluate left ventricular dyssynchrony before and after biventricular pacing in patients with idiopathic dilated cardiomyopathy. Am J Cardiol 2003;91:94–97.

38. Alonso C, Leclercq C, Victor F, et al. Electrocardiographic predictive factors of long-term clinical improvement with multisite biventricular pacing in advanced heart failure. Am J Cardiol 1999; 84:1417–1421.

39. Yu CM, Chau E, Sanderson JE, et al. Tissue Doppler echocardiographic evidence of reverse remodeling and improved synchronicity by simultaneously delaying regional contraction after biventricular pacing therapy in heart failure. Circulation 2002;105:438–445.

40. Duncan A, Wait D, Gibson D, Daubert JC. Left ventricular remodelling and haemodynamic effects of multisite biventricular pacing in patients with left ventricular systolic dysfunction and activation disturbances in sinus rhythm: substudy of the MUSTIC (Multisite Stimulation in Cardiomyopathies) trial. Eur Heart J 2003;24:430–441.

41. Saxon LA, Ellenbogen KA. Resynchronization therapy for the treatment of heart failure. Circulation 2003;108:1044–1048.

42. Hamdan MH, Barbera S, Kowal RC, et al. Effects of resynchronization therapy on sympathetic activity in patients with depressed ejection fraction and intraventricular conduction delay due to ischemic or idiopathic cardiomyopathy. Am J Cardiol 2002;89:1047–1051.

43. Silverberg DS, Wexler D, Sheps D, et al. The effect of correction of mild anemia in severe, resistant congestive heart failure using subcutaneous erythropoietin

and intravenous iron: a randomized controlled study. J Am Coll Cardiol 2001;37:1775–1780.

44. Moss AJ, Zareba W, Hall WJ, et al. Prophylactic implantation of a defibrillator in patients with myocardial infarction and reduced ejection fraction: Multicenter Automatic Defibrillator Implantation Trial II. N Engl J Med 2002;346:877–883.

45. Kadish A, Dyer A, Daubert JP, et al. Prophylatic defibrillator implantation in patients with nonischemic dilated cardiomyopathy. N Engl J Med 2004;350:2151–2158.

46. Sachs GA, Ahronheim J, Rhymes JA, et al. Good care of dying patients: the alternative to physician-assisted suicide and euthanasia. J Am Geriatr Soc 1995;43:553–562.

CHAPTER 2

DISORDERS OF VENTRICULAR FILLING: DIASTOLIC HEART FAILURE, RESTRICTIVE CARDIOMYOPATHY, AND PERICARDIAL DISEASE

Abbreviations

ACE	angiotensin converting enzyme	IHSS	idiopathic hypertrophic subaortic stenosis
AS	aortic stenosis		
BNP	brain natriuretic peptide	LV	left ventricle (ventricular)
CHF	congestive heart failure	LVEDP	LV end diastolic pressure
DHF	diastolic heart failure	LVEF	LV ejection fraction
ECG	electrocardiogram	LVH	LV hypertrophy
EF	ejection fraction	S4	fourth heart sound
HCM	hypertrophic cardiomyopathy	SAM	systolic anterior motion (of the mitral valve)
ICD	implantable cardioverter-defibrillator	SCD	sudden cardiac death

Diastolic Heart Failure

Congestive heart failure (CHF) is the most common reason for hospital admission for elderly people. Many physicians are unaware that left ventricular diastolic dysfunction is the predominant mechanism of heart failure for more than half of these patients.[1] One reason is that cardiac physiology focused on contractile function, treating the heart in diastole as a passive balloon. We now realize that failure to adequately inflate this balloon leads to low cardiac output and CHF.

The word *diastole* is Greek and means to dilate or expand. Diastolic dysfunction is an inability to inflate the ventricle to a normal end-diastolic volume without increasing the end-diastolic pressure (EDP). It is like inflating a stiff, thick-walled balloon. Thus, a patient with diastolic CHF has normal left ventricular ejection fraction (LVEF) but elevated LVEDP. The heart ejects blood easily, but cannot fill during diastole because it is too stiff.

It is useful clinically to identify the mechanism of CHF as either systolic or diastolic dysfunction. The two conditions are treated differently, and the prognosis is better with diastolic CHF.[2] Most patients with diastolic heart failure (DHF) have an element of systolic dysfunction. However, when the predominant mechanism of disease is diastolic dysfunction, and the pattern of LV remodeling is concentric LV hypertrophy (LVH), or diastolic CHF is the proper diagnosis.[3]

Etiology and Natural History

Illnesses that provoke LVH result in increased LV stiffness, and may cause DHF. The most common of these is hypertension, a comorbidity in about half of those with diastolic dysfunction. Aortic stenosis (AS) with associated LVH causes obvious problems with diastolic filling, although the reduction in stroke volume is primarily the result of LV outflow obstruction.

Myocardial ischemia also causes diastolic dysfunction, as myocardial relaxation is an energy requiring process. Recall that the usual gallop heard in patients with ischemic heart disease is the S_4, reflecting the atrial kick into a stiff ventricle. An occasional patient with coronary artery disease presents with exertional dyspnea as a manifestation of ischemia. Transient diastolic dysfunction is a mechanism of this anginal equivalent, pulmonary congestion but no pain. In others with chronic diastolic dysfunction, transient ischemia may aggravate symptoms.

Diastolic heart failure is frequently a condition of advanced age. Old people get stiff hearts well as stiff joints. It is more common in women as well—a majority of patients in large studies of DHF are women.[4,5] Both hypertension and diabetes mellitus confer a greater risk of heart failure for women compared with men, suggesting a fundamentally different biologic response.[6] Diastolic failure accounts for 10% of all cases of CHF at age 60 years, but for 50% at age 80 years. In nursing homes, where the ratio of women to men is seven to one, most of those with new CHF have diastolic failure.

DHF is less malignant than systolic heart failure. In general, the best predictor of survival in adults with heart disease is LVEF. The 5-year mortality rate for systolic (low EF) heart failure is approximately 50%, for diastolic (normal EF) CHF, about 25%, and for age-matched controls without CHF, about 5%. The mortality risk with both forms of CHF is higher with advanced age and coronary artery disease. On the other hand, aymptomatic diastolic dysfunction is not a benign condition. Poor long-term prognosis has been documented in those with diastolic dysfunction but no other cardiac illness.[7] That may be because these patients tend to have poorly controlled hypertension. Also recall that LVH is an independent indicator of poor prognosis regardless of the underlying cardiac illness.[8]

Pathophysiology

Diastolic function—When considering ventricular function, it is natural to think primarily of the contractile process. There often is confusion about diastolic function and ventricular compliance. These terms relate to how easily the ventricle fills during diastole, when it is relaxed, and have nothing to do with contraction. But diastolic compliance of the ventricle determines *preload* and therefore affects stroke volume (Figure 2.1). Students are often confused by preload, because we describe it using two different measurements. In reality, preload is the length of the muscle fiber just before contraction, or in the case of the intact heart, the volume of the LV at the end of diastole. Unfortunately, it is hard to measure LV volume precisely; a 20 to 30 mL increase in diastolic volume provides enough extra stretch to increase stroke volume, but current techniques are not accurate enough to measure it.

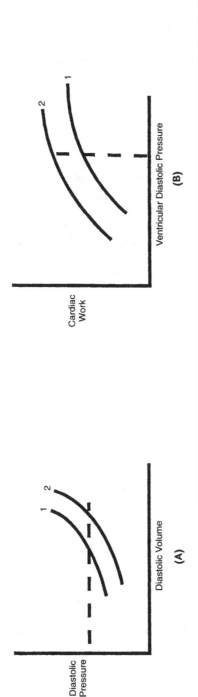

Figure 2.1 (A) Compliance of the ventricle during diastole influences ventricular filling. At a given ventricular diastolic pressure, patient 1 has a lower ventricular volume (and therefore muscle fiber length) than patient 2. Patient 1 has a stiffer, less compliant ventricle. (B) In practice, it is easier to measure ventricular diastolic pressure than volume. Because the two are roughly proportional, pressure is substituted for volume on the ventricular function curve. Patient 1 appears to have worse ventricular function than Patient 2, and that would be the case if diastolic compliance is the same for both. But if Patient 1 has a stiffer ventricle (as in A), end–diastolic volume may be lower than it is for Patient 2. In this case, at equal ventricular volumes, the two might have identical systolic function and therefore identical ventricular function curves. This illustrates the potential problem of substituting diastolic pressure for diastolic volume on the abscissa of the LV function curve. (Reprinted with permission from Taylor GJ. The Cardiology Rotation. Malden, MA: Blackwell Science, 2001:8–9.)

Also, volume is impossible to monitor continuously. For this reason, you do not see end-diastolic volume on the abscissa of the LV function (Starling) curve (Figure 2.1, Panel B). Instead, we substitute the more easily monitored end-diastolic pressure. That works most of the time, because diastolic pressure and volume are proportional.

A compliant ventricle fills easily, allowing adequate preloading of the ventricle (stretching of muscle fibers) to generate stroke volume. A stiff (e.g., noncompliant) ventricle does not allow adequate ventricular filling, and with less myocyte stretch, stroke volume suffers (Figure 2.1). Abnormal stiffness, or diastolic dysfunction, may result from hypertrophy, fibrosis, ischemia, or infiltrative disorders (i.e. amyloidosis, hemachromatosis).

The problem is that a fall in LV compliance (diastolic dysfunction) changes the pressure-volume relation. Higher pressure is needed to inflate the LV to an adequate volume (or preload). The ventricle must operate with a much higher than normal diastolic pressure to maintain stroke volume and cardiac output. Higher LV diastolic pressure is accomplished by volume expansion, the same neurohormonal and renal responses to low cardiac output that occur with systolic heart failure. Remember that during diastole, with the mitral valve open, high LV pressure is transmitted to the left atrium and pulmonary capillary bed, leading to pulmonary congestion.

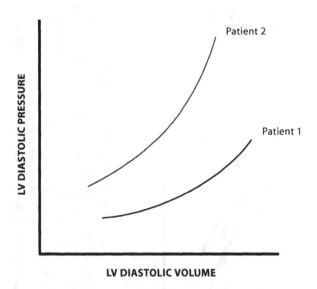

Figure 2.2 LV diastolic pressure-volume curves from two patients. Patient 1, normal. Patient 2, hypertensive heart disease with LV diastolic dysfunction. For a given volume, patient 2 has higher diastolic pressure (the balloon is stiffer). Furthermore, the curve is steeper, as is usually the case with diastolic dysfunction. For this reason, small changes in diastolic volume lead to much greater changes in pressure. (And the LV diastolic pressure is transmitted to the left atrium and pulmonary capillary bed, leading to congestion.)

The steeper pressure-volume curve—Increased stiffness means that the pressure-volume curve is shifted up and to the left (Figure 2.2). In addition, the curve is steeper, so that a small increase in volume leads to much greater increases in LV diastolic pressure. This is the explanation for flash pulmonary edema, or the rapid development of pulmonary congestion after a relatively modest increase in salt intake (i.e., the nursing home resident who has a couple beers with chips when watching the Super Bowl with her chums).

The reverse is true as well, and over-diuresis may cause hypotension. Consider a patient with hypertensive and coronary heart disease who has had cardiac catheterization. The patient has had little to drink, and the contrast agent functions as an osmotic diuretic. Hypotension may develop in the hours after angiography with volume depletion. In such cases we pay careful attention to hydration for 12 hours after the procedure.

Atrial contraction—Think about the role of the atrial kick. Contraction of the atria at the end of diastole provides the last increment of ventricular filling, increasing preload and, therefore, stroke volume.

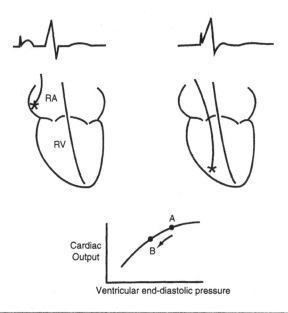

Figure 2.3 This simple study is easily repeated in the cardiac catheterization laboratory. The heart is paced at a rate just above its baseline, and cardiac output is measured. (A) When the pacemaker is in the right atrium, atrial contraction is preserved (a P wave follows the pacing spike). (B) Pacing from the right ventricle leads to a loss of the P wave and atrial contraction. Ventricular diastolic pressure and volume decline—a drop in preload—and cardiac output falls. On the LV function curve, the patient shifts from point A to point B (bottom). (Reprinted with permission from Taylor, GJ. The Cardiology Rotation. Malden, MA: Blackwell Science, 2001:10.)

The simple and interesting experiment that defined the contribution of atrial contraction to cardiac output is illustrated in Figure 2.3. A person with normal diastolic function may have a 10% drop in cardiac output when atrial contraction is bypassed with ventricular pacing. But another with diastolic dysfunction may have cardiac output fall 25% or more with loss of the atrial kick.

Patients with stiff ventricles are said to be *preload dependent* and are especially susceptible to loss of atrial contraction or volume depletion. This explains why a patient with LVH may experience a fall in blood pressure with the development of atrial fibrillation. It is also the explanation for the *pacemaker syndrome*, an abrupt onset of fatigue or dyspnea when a ventricular pacemaker turns on. It is avoided with dual chamber, atrio-ventricular pacing, which maintains atrial contraction.

Heart rate—"Tachycardia robs diastole." The duration of systole on the LV pressure tracing is constant, regardless of the heart rate. With an increase in heart rate, the total duration of diastole thus declines, and there is less time for ventricular filling. Those with stiff ventricles need as much time in diastole as possible for ventricular filling.

Consider a patient with AS and LVH who develops rapid atrial fibrillation and has a drop in blood pressure. There is a double insult to LV filling and stroke volume: loss of atrial contraction plus tachycardia. If hypotension is so severe that the patient appears to be in shock, the atrial fibrillation is a medical emergency and requires immediate DC cardioversion. Do not wait for a cardiology consultation or take time to push rate-lowering drugs. You must act promptly to resuscitate the patient when a tachyarrhythmia causes shock, even when it is an atrial tachyarrhythmia.

History and Physical Examination

Diastolic heart failure may be mild, with effort intolerance or dyspnea with exertion the only symptoms. Diastolic dysfunction is often diagnosed from the echocardiogram in asymptomatic patients with hypertension, but the heart failure syndrome is needed to call it diastolic CHF.

At the other end of the spectrum is flash pulmonary edema, mentioned previously. This may occur in a person with no history of CHF or heart disease, who gives no history of gradually increasing exertional dyspnea or orthopnea. In contrast, CHF from systolic dysfunction develops slowly and progressively. Flash pulmonary edema illustrates an important clinical feature of DHF, the narrow window between volume overload (congestion), and depletion (hypotension).

Features of the history that point to diastolic dysfunction as the cause of CHF include advanced age, hypertension, and female gender. Both the history and physical examination should screen for other conditions that may cause LVH such as AS or hypertrophic subaortic stenosis. Look carefully for any evidence of coronary artery disease. Myocardial relaxation is an active, energy-requiring process, and ischemia has an immediate negative effect on diastolic function. Those with ischemic cardiomyopathy often have an element of diastolic dysfunction, although low LVEF is the predominant mechanism.

Most patients with diastolic CHF have just pulmonary congestion. Right heart failure may occur, but is uncommon. Thus, jugular venous distension and peripheral edema are not usually present. The physical findings of left heart congestion are typical.

The cardiac examination may allow you to differentiate diastolic from systolic failure at the bedside. With diastolic CHF the heart is usually small, so the point of maximum impulse is in the mid-clavicular line. It is not diffuse and sustained. If there is LVH, it may be forceful. There is no S_3 gallop. Instead, increased LV diastolic stiffness causes an S_4 gallop, the result of the atrium forcing blood into the stiff ventricle at the end of diastole.

An especially useful physical finding is a palpable S_4, the *apical A wave* (Figure 2.4). To detect the A wave, have the patient roll to the left and carefully feel the apex impulse. Normally its upstroke is smooth. The A wave is felt as a glitch or shudder. Practice feeling for it in patients with hypertension and LVH; it is not that subtle a finding. Describing an apical A wave indicates advanced

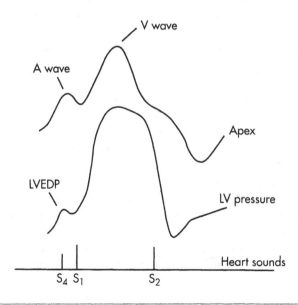

Figure 2.4 The contour of the apical impulse (top tracing) mirrors the LV pressure tracing. Just before ventricular systole, atrial contraction causes a small rise in LV pressure that is measured as the LV end-diastolic pressure (LVEDP). This is elevated in conditions that increase LV stiffness. When the apical A wave is greater than 15% of the total apical excursion, it is palpable as a shudder or glitch on the upstroke of the impulse. This is a reliable indicator of elevated LVEDP and is audible as the S_4 gallop.

understanding and physical diagnosis skills (and is very cool). More importantly, the A wave is the most specific physical finding for increased LV stiffness, and its presence reliably indicates elevated LV diastolic pressure. Remember that the A wave and S_4 gallop disappear with atrial fibrillation and the loss of atrial contraction (medical residents *always* ask students if they hear the S_4 in patients with atrial fibrillation—don't be fooled).

We have become accustomed to using brain natriuretic peptide (BNP) as an indicator of heart failure. It is less sensitive in patients with diastolic than in those with systolic failure. However it is still useful. Patients with LVH and CHF have elevation of BNP, while others with LVH and no heart failure do not.[3]

Laboratory Examination

There are just two things needed to make the diagnosis of diastolic failure. The first is to establish the diagnosis of CHF. Ralesora chest x-ray showing congestion that subsequently responds to diuresis is adequate evidence. Type B natriuretic peptide (BNP) is elevated with diastolic failure, but less so than with systolic heart failure where there is more LV stretch.

The second step is documentation of LVEF. If the LVEF is above 50%, then it is DHF.[3] Some studies use 40% as the criterion for diastolic dysfunction; in practice, most patients have normal or even hyperdynamic LV contraction, and the ventricle is small.

Supporting evidence includes LVH on the ECG or echocardiogram. Remember that only half of those with increased LV thickness on the echo meet ECG criteria for LVH. Diastolic dysfunction is about abnormal LV filling, and the echo-Doppler study allows assessment of flow across the mitral valve during diastole (Figure 2.5). Normally flow into the ventricle is highest in early diastole, but with increased LV stiffness the velocity of flow caused by atrial contraction—the A wave—increases. These Doppler measures are confirmatory, and not necessary for making the diagnosis.[3]

The echocardiogram may not be technically adequate to assess LV size and function (in a setting of obesity or emphysema). The other noninvasive tool for measuring LVEF is the radionuclide angiogram. Using the first-pass technique, the radionuclide angiogram can also provide information about LV filling. In the absence of CHF, echo-Doppler findings of abnormal diastolic filling identify pre-clinical diastolic dysfunction, strong evidence for treatment aimed at regression of LVH.

It is important to exclude ischemic heart disease, especially for a younger patient. In addition to controlling symptoms caused by transient ischemia in an already stiff ventricle, you want to intervene before the patient has a myocardial infarction. Combined systolic and diastolic dysfunction—often the case with ischemic cardiomyopathy—is the worst of all possible worlds. In the absence of anginal symptoms and risk factors, a screening perfusion study may be adequate.

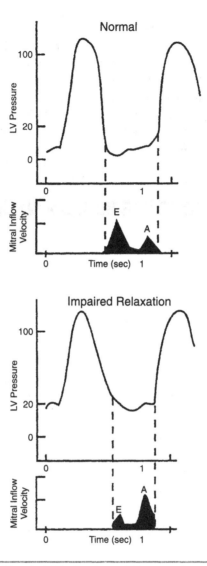

Figure 2.5 The effect of impaired LV relaxation on LV pressure (measured at cardiac catheterization) and flow across the mitral valve (measured from the echo-Doppler study). Normally, maximal flow into the ventricle occurs in early diastole, the E wave. With impaired relaxation in early diastole, atrial contraction produces a higher flow velocity, and the A wave is larger than the V wave. Note that with the stiffer ventricle the LV diastolic pressure is higher. (Reprinted with permission from Taylor, GJ. The Cardiology Rotation. Malden, MA: Blackwell Science, 2001:36.)

If the symptoms are suggestive, consider cardiac catheterization. This is also useful when there is uncertainty about the diagnosis (is CHF causing the patient's symptoms?). A normal LV end-diastolic pressure at rest and with arm exercise in the catheterization lab indicates normal diastolic function.

Treatment of Diastolic Heart Failure

Unlike systolic heart failure, there have been no large clinical trials of therapy for diastolic failure.[3] The strategy outlined in Table 2.1 is a reasonable approach based upon experience and the pathophysiology of the illness.

Congestion is relieved by lowering preload. Small doses of furosemide are usually sufficient, as the pressure–volume curve is steep (Figure 2.2), and there is a narrow difference between congestion and volume depletion. It is common to overshoot with diuretics. We usually begin with 20 mg furosemide daily, and carefully titrate the dose. Stable patients may be controlled with 12.5–25 mg hydrochlorothiazide per day. Nitrates may also be used to reduce preload, especially

Table 2-1 The Treatment Strategy for Diastolic CHF		
Goal of Treatment	Intervention/Drug	Comment
Reduce preload and congestion	Diuretics, occasionally nitrates	The LV pressure volume curve is steep with diastolic failure; small changes in volume lead to big changes in pressure. Thus, *low-dose* diuretics usually works
Treat hypertension and reduce LVH	First choice: ACE inhibitors. Calcium channel blockers, beta-blockers, and central alpha-blockers also work.	Short-term benefit: lower afterload favorably affects LV relaxation. Long-term benefit: regression of LVH. There is no need to slowly titrate beta-blockers (as there is with systolic heart failure).
Treat ischemia	Revascularization when possible. Beta blockade and calcium channel blockade.	Ischemia directly impairs LV relaxation. New onset, episodic, exertional dyspnea may be an anginal equivalent.
Lower the heart rate to 60–70 beats/minute.	Beta-blockers (metoprolol works and is cheap), verapamil or diltiazem.	At higher heart rates, the total diastolic time is reduced, so there is less time for LV filling. These drugs may be used even when blood pressure is normal to blunt exercise-induced tachycardia.
Maintain atrial booster function.	Correct atrial fibrillation.	The stiff LV is especially dependent on atrial contraction for adequate filling.
Avoid inotropes and use caution with pure arterial dilators.	Avoid digoxin.	Hydralazine, and calcium blockers that are pure vasodilators (nifedipine) may provoke reflex tachycardia (when tachycardia is prevented, vasodilators are okay).

when there is ischemia. Again, start with a low dose, such as 15–30 mg isosorbide mononitrate (Imdur).

Reducing blood pressure has an immediate benefit, because the excessive after-load of hypertension slows relaxation. Over the long run, control of blood pressure leads to regression of LVH and improved diastolic function. Angiotensin-converting enzyme (ACE) inhibitors appear to be the most effective for regression of hypertrophy, and they may have a direct myocardial effect. Calcium channel blockers, beta-blockers, and centrally acting sympatholytic agents also work. Early data suggest a role for aldosterone antagonists (spironolactone), which may prevent or reduce myocardial fibrosis.

As noted, tachycardia is a major problem when there is diastolic disease. Drugs that lower the sinus rate (beta-blockers, verapamil, or diltiazem), or that control the ventricular rate with atrial fibrillation will improve exercise tolerance. This is the only indication for digoxin in DHF. When using arterial dilators—including ACE inhibitors, angiotensin receptor blockers, and calcium blockers—watch for reflex tachycardia.

I have emphasized the importance of atrial contraction in the patient with a stiff LV. Unfortunately, atrial fibrillation is a common complication of diastolic failure, because there is elevation of the left atrial pressure. Every effort should be made to restore sinus rhythm.

Hypertrophic Cardiomyopathy

Hypertrophic cardiomyopathy (HCM) is a unifying diagnosis for a number of illnesses with a common pathophysiology: LVH in the absence of pressure overload. Approximately 60% of the cases are inherited, with the remainder sporadic. A single pattern of inheritance is not characteristic, an observation that suggests that several genetic defects may contribute to the pool of patients with familial HCM.

The most common HCM is idiopathic hypertrophic subaortic stenosis (IHSS). The anatomic defect is hypertrophy of the interventricular septum; the thickened lump of septal muscle is histologically abnormal, with disorientation of muscle fibers. Diastolic dysfunction is one of four mechanisms that contribute to symptoms in IHSS. The others are aortic outflow tract obstruction, myocardial ischemia and arrhythmias.[9]

Pathophysiology and Physical Examination

Valvular AS causes a pressure gradient across the valve; systolic pressure in the LV is higher than aortic pressure. With IHSS, the level of obstruction—also the level of the gradient—is subvalvular (Figure 2.6). It is attributed to crowding of the outflow tract by the hypertrophied septum and to movement of the mitral valve leaflet into the outflow tract. High velocity flow across the narrowed space creates a Venturi effect, pulling the mitral leaflet into the outflow tract toward the septum, the so-called systolic anterior motion (SAM) of the mitral valve that is one of the diagnostic features of IHSS. SAM contributes to the gradient, and when there is no

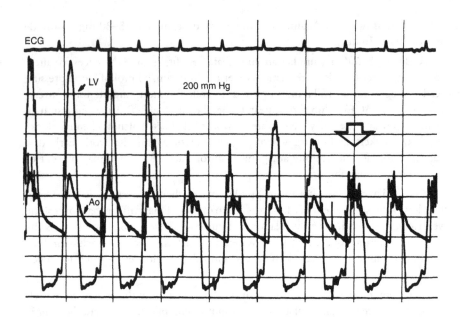

Figure 2.6 Hypertrophic cardiomyopathy with left ventricular outflow tract obstruction. These are simultaneous pressures from the left ventricle (LV) and aorta (Ao). Left ventricular pressure is initially measured at the LV apex, the left side of the tracing. As the catheter is withdrawn toward the aortic valve (right side of the tracing), a point is reached just below the valve (arrow) where there is no difference, or gradient, between left ventricular and aortic pressure. This indicates that the level of obstruction is subvalvular, in the body of the ventricle, rather than valvular. (Reprinted with permission from Kern, MJ. The Cardiac Catheterization Handbook. St. Louis: Mosby, 1991.)

SAM on the echocardiogram, there usually is no gradient. The semantics of this condition may be confusing, and without a gradient some describe it as asymmetric septal hypertrophy—ASH—rather than IHSS.

The outflow tract gradient and murmur increase with lower LV volume. It is a matter of geometry. Less filling of the ventricle means that the outflow tract is narrower, flow velocity, and the Venturi effect are heightened, and there is more SAM. Standing after squatting and the strain phase of the Valsalva maneuver lower venous return and accentuate the systolic murmur. In the echo laboratory, amyl nitrite, a venodilator, does the same thing, provoking SAM, the gradient, and murmur.

The systolic murmur is the key diagnostic finding. Unlike valvular AS, there is little radiation of the murmur to the neck (the murmur is generated by mitral regurgitation and outflow tract turbulence). The peripheral pulse also helps differentiate IHSS and AS. With IHSS, initial LV emptying is normal, as obstruction to outflow worsens in mid-systole, as the ventricle empties and is smaller. Thus, the pulse upstroke is brisk (with valvular AS the pulse upstroke is delayed). In both conditions, the stiff ventricle produces an S_4 gallop and an apical A wave.

The diagnosis is made by the echocardiogram-Doppler study. The pattern of hypertrophy is well visualized using the transthoracic echo, and the muscle may appear qualitatively abnormal. Tissue Doppler echocardiography, not widely available, allows identification of this abnormal muscle even before hypertrophy develops. Using conventional techniques, the Doppler examination allows measurement of flow velocity across the outflow tract and calculation of the pressure gradient between the LV and aorta.

Treatment

None of the treatments for IHSS have been shown to improve survival, although many relieve symptoms. The principles of treating diastolic dysfunction apply (Table 2.1). In addition, medical therapy is directed at increasing space in the outflow tract. Drugs that block contractility (verapamil, beta-blockers, and disopyramide) cause ventricular dilatation, widening the outflow tract and reducing flow velocity, which minimizes SAM. The outflow tract gradient is thus reduced.

Dual-chamber, atrio-ventricular pacing has been used. Pacing the right ventricle creates a left bundle branch block pattern on the ECG. Septal activation is thus later in systole, and this septal dyskinesis has been shown to reduce the outflow tract gradient. It is the reverse of resynchronization therapy for systolic heart failure (see Chapter 1). One randomized trial showed no long-term benefit with pacing, but there are small series that described symptomatic benefits.[10]

The newest therapy is ablation of septal muscle with local infusion of alcohol through a coronary catheter positioned in a small septal perforating artery.[11] Alcohol kills septal muscle. There is immediate reduction of septal contractility, then regression of septal hypertrophy over a period of weeks. This technique is replacing surgical myotomyectomy for patients whose symptoms are not adequately controlled with medical therapy. There is sustained improvement in symptoms, exercise capacity, and LV outflow tract gradient. Heart block requiring pacemaker therapy is a possible complication.

Sudden Cardiac Death

The annual mortality with HCM is relatively low, estimated at 2% to 3%. About half the deaths are sudden and unexpected, and sudden cardiac death (SCD) may be the initial symptom. Risk factors for sudden death include extreme LVH, a family history of sudden death, a history of ventricular tachycardia or syncope, and a failure of blood pressure to rise during exercise.[12] Recently, evaluation of a large cohort (1101 patients) found that a resting outflow tract gradient of 30 mm Hg or greater is a predictor of progression to severe symptoms of heart failure and of death.[13] On the other hand, therapies that lower the outflow gradient and relieve symptoms have not been shown to prevent SCD.

Because SCD may be a presenting symptom of HCM, screening echocardiograms in first-degree relatives can be justified. HCM is one of the causes of SCD in young athletes, a consideration when doing pre-sports physical examinations. A murmur that increases after squatting or with Valsalva would be an indication for an echocardiogram. The illness is rare enough that a screening echocardiogram is not justified for a young athlete with no family history and a normal physical examination.

Antiarrhythmic drug therapy is of no benefit. The implantable cardioverter-defibrillator (ICD) is indicated for secondary prevention—that is to say, as treatment for one who has experienced syncope caused by ventricular tachycardia or fibrillation. More recently, ICD therapy is being recommended for primary prevention in patients with risk factors for sudden death. Patient selection—how many and which risk factors justify an ICD—is uncertain at this time.[12]

Restrictive Cardiomyopathy

Restrictive cardiomyopathies may or may not lead to reduction in LVEF. All of them cause an increase in LV stiffness, and diastolic dysfunction contributes to the CHF syndrome. The general principles of treatment are those outlined for other forms of DHF (Table 2.1). In addition, some of the conditions respond to disease-specific therapy.

The restrictive illnesses have a characteristic ventricular filling pressure. Initial filling is rapid, but filling quickly hits the wall of the restrictive process. This leads to the square root sign: an early dip in LV diastolic pressure followed by a plateau, without the gradual rise in pressure that is normally observed through the rest of diastole.

Amyloidosis

When amyloidosis causes DHF, the usual etiology is a plasma cell disorder such as multiple myeloma.[14] Senile amyloidosis may involve the heart, but usually causes dilated cardiomyopathy and systolic heart failure. The other forms of amyloidosis, familial and the secondary form that accompanies chronic inflammation, are rare and usually do not affect the heart.

The fibrillar protein is deposited throughout the myocardium, leading to a rubbery consistency and concentric hypertrophy. Both the right and left ventricles are thickened, an infrequent finding with the usual causes of LVH. Perhaps the most useful diagnostic finding is an absence of high QRS voltage on the ECG; the amyloid infiltrate is not depolarized and therefore does not generate voltage. Think of amyloid heart disease when there is a combination of increased LV thickness on the echo, but low voltage on the ECG (this may be a board question).

The diagnosis of amyloid heart disease is supported by fat pad aspirate or rectal biopsies indicating systemic amyloidosis. Endomyocardial biopsy is required for a definite diagnosis. In addition to concentric hypertrophy with normal or reduced chamber size, the echocardiogram often shows a qualitative abnormality of muscle described as granular or sparkling. LVEF may or may not be reduced, and there is usually evidence for diastolic dysfunction.

The prognosis with amyloid heart disease is poor; the severity of LVH predicts mortality. Doppler measures of diastolic dysfunction also indicate early mortality. Systemic amyloidosis is considered a contraindication for heart transplantation, primarily because of disease progression in other organ systems. It is not certain whether the transplanted heart is at risk.

Hemochromatosis

This iron storage disorder primarily affects the liver, and should be considered with the clinical triad of diabetes mellitus, hyperpigmentation, and liver disease. Iron deposition in the heart is in the myocardial cells, not interstitial. It tends to affect the subepicardium primarily, with less subendocardial involvement. The heart is dilated, with or without hypertrophy (distinguishing it from amyloid heart disease). LVEF is reduced, and there usually is diastolic dysfunction. Endomyocardial biopsy is needed to make the diagnosis of cardiac hemochromatosis. Most patients die from liver failure, not from heart disease.

Loeffler's Endocarditis

The illness begins with eosinophilia, either idiopathic or in response to chronic infection. Myocardial fibrosis develops in approximately 80% of those with chronic eosinophilia within 5 years.[14] Eosinophils invade the subendocardium, degranulate and thus provoke tissue damage, necrosis, and then fibrosis. Mural thrombus often forms over the necrotic myocardium, and systemic or pulmonary embolism is a feature of the illness.

The ventricular inflow tracts and apices are preferentially involved, and this may include tricuspid and mitral valves leading to regurgitation. It affects both right and left ventricles, so right and left heart failure are common.

Suspect the diagnosis when there is heart failure plus eosinophilia. About 20% of patients do not have eosinophilia at the time of diagnosis; presumably, they had it at one point. When eosinophilia is present, prednisone and hydroxyurea may be effective. Anticoagulation should be considered, especially when there is suspicion of mural thrombus.

Pericardial Effusion, Tamponade, and Constriction

Although the pericardium is external to the heart, tamponade and constriction compress the heart and limit cardiac filling. This inadequate preload—as that is what it is—results in lower stroke volume.[14]

Pericardial Tamponade

Clinically, acute tamponade causes a precipitous fall in blood pressure. Think of it when there is low blood pressure unresponsive to intravenous fluids plus jugular venous distension.

Tamponade occurs when pericardial fluid accumulates quickly and the pericardium has no time to stretch. Slowly accumulating effusions (as with

Table 2-2 Causes of Pericardial Effusion

Idiopathic
Viral (Coxsackie, adenovirus, HIV, mononucleosis)
Bacterial (tuberculosis, staphylococcus, pneumococcus, brucella, salmonella, mycoplasma)
Neoplastic (breast and lung cancer)
Collagen vascular disease (systemic lupus erythematosus, rheumatoid arthritis)
Drugs (procainamide, hydralazine)
Hypothyroidism*
Uremia
Post myocardial infarction (Dressler's syndrome)
Post heart surgery (postpericardiotomy syndrome)
Radiation exposure
Aortic dissection

* Any of these illnesses may cause tamponade, but it is a rare complication of hypothyroid effusion (which can be massive, but which accumulate slowly).

hypothyroidism—a board question) allow time for the pericardium to expand with no increase in pericardial pressure. Causes of effusion are reviewed in Table 2.2, and most of them can cause tamponade. However, the most common cause is malignancy (more than half the cases), followed by viral and uremic pericarditis. Anticoagulation increases the risk.

Pathophysiology and physical examination—The pathophysiology of tamponade is illustrated in Figure 2.7. Inflation of the atria and ventricles is determined

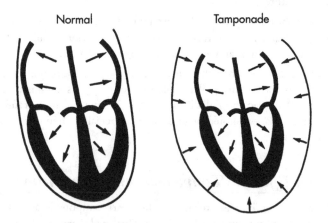

Normal   Tamponade

Figure 2.7 The physiology of cardiac tamponade. In the normal state, pericardial pressure is near zero and intracardiac pressures, in effect, inflate the cardiac chambers. With tamponade, pericardial pressure increases and tends to compress the heart. Intracardiac pressure is the sum of pericardial pressure plus that pressure generated by volume within the cardiac chambers. During diastole, the pericardial pressure is sufficiently high to be the major determinant of intracardiac pressure, and pressures in the four chambers tend to equalize. External compression of the atria also retards venous return to the heart, lowering cardiac output and blood pressure. (Reprinted with permission from Taylor GJ. Primary Care Management of Heart Disease. St. Louis: Mosby, 2000:343.)

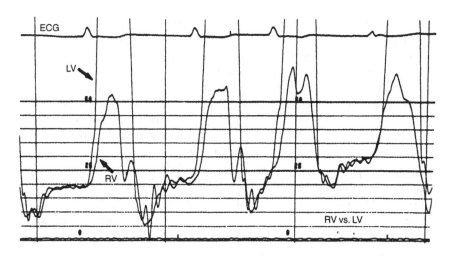

Figure 2.8 Simultaneous left and right ventricular (LV and RV) pressures in a patient with constrictive pericarditis. Normally, the left ventricular pressure is much higher than right ventricular pressure during diastole, and identical pressure during diastole is a hallmark of both constriction and pericardial tamponade. In addition, this patient has the early diastolic pressure dip and then plateau that is typical of constriction (best seen in the first and last beats). (Reprinted with permission from Kern MJ. The Cardiac Catheterization Handbook. St. Louis: Mosby, 1999:203.)

by transmural pressure, or the difference between the internal (inflating) pressure, and external (deflating) pressure. Normally, the pericardial pressure is zero, and the diastolic, inflating pressure within the cardiac chambers is unopposed. Rapidly accumulating effusion increases pericardial pressure, so the transmural pressure declines. This limits diastolic filling. With tamponade, pericardial pressure is so high that it exceeds intracardiac diastolic pressure. This leads to the key diagnostic feature: equalization of the diastolic pressure in all four cardiac chambers (Figure 2.8). Normally the thicker LV has a higher diastolic pressure than the right ventricle (RV). Diastolic pressures in the atria and RV are higher than usual because of the external pressure, not because of increased filling of the chambers. Filling is actually lower, and the echocardiogram may shows collapse of the atria and/or RV.

The external pressure blocks blood return to the heart. With reduced cardiac filling, stroke volume and cardiac output fall. The consequence is hypotension. The key findings on physical examination are jugular venous distension and pulsus paradoxus.

I find nothing paradoxical about pulsus paradoxus, and consider the term misleading.[15] Normally the systolic blood pressure falls during inspiration, by less than 10 mm Hg. With pulsus paradoxus it falls more; if severe, there may be an appreciable diminution of the arterial pulse with inspiration.

The mechanism may seem complex, but like most of cardiology, it is easily understood. Normally intrathoracic and intrapericardial pressures become negative during inspiration; this sucks blood (as well as air) into the chest and increases venous return to the right heart. Right ventricular volume increases. The expanded RV pushes the interventricular septum toward the LV, reducing LV volume. In addition, pulmonary venous return to the left atrium is decreased during inspiration. Physiologists speak of *respiratory preload variation*: RV preload rises and LV preload falls. The net effect is a smaller LV during inspiration, leading to lower stroke volume and systolic blood pressure.

Cardiac tamponade exaggerates these changes. Both ventricles are smaller than usual because of elevated pericardial pressure. With inspiration there is still an increase in flow to the RV. Bowing of the septum toward the LV has an even greater effect on LV stroke volume because the LV is already small—and systolic blood pressure falls by more than 10 mm Hg.

Pulsus paradoxus is measured with the patient breathing normally. The best method is to inflate the blood pressure cuff and then have it deflate very, very, very slowly. You will initially hear the Korotkoff sounds during expiration but not during inspiration; record that blood pressure as pressure-1. As the cuff continues to deflate slowly, at some point you will hear the sounds during both inspiration and expiration. Record that as pressure-2. The difference between pressures 1 and 2 is the pulsus paradoxus. When there is a large pulsus, you may feel a reduction in the radial pulse volume with inspiration.

Laboratory diagnosis and treatment or pericardial effusion—The ECG may show ST segment elevation with pericarditis, but in most cases of effusion and tamponade, there is no ST elevation. With large effusions, QRS voltage may be low. Electrical alternans, a rise and fall in QRS voltage, may occur with the heart swinging in the enlarged pericardial space (and is referred to as the *swinging heart syndrome*).

The echocardiogram is able to detect even small effusions.[16] With tamponade there may be apparent collapse of the atria or right ventricle. Hemodynamic instability is an indication for urgent pericardiocentesis. When done at the bedside as an emergency procedure, the complication rate is about 20%. With echocardiographic guidance, usually in the catheterization laboratory, the complication rate is less than 5%.

An occasional patient with a large effusion does not have tamponade, and may be asymptomatic, indicating that the accumulation of fluid was slow enough for the pericardium to expand. This is often the case with hypothyroidism (a board question). Diagnostic pericardiocentesis is of little use when viral pericarditis is likely. It is not usually needed to make a diagnosis for those with collagen vascular disease.

On the other hand, pericardiocentesis may be diagnostic in a patient with suspected malignancy. This usually involves an older patient with no history indicating pericarditis (no fever or pain, and a normal sedimentation rate). The effusion may be an incidental finding on a chest x-ray or echocardiogram.

A bloody pericardial effusion in the absence of anticoagulant therapy points to tumor, and cytology is usually positive.

Constrictive Pericarditis

Chronic inflammation and thickening of the pericardium may lead to constriction, which limits diastolic filling.[17,18] The usual clinical presentation is isolated right heart failure. Hepatomegaly and ascites are common, and constriction is one of the causes of cryptogenic cirrhosis. We see one or two cases each year when evaluating patients for liver transplantation, and surgical correction of constriction cures the liver disease.

Like tamponade, there is equalization of right and left heart diastolic pressures. Unlike tamponade, early diastolic filling is normal, but it is limited in later diastole. This leads to the characteristic dip-and-plateau, or square-root wave form of the ventricular pressure tracing. This may be similar to the pressure waveform of restrictive cardiomyopathy. One way to differentiate the two is to infuse saline; with restrictive myopathy, the LV diastolic pressure rises more than RV pressure, and with constriction, equalization of diastolic pressures persists.

There is elevation of jugular venous pressure, but constriction prevents a fall with inspiration. Instead, venous pressure may increase with inspiration (Kussmaul's sign). Elevated pulsus paradoxus is uncommon with constriction, and always present with tamponade. A rare patient will have an extra heart sound in early diastole, a *pericardial knock*. Pericardial calcification on an over-penetrated chest x-ray supports the diagnosis. Most texts recommend magnetic resonance imaging to measure pericardial thickness. I have rarely found it helpful; a normal study does not exclude constriction.

When suspected, left and right heart catheterization is needed to make a diagnosis. Equalization of pressures, even with fluid infusion, is the usual indication for surgical stripping of the pericardium. But this is a tough diagnosis to make. Even when all studies point to constriction, a fair number of patients are found to have no pericardial disease at operation. I tell patients this before surgery, indicating that the procedure is, in a sense, an exploratory operation. The possibility of a surgical cure justifies it.

Effusive-constrictive pericarditis—An occasional patient has concomitant tamponade and constriction.[19] In this case, constriction comes from a thickened visceral pericardium (the layer of pericardium that is attached to the epicardial surface). Measuring pericardial pressure at the time of pericardiocentesis, and at the same time measuring right atrial, RV, and LV pressure makes the diagnosis. As the fluid is drained, pericardial pressure decreases, but there is little if any fall in intracardiac diastolic pressure. The dip and plateau morphology of the ventricular diastolic pressure remains.

Effusive-constrictive disease is possible with all types of pericarditis. It is more common with radiation and neoplasm. Effective therapy requires both pericardiocentesis and surgical removal of the visceral pericardium. Consider this if draining the pericardium does not relieve the patient's symptoms.

References

1. Angeja BG, Grossman W. Evaluation and management of diastolic heart failure. Circulation 2003;107:659–663.

2. Smith GL, Masoudi FA, Vaccarino V, et al. Outcomes in heart failure patients with preserved ejection fraction: mortality, readmission, and functional decline. J Am Coll Cardiol 2003;41:1510–1518.

3. Zile MR. Heart failure with preserved ejection fraction: Is this diastolic heart failure. J Am Coll Cardiol 2003:41:1519–1522. Also note, Yamaguchi H, Yoshida J, Yamamoto K, et al. Elevation of plasma brain natriuretic peptide is a hallmark of diastolic heart failure independent of ventricular hypertrophy. J Am Coll Cardiol 2004;43:55–60.

4. Masoudi FA, Havranek EP, Smith G, et al. Gender, age, and heart failure with preserved left ventricular systolic function. J Am Coll Cardiol 2003;41:217–223.

5. Jessup M. The less familiar face of heart failure. J Am Coll Cardiol 2003;41:224–226.

6. Petrie MC, Dawson NF, Murdoch DR, et al. Failure of women's hearts. Circulation 1999;99:2334–2341.

7. Schillaci G, Pasqualini L, Vaudo G, et al. Importance of diastolic dysfunction in essential hypertension. Cardiol Rev 2003;20:29–33.

8. Messerli FH, Ventura HO, Elizardi DJ, et al. Hypertension and sudden death. Increased ventricular ectopic activity in left ventricular hypertrophy. Am J Med 1984;77:18–22.

9. Nishimura RA, Holmes DR. Hypertrophic obstructive cardiomyopathy. N Engl J Med 2004;350:1320–1327.

10. Maron BJ, Nishimura RA, McKenna WJ, et al. Assessment of permanent dual-chamber pacing as a treatment for drug-refractory symptomatic patients with obstructive hypertrophic cardiomyopathy. A randomized, double-blind, crossover study. Circulation 1999;99:2927–2933.

11. Shamim W, Yousufuddin M, Wang D, et al. Nonsurgical reduction of the inter-ventricular septum in patients with hypertrophic cardiomyopathy. N Engl J Med 2002;347:1326–1333.

12. Maron BJ, Estes NA, Maron MS, et al. Primary prevention of sudden death as a novel treatment strategy in hypertrophic cardiomyopathy. Circulation 2003;107;2872–2875.

13. Maron MS, Olivotto I, Betocchi S, et al. Effect of left ventricular outflow tract obstruction on clinical outcome in hypertrophic cardiomyopathy. N Engl J Med 2003;348:295–303.

14. Kabbani SS, LeWinter MM. Diastolic heart failure. Constrictive, restrictive, and pericardial. Cardiol Clin 2000;18:501–509.

15. Swami A, Spodick DH. Pulsus paradoxus in cardiac tamponade: a pathophysio-logic continuum. Clin Cardiol 2003;26:215–217.

16. Tsang TS, Oh JK, Seward JB. Diagnosis and management of cardiac tamponade in the era of echocardiography. Clin Cardiol 1999;22:446–452

17. Garcia MJ. Constriction vs. restriction: how to evaluate. ACC Curr J Rev 2003;12:49–52.

18. Mehta A, Mehta M, Jain AC. Constrictive pericarditis. Clin Cardiol 1999;22:334–344.

19. Sagrista-Sauleda J, Angel J, Sanchez A, et al. Effusive–constrictive pericarditis. N Engl J Med 2004;350:469-475.

CHAPTER 3

ATHEROSCLEROSIS: MECHANISMS, LIPID DISORDERS, AND SCREENING FOR PRECLINICAL DISEASE

Abbreviations			
ACE	angiotensin-converting enzyme	IDL	intermediate-density lipoprotein (cholesterol)
AHA	American Heart Association	LDL	low-density lipoprotein (cholesterol)
ASCVD	atherosclerotic cardiovascular disease	MI	myocardial infarction
CAC	coronary artery calcium	NCEP	National Cholesterol Education Program
CAD	coronary artery disease		
CRP	C-reactive protein	NSAIDs	nonsteroidal anti-inflammatory drugs
CT	computed tomography		
ESRD	end-stage renal disease	PUFAs	polyunsaturated fatty acids
HDL	high-density lipoprotein (cholesterol)	SCD	sudden cardiac death
		VLDL	very-low-density lipoprotein (cholesterol)
HRT	hormone replacement therapy		

Atherosclerotic cardiovascular disease (ASCVD) is the most common cause of death in the United States, with almost 1 million dying each year.[1] Coronary artery disease (CAD) causes a majority of these deaths. About 150,000 people with no history of ASCVD die suddenly.

Women are not immune; ASCVD is their leading cause of death. ASCVD tends to develop in women about a decade later than in men. The chance of a woman dying with heart disease is 10 times greater than it is with breast cancer.

ASCVD is a disease of middle and older age; just 45% of myocardial infarction (MI) occurs in people younger than 65 years old. Almost 40% of men and 30% of women who die of CAD are younger than 55.

Risk Factors for Atherosclerotic Cardiovascular Disease

Fifty years ago, the Framingham Study established the concept of risk factors for premature ASCVD.[2] It is still clinically useful. A recent trial calculated the risk of coronary events over 10 years of follow-up. In descending order of importance, the risk was influenced by age, low-density lipoprotein (LDL) cholesterol, smoking, high-density lipoprotein (HDL) cholesterol, systolic blood pressure, family history, diabetes mellitus, and triglycerides.[3] Table 3.1 reviews known risk factors for ASCVD, plus a few of the more than 200 that have been suggested.

Epidemiologists emphasize that risk factors are useful for predicting who will get disease, but do not prove causality. This requires showing that treatment of a risk factor prevents disease (*primary prevention*) or halts progression of established disease (*secondary prevention*). Such proof is available with a number of risk factors, and their modification is the cornerstone for prevention and treatment of ASCVD.[9] For example, the Nurses Health Study found that women who maintain ideal body weight, exercise regularly, use alcohol in moderation, and do not smoke lower their risk of ASCVD by 84%.[10]

Smoking

More American teenagers are smoking now than in 1970, despite clear information about its role in causing disease. Half of all smokers die of smoking-related causes, and they lose an average of 23 years of life. ASCVD accounts for 38% of those deaths.[11,12] For every 10 cigarettes smoked per day, cardiovascular mortality increases by 18% in men, and 31% in women.[13] Continued smoking after MI halves life expectancy. Low tar cigarettes do not appear to lower the risk of ASCVD.[14]

Smokeless tobacco also increases vascular risk, although not as much as smoking. The relative risk of developing ASCVD is 1.8 higher smoking 15 cigarettes per day, and 1.4 higher dipping snuff.[15] Passive, second-hand smoking increases the relative risk of ASCVD by 20%, and of lung cancer by 30%.

Smoking has multiple actions that promote atherosclerosis. It lowers HDL cholesterol, adversely affects endothelial function (vide infra), promotes vasospasm, increases fibrinogen levels, and enhances platelet aggregation. A potential mechanism for these actions is increased insulin resistance; smokers have higher insulin levels than nonsmokers.[16] In addition, there is an acute effect. The carbon monoxide from burning cigarettes increases carboxyhemoglobin levels, reducing the oxygen-carrying capacity of blood, and thus reduces the level of exercise that provokes ischemia (the angina threshold). I often mention this to patients, indicating that there will be an immediate benefit from stopping tobacco use. As a risk factor for ASCVD, smoking no longer counts 10 to 12 years after stopping.

The current approach to treating tobacco addiction is outlined in Table 3.2. Using it you may expect sustained (6 months) abstinence in 20% to 40% of patients, depending on the effectiveness of behavioral therapy. Many go through multiple quit-attempts before they are successful, so never give up. Your role is critical. Repeated mention of smoking by the practitioner has been shown to double the chance of a patient quitting. Consider making smoking status a vital sign that is recorded at each clinic visit.

Obesity, Diabetes Mellitus, and the Metabolic Syndrome

Despite a culture that emphasizes fitness and appearance, we've become increasingly fat during the past four decades. Presently, almost one third of American adults are obese, and another one third are overweight.[9] Most of them have hypertension.

Table 3.1 Risk Factors for Atherosclerotic Cardiovascular Disease

Risk Factor	Examples of Available Data
Dyslipidemia*	Lowering total cholesterol by 1% reduces the incidence of CAD by 2%. Raising HDL also prevents disease.
Hypertension*	≥140/90 mm Hg. SHEP showed that control of systolic pressure lowers the risk of 1) fatal and nonfatal stroke, 2) nonfatal MI and coronary death, 3) combined ASCVD outcomes.[4] A meta-analysis showed that lowering blood pressure 6 mm Hg reduces the CAD rate 14%.[5]
Diabetes mellitus*	A risk factor for all, but with greater influence in women. In addition to more ASCVD it is a risk factor for heart failure. With diabetes there is also worse prognosis.
Abdominal obesity	The central element of the metabolic syndrome (see text), and an independent risk factor for ASCVD in the Framingham study.
Cigarette smoking*	See text. There is a dose-response curve, with the number of cigarettes smoked each day proportional to MI, stroke, and death.
Family history*	Definite MI or sudden death in first-degree relative <65 yr old (for male patients), or <55 (female). After stratifying for other risk factors, a positive family history increases risk two- to fourfold.
Male gender	Premature disease is more common in men. Women develop ASCVD about 10 years later.
Age*	≥ 45 yr for men, 55 yr for women. About four fifths of fatal MI occur over age 65.
Left ventricular hypertrophy	An independent predictor of CAD, especially for older people. Also predisposes to heart failure and sudden cardiac death.
Physical inactivity	In the MRFIT study those who exercised had a 27% lower CAD mortality rate.[6]
Stress, mood, and personality type	Proposed risk factors include negative affectivity, social inhibition, and type A personality. Evidence is mixed. Anger is associated with onset of MI, and both MI and sudden death are more common on Monday morning. Depression predicts poor outcome after MI. Effects of treatment are mixed, with two random trials showing little survival benefit with nonspecific intervention for depression after MI.[7]
Hemostatic factors	Fibrinogen, factor VII, and plasminogen activator inhibitor 1 may be elevated in patients with CAD, and fibrinolytic activity reduced.[8]
Inflammation: elevated CRP	Higher risk for developing CAD, plus a risk factor for becoming unstable (see text).
Chlamydia pneumoniae	Bacteria have been isolated from plaque, but an infectious mechanism for atherogenesis is not established (see text).
Homocysteine	Elevated in 20% to 30% with ASCVD, and treatable with vitamins. See text.
Negative risk factor: HDL cholesterol >60 mg/dL*	With high HDL, you may subtract one other risk factor

ASCVD, atherosclerotic cardiovascular disease; CAD, coronary artery disease; MI, myocardial infarction; CRP, C-reactive protein.

*The National Cholesterol Education Program uses these risk factors when deciding whether to begin LDL lowering therapy for primary prevention.

Table 3.2 An Approach to Smoking Cessation	
Behavioral modification	There are various elements: 1. The practitioners should mention tobacco at every visit (one survey found that half of us fail to comment on continued smoking). 2. Smoking cessation clinics; this intense approach helps patients develop techniques (i.e., using substitute behaviors, making the home-car-office smoke free, avoiding alcohol while stopping). 3. Social support—enlist family, friends, and a medical team to help with positive reinforcement.
Nicotine replacement	There is usually a preference for gum, nasal spray, or patch. Consider starting with a kit containing all three, and encourage the patient to experiment (although staying in the recommended dose range). Start replacement the day of the last cigarette. Do not reduce the nicotine dose until the new behavior (nonsmoking) is well entrenched. The patient should not smoke while using replacement therapy.
Antidepressant therapy	Smoking has an antidepressant effect, and there is mild rebound depression with cessation that is blocked by bupropion (Zyban or Wellbutrin, 150 mg once—and after 3 days—twice daily). Start it a week before the cessation; attempt to reach a steady-state blood level. Continue therapy for 7 to 12 weeks. If still smoking at 7 weeks, this will not be a successful quit attempt, and the drug can be stopped.

Obesity is the initiating element of the metabolic syndrome, thought to affect one fourth of American men and postmenopausal women. The consequence of this is an epidemic of diabetes mellitus, with a remarkable increase in diabetes-related mortality (Figure 3.1).[17]

Diagnostic criteria for the metabolic syndrome are summarized in Table 3.3.[18] It begins with abdominal obesity, which causes insulin resistance. That is to say, for a given level of glucose, the insulin level is elevated. Not all obese people with insulin resistance develop diabetes, but those with a family history of beta cell dysfunction eventually do.[19] These obese offspring of diabetic parents have high insulin levels for more than a decade before their beta cells wear out, serum glucose increases, and they are diabetic.

Most obese people, and all of those with diabetes, thus have elevated insulin levels. Hyperinsulinemia is toxic, and is a risk factor for early vascular disease in those who are not diabetic.[20] It causes endothelial dysfunction, possibly by increasing oxidative stress. Most patients with elevated insulin levels are hypertensive; whether this is from associated obesity or a pressor effect of insulin is uncertain. The hypertension contributes to endothelial dysfunction. Interaction with other risk factors has been described. Smoking provokes insulin resistance, and smokers' hyperinsulinemia may contribute to their premature ASCVD.[16]

Obesity is also associated with elevated free fatty acids, an increase in hepatic lipase, reduced HDL cholesterol, and high triglycerides. The LDL cholesterol level is less affected, but there is a qualitative shift to small, dense LDL particles that are more atherogenic.

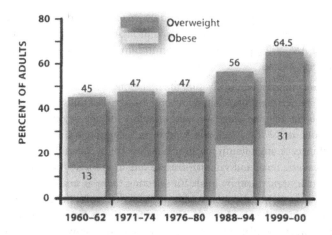

Figure 3.1 Prevalence of overweight and obese adults in the USA, 1960–2000. Data from the National Center for Health Statistics.

Clinical course and treatment—A nondiabetic patient may have the metabolic syndrome. Most obese people meet diagnostic criteria, even without diabetes (Table 3.3). They may be assumed to have insulin resistance and hyperinsulinemia, and most of them have high triglycerides and low HDL cholesterol.

Premature vascular disease is one consequence of the metabolic syndrome. It is so prevalent that type 2 diabetes is considered a surrogate for established CAD. Studies of treatment have shown that diabetic patients benefit from a

Table 3.3 The Metabolic Syndrome[10]	
Diagnostic criteria (those with three or more have the metabolic syndrome)	
1	Abdominal obesity: Waist circumference >40 in (men), or >35 in (women)
2	Plasma triglycerides ≥150 mg/dL
3	HDL cholesterol <40 mg/dL (men), or <50 mg/dL (women)
4	Blood pressure ≥130/85 mm Hg
5	Fasting glucose ≥110 mg/dL (or diabetes)
Other conditions observed with the metabolic syndrome that may contribute to premature vascular disease	
1	Prothrombotic state (increased fibrinogen and platelet activator inhibitor-1)
2	Abnormal endothelial and smooth muscle function
3	Increased inflammation (increased leukocyte adhesion to endothelium)

secondary—rather than primary—prevention strategy. Anecdotally, we performed screening stress perfusion scans on 100 asymptomatic patients with diabetes with no history of ASCVD (age over 45 and on insulin for at least 10 years); 70 of the 100 had a positive scan.

Weight loss and exercise usually cure the metabolic syndrome, and I point this out to patients. The treatment of obesity is beyond the scope of this review.[21] Despite best efforts, long-term success is rare. We must therefore include treatment of each of the other components of the metabolic syndrome.[22] Angiotensin-converting enzyme (ACE) inhibitors or angiotensin receptor blockers are of special benefit for the prevention of diabetic renal and vascular disease, and are indicated for all patients with diabetes.[23] An argument can be made for selecting them as treatment for hypertension in non-diabetic obese patients who probably have insulin resistance. There is uncertainty whether the benefit of ACE inhibition comes from blood pressure control, or is a direct vascular effect.[20] Current data favor lowering the pressure to 120/80 mm Hg for diabetic patients, a goal that is seldom achieved in clinical practice, but that is possible with available therapy.[20] Aggressive treatment of dyslipidemia is critical, with treatment goals similar to those for patients with known CAD.[18] Antiplatelet therapy is indicated, even in the absence of known ASCVD.[23] Glycemic control is helpful, but probably has less effect on macrovascular disease than lifestyle changes—weight loss, exercise, and smoking cessation.

I will not attempt to review management of diabetes. Of special interest to those treating vascular disease is the modulation of insulin resistance with metformin and thiazolidinediones (either rosiglitazone or pioglitazone). This therapy is being actively studied, because it lowers insulin levels and favorably affects inflammation, endothelial function, and fibrinolysis. It also increases HDL and increases LDL particle size.[23] On the other hand, it may cause fluid retention and is contraindicated with class 3 to 4 heart failure.

Dyslipidemia

It is important to understand the difference between *primary* and *secondary* prevention. Stopping the progression of disease in a patient who already has it (secondary prevention) justifies more aggressive treatment that preventing disease in one who does not have it (primary prevention). Current treatment recommendations by the National Cholesterol Education Program (NCEP) are summarized in Table 3.4.

Lipoprotein Metabolism

Oil and water do not mix. Cholesterol and triglycerides are hydrophobic, like other oils, and do not go into solution into aqueous media, such as blood. To get fats to dissolve in water requires a chemical that works like a detergent: a molecule that binds to fat on one side and to water on the other.

Lipoprotein particles have a core of fat packaged with a specialized protein that works like a detergent. This protein molecule, called an apoprotein, has regions

Table 3.4 The National Cholesterol Education Program (NCEP), Adult Treatment Panel III Guidelines		
Patient Profile	Initiate Drug Therapy if the LDL-C Is:*	Target LDL-C
0–1 CAD risk factors, no ASCVD	≥190 mg/dL after 6 mo of diet therapy	<160 mg/dL
≥2 risk factors, no ASCVD	≥130 mg/dL	<100 mg/dL
Known ASCVD or diabetes	>100 mg/dL	<70 mg/dL†

CAD, coronary artery disease; LDL-C, low-density lipoprotein cholesterol; ASCVD, atherosclerotic cardiovascular disease (including coronary, cerebrovascular and peripheral vascular disease).
*This version of the guidelines is based on an update from the NCEP (see text).

that are nonpolar (hydrophobic) that bind with lipids, and other regions that are polar (hydrophilic) that face the surrounding aqueous phase and form hydrogen bonds with water. The lipid-apoprotein package is thus water-soluble.

Another useful property of apoproteins is binding sites that regulate steps in lipid metabolism. For example, the apoB-100 protein on the surface of the LDL cholesterol particle is recognized by the liver's LDL receptor, allowing hepatic uptake of LDL. Other apoproteins are cofactors for enzymes that interact with lipoproteins, such as lipoprotein lipase.

The core of fat in the lipoprotein particle includes fatty acids, cholesterol esters, phospholipids, and triglycerides. Lipoproteins vary in density, and the first measurement techniques and classification schemes used ultracentrifugation. Larger, less dense particles contain more triglyceride and do not migrate as far in the centrifuge. Very-low-density lipoprotein (VLDL) has 55% triglyceride, 19% cholesterol, and only 8% protein by weight—this fluffy particle migrates the least. The highest density lipoprotein (HDL) has just 5% triglyceride and a higher proportion of protein (40%) and cholesterol (22%), and it migrates the farthest in the centrifuge. Between the two is the LDL particle, which has the largest percentage of cholesterol (50%), 6% triglyceride, and 22% protein.

Newer antibody techniques allow measurement of surface apoproteins. ApoA is found on HDL, and apoB-100 primarily on LDL. Thus, a patient with a high apoB level will also have high LDL cholesterol.

It helps to know just what your clinical laboratory is measuring. Most common is the centrifugation technique that isolates the entire lipoprotein molecule (fat core plus the apoprotein envelope), and then measures just the lipid component. Thus, when the laboratory reports the LDL cholesterol level, it is understood that the LDL component has been isolated from other lipoproteins by centrifugation, the apoprotein envelope separated from the lipid core, and the cholesterol contained in the lipid core measured and reported as milligrams cholesterol per deciliter. This is what you usually get from the clinical laboratory, although you will encounter research studies that refer to apoprotein levels.

Metabolic Pathways

The plasma lipoproteins are constantly being remodeled. Influenced by several enzymes, core lipids and apoprotein can be transferred from or among particles, altering their density (and therefore the lipoprotein class). Some particle alteration occurs in the liver, but much of it takes place in circulating plasma or in peripheral tissue. There are parallel systems that transport lipids: *exogenous transport* involves movement of lipid from the intestinal lumen, and uses a transport system distinct from *endogenous transport*, which handles either stored or synthesized fat. The two systems have a lot in common (and here is the big picture). Both begin by packaging lipid, predominantly triglyceride but some cholesterol as well, into large, fluffy particles. The large particles circulate, and are subjected to a series of lipolytic reactions, with hydrolysis of triglyceride to fatty acids that melt away from the particle. The remodeled particle is smaller and denser, contains less triglyceride, and therefore has proportionately more cholesterol. Small particles are cleared from the circulation by the liver through the action of specialized receptors on the hepatic cell membrane.

Genetic defects may affect any of these metabolic steps, accounting for the familial nature of CAD. When reviewing the pathways (subsequent sections), also follow Table 3.5 to understand the genetics of hyperlipidemia.

Exogenous fat transport—Dietary fats are absorbed by the intestinal epithelial cell. In the cell, cholesterol is esterified into long-chain fatty acids (Figure 3.2). Apoprotein is added, and the particle is secreted as a *chylomicron*. Most of the fat in the chylomicron is triglyceride. *Lipoprotein lipase* located in vascular endothelial cells—especially in muscle and adipose tissue capillary beds—hydrolyzes the triglyceride to free fatty acid, either for storage or as a source of energy. What is left is the chylomicron remnant, which is cleared by liver cells.

This process is rapid with most chylomicrons cleared from the circulation a couple hours after eating. The lipid profile measured after 12 hours of fasting thus does not reflect exogenous fat transport.

Endogenous fat transport—A 70-kg person has approximately 10 kg of triglyceride stored in adipose tissue (Figure 3.3). Lipases, inhibited by insulin and stimulated by epinephrine, hydrolyze stored triglyceride and release free fatty acid from adipose tissue into the circulation. It is bound to albumin and then cleared from the circulation by the liver.

Some of the free fatty acid is burned as fuel. The remainder is converted to triglyceride, which is packaged by the liver into VLDL. Again note the parallel between exogenous and endogenous pathways: the bulk of lipid at the origin of the cascade is triglyceride, and the lipoprotein particle carrying it is large and has low density.

The triglyceride in VLDL, like that in chylomicrons, is hydrolyzed by lipoprotein lipase to free fatty acids that melt away from the particle. As with the exogenous pathway, apoC-II acts as a cofactor for lipoprotein lipase (Figures 3.2 and 3.3, Table 3.5). The resulting particle is smaller, has less triglyceride, and proportionately

Table 3.5 Familial Dyslipidemia		
Syndrome	Mechanism	Clinical Features
LDL Disorders		
Familial hyper-cholesterolemia	Abnormal, ineffective LDL receptor. High LDL, normal HDL, and triglycerides. Heterozygous carriers have approximately 50% ineffective receptors. The rare homozygote dies in the second decade of life.	Autosomal dominant. Incidence of heterozygous state is 1 in 500. CAD is common. Examination: arcus and tendonous xanthoma.
Familial defective apoB-100	The defective apoprotein fails to bind to the LDL receptor.	Uncommon. The clinical syndrome and laboratory findings are similar to familial hypercholesterolemia.
Disorders of Triglycerides		
Familial combined dyslipidemia (FHC)	Overproduction of apoB-100 leading to an excess of VLDL particles. LDL particles are small and dense (more atherogenic). The apoB-100 to serum LDL ratio is >1.	High triglycerides and LDL, low HDL. A common cause of CAD. There is usually a family history of CAD *plus hypertriglyceridemia*. Examination: corneal arcus and tuberoeruptive xanthoma (when triglycerides are very high).
Chylomicronemia	Deficiency in lipoprotein lipase or an abnormal apoC-II (the cofactor).	Rare. There is no increase in vascular disease. Examination: tuberoeruptive xanthoma and xanthelasma.
Familial hypertriglyceridemia	The liver makes an excess of large, fluffy VLDL particles. The ratio of apoB-100 to LDL is <1.	Little increase in vascular disease. Tuberoeruptive xanthoma. With high triglycerides there is a risk of pancreatitis.
Type III dyslipidemia	Combination of FHC (above) plus abnormal apoE, which binds to the chylomicron remnant receptor. There is accumulation of IDL, which has equal quantities of triglyceride and cholesterol.	Rare. There is a higher incidence of CAD. Deposition of IDL leads to orange creases on the palms. It improves with a low fat diet.

CAD, coronary artery disease; HDL, high-density lipoprotein; IDL, intermediate-density lipoprotein; LDL, low-density lipoprotein; VLDL, very-low-density lipoprotein.

more cholesterol, and it is called intermediate-density lipoprotein (IDL). This can be cleared by the liver, which has receptors for the apoE surface protein of IDL. Those IDL particles that are not removed undergo further hydrolysis to become LDL.

LDL has almost no triglyceride, and its lipid core is composed predominantly of cholesterol esters. The surface protein molecule is apoB-100. LDL is the lipoprotein most commonly linked to premature ASCVD.

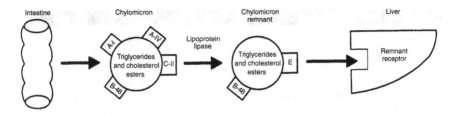

Figure 3.2 Exogenous fat transport. A-1, A-IV, B-48, C-II, and E are apolipoproteins. C-II functions as a cofactor for the enzyme lipoprotein lipase, and E interacts with the remnant receptor on the hepatocyte.

Regulation of LDL levels depends on the balance between production (via the lipolytic cascade described) and clearance. Clearance of LDL is governed by the number of hepatocyte LDL receptors. ApoB-100 on the LDL particle surface binds to the LDL receptor, and the LDL particle is thus absorbed by the hepatocyte.

An excess of free cholesterol within the liver cell blocks production of LDL receptors, so that less LDL cholesterol is cleared from the circulation. A deficiency of intracellular cholesterol provokes a compensatory *increase in the number of LDL*

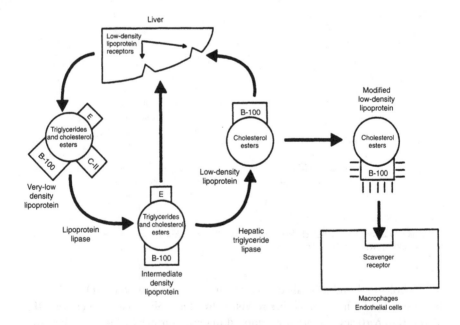

Figure 3.3 Endogenous fat transport. B-100 and E are apolipoproteins and bind with specific liver receptors. The liver uses large amounts of cholesterol for the manufacture of bile. Any condition or therapy that reduces the liver's supply of cholesterol provokes an increase in the number of LDL receptors, so that cholesterol-rich LDL is removed from the circulation, thus meeting the liver's needs.

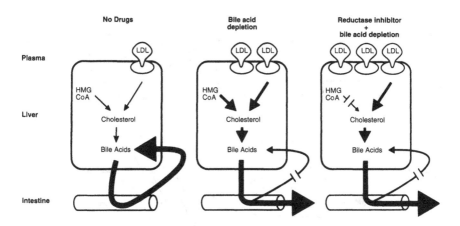

Figure 3.4 How cholesterol-lowering therapy works. The final common pathway is reduced cholesterol availability to the liver, which increases the number of hepatocyte LDL receptors so that the cholesterol can be extracted from the circulation. This happens with a low-cholesterol diet. Bile acid binding resins block the enterohepatic circulation of bile, a cholesterol-rich substance (middle panel). Reductase inhibitors block cholesterol synthesis in the hepatocyte. The combination of reductase inhibitors with either resins or diet therapy is synergistic. (Reprinted with permission from Brown MS, Goldstein JL. A receptor-mediated pathway for cholesterol homeostasis. Science 1986;232:34–47. Copyright © 1985, The Nobel Foundation.)

receptors (upregulation of receptors). More receptors are able to react with LDL particles, increasing clearance of LDL from the circulation.

The final common pathway for treatment to reduce LDL cholesterol is the upregulation of hepatocyte LDL receptors (Figure 3.4). For example, decreasing cholesterol availability by dietary restriction or by blocking an enzyme in the cholesterol synthetic pathway (HMG-CoA reductase) causes a deficiency of intracellular cholesterol. The hepatocyte compensates by upregulating LDL receptors, and there is increased clearance of LDL particles from the circulation. This is a desirable effect, because it is *circulating* LDL cholesterol that is atherogenic.

The liver processes a large amount of cholesterol for a variety of purposes. The greatest proportion is used to manufacture bile. Some of the bile is recycled, and blocking its enterohepatic circulation with resins that bind bile salts in the gut creates a need for more bile production, and a relative deficiency of hepatocyte cholesterol. The result: generation of more LDL receptors and lowering of circulating LDL cholesterol.

HDL and reverse cholesterol transport—Cholesterol that is not metabolized by peripheral tissue is excreted by the liver in bile (Figure 3.5). The reverse cholesterol transport system is responsible for moving excess cholesterol from the periphery to the liver so that it can be converted to bile. HDL is the transport vehicle.

Production of HDL begins with secretion of apoA-I by both the liver and intestine. Apo A-I complexes with phospholipids, forming a disk-like structure

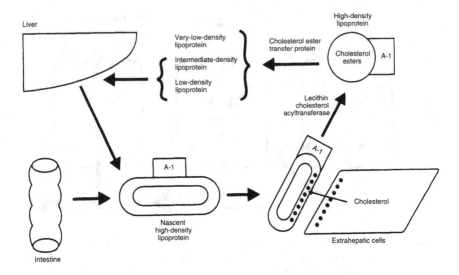

Figure 3.5 Reverse cholesterol transport. The nascent HDL particle draws cholesterol from extrahepatic cells (including the vascular endothelium) and transfers it to VLDL and then LDL particles, which are taken up by the liver.

called *nascent HDL*. This particle attracts free cholesterol from the cell membranes of peripheral tissue or from other lipoprotein particles. Free cholesterol contained in early atherosclerotic plaque may be absorbed by the nascent HDL particle.

At this stage an important enzyme, lecithin cholesterol acyltransferase, esterifies the free cholesterol. The cholesterol ester is less soluble than free cholesterol and moves to the inside of the phospholipids disk, which then assumes a spherical shape, is more stable, and is known as HDL. The HDL particle continues to accumulate cholesterol, not just from peripheral tissue but also from the surface of chylomicrons and from VLDL.

The liver does not have an HDL receptor. Instead, cholesterol is transferred from HDL to either LDL or to intermediate density lipoprotein, which are removed by the liver, or to VLDL, which is subsequently converted to LDL. Freed of its cholesterol load, the HDL particle moves on to scavenge more cholesterol from the periphery.

The level of HDL, expressed as milligrams per deciliter cholesterol by your clinical laboratory, is much lower than the level of LDL cholesterol. This gives the impression that the cholesterol removal system is comparatively small. But the HDL particle is composed of just 22% cholesterol, and remember that the laboratory measures just the cholesterol component of HDL. Furthermore, the HDL particle is small, weighing about one tenth of the LDL particle. In reality, the number of HDL particles (the molar concentration) exceeds that of LDL. The total surface area of HDL particles is greater than that of all other lipoproteins. The cholesterol removal system is thus quite large.

Treatment of Hyperlipidemia

Table 3.4 summarizes the most recent update of the NCEP treatment guidelines.[25] The language is a bit wishy-washy, stating that lowering LDL below 100 mg/dL is the recommended goal, but that pushing it below 70 mg/dL is a therapeutic option supported by multiple clinical trials. Suffice it to say that most cardiologists consider the optimal LDL to be less than 70 mg/dL for those with established ASCVD (secondary prevention) or diabetes (an ASCVD surrogate).[25] For moderately high risk patients with at least 2 risk factors but no clinically apparent ASCVD (primary prevention), the LDL should be less than 100 mg/dL. Weight reduction is still a critical element of treatment; drug therapy is no substitute.

In addition to the long-term effects of low LDL on atherogenesis, there are fewer acute vascular events in the short term, before there can be much effect on plaque accumulation. Furthermore, the degree of lipid alteration in large statin trials accounted for just two thirds of the clinical benefit (reduced MI and death from CAD), indicating plaque-stabilizing benefits from statins independent of cholesterol-lowering.[24]

The atherogenic effect of LDL cholesterol is strong enough that its reduction minimizes the risk of associated lipid disorders. Thus, for a patient with ASCVD who has low HDL or elevated triglycerides, the first goal of treatment is lowering the LDL to the target range. This makes the treatment of dyslipidemia fairly straightforward. If you remember nothing else, you will usually be right if your first step is to recommend LDL lowering for any high-risk patient. Then the guidelines recommend adding HDL raising therapy once LDL is at goal, particularly for those with the metabolic syndrome.

The familial dyslipidemias are of scientific interest, but are hard to remember since their diagnosis is not required in clinical practice (Table 3.5). We usually treat dyslipidemia without a genetic diagnosis. Treatment is determined by the lipid fraction that is elevated, and the principles of drug therapy are summarized in Table 3.6.

LDL lowering—Statins have emerged as the most useful. Clinical trials have established the importance of LDL lowering to halt the progression of ASCVD—secondary prevention—and almost all patients with any vascular disease are on therapy to push LDL below 70 mg/dL.[25,26]

How low is low enough has been debated. Many have contended that whatever the LDL level, it is too high for a person who has developed ASCVD. A series of clinical trials compared moderate LDL lowering (pravastatin 20 mg/day) with more aggressive therapy (atorvastatin 80 mg/day), and have confirmed a better outcome with an LDL level below 70 mg/dL.[26]

Raising HDL and lowering triglycerides—An occasional patient has low HDL and high triglycerides, and LDL is already below 100 mg/dL. When LDL lowering is not an issue the first step for lowering triglycerides and raising HDL is weight loss. I tell patients that triglyceride is the lipid fraction most sensitive to weight. An obese person who loses just 10 to 20 pounds may have a significant reduction

Table 3.6 Drug Treatment of Hyperlipidemia	
Lipid Abnormality	Treatments
High LDL cholesterol	1. Reductase inhibitor—blocks cholesterol synthesis, and the liver increases the number of LDL receptors to pull cholesterol from the circulation. 2. Niacin—highly effective, as it lowers both LDL and triglycerides, and raises HDL (see text). Problematic side effects limit use of this "perfect" drug. 3. Ezetimibe—blocks intestinal absorption of cholesterol with 20% reduction in LDL. Safe in combination with other drugs. 4. Resins—minimal reduction of cholesterol, though effective in clinical trials. Safe in combination with other drugs.
High triglycerides	When isolated, specific therapy may not be needed. If very high (>700) treat with fibric acid derivatives to prevent pancreatitis. Other effective drugs: niacin and fish oil. Many cases are secondary to high alcohol intake, diabetes mellitus, or obesity. Weight loss often works.
Low HDL cholesterol	Without vascular disease or risk factors for ASCVD, therapy is not required by the NCEP. First try exercise, weight loss, and a glass of wine a day.
Combined hyperlipidemia	The first goal is reduction of LDL (reductase inhibitors, niacin, ezetimibe). Add aggressive diet therapy for high VLDL (meaning high triglycerides), and exercise to raise HDL. Combination drug therapy—see text.
High Lp(a)	The first step is reduction of LDL. An occasional patient will have Lp(a) fall with niacin.

ASCVD, atherosclerotic cardiovascular disease; HDL, high-density lipoprotein; LDL, low-density lipoprotein; NCEP, National Cholesterol Education Program.

in triglycerides. Many are encouraged to learn they will benefit from any increment of weight loss, and do not have to reach ideal body weight for it to help. When triglycerides fall, the HDL increases.

Exercise has an effect on HDL that seems independent of its weight control benefit. The moderate use of alcohol, about 2 ounces of spirits a day, also increases HDL. Excessive drinking, on the other hand, tends to raise triglycerides, lower HDL, and provoke an increase in blood pressure.

Fibrates are often prescribed; they increase HDL about 5% to 15% and decrease triglycerides by 31%.[26] They are used for hypertriglyceridemia to prevent pancreatitis (that will be a board question). Niacin has a greater effect on HDL, increasing it 30%, and it has the additional benefit of lowering LDL cholesterol.[26]

Combined hyperlipidemia—Patients with the metabolic syndrome and early vascular disease usually have LDL above 120 to 130, plus high triglycerides–low HDL. Although the triglyceride-HDL abnormality seems the primary condition, the first goal is still to lower LDL to below 70 mg/dL. Two-drug therapy with a statin plus gemfibrozil has been popular, but I am concerned about the increased risk of myositis with this combination. Fenofibrate (Tricor), a newer fibrate, does not cause myositis when combined with statin therapy (vide infra). Another alternative is niacin, alone, which works for each of the lipid abnormalities. More recently, combination therapy using a statin plus niacin is being promoted, with the dose of niacin limited to 1.5 to 2 g/day.[26]

Homocysteine—There is a three-fold increase in ASCVD with homocysteine levels exceeding the 95th percentile (above 16 μmol/L for men and postmenopausal women). Retrospective, pooled data suggest that decreasing homocysteine by 25% lowers the risk of coronary heart disease 11%, and stroke 19%.[27] Vitamin therapy lowers the level of homocysteine, but as yet there has not been a randomized trial demonstrating a favorable effect. Furthermore, even the meta-analysis data do not favor routine homocysteine screening.[27] Ongoing clinical trials will sort this out.

Methionine is an amino acid that is demethylated to yield adenosine and homocysteine. This reaction and the further metabolism of homocysteine require vitamin cofactors, B_6, B_{12}, and folate. Two thirds of patients with homocystinemia have vitamin deficiency, and the rest have a genetic defect. Homocystinuria—a rare condition—is the worst of these, leading to death from vascular and thromboembolic disease early in life.

Elevated homocysteine levels promote atherosclerosis by at least three mechanisms: (1) endothelial cell toxicity, (2) increased platelet adhesiveness, and (3) modification of clotting factors.

Uremia merits special mention, as the plasma homocysteine level parallels serum creatinine. The defect is impaired metabolism of homocysteine with uremia, rather than decreased excretion. Levels improve, but do not normalize with dialysis. Those with end-stage renal disease (ESRD) plus elevated homocysteine have a five- to tenfold increase in MI and stroke. In fact, MI is the most common cause of death with ESRD. Routine measurement of homocysteine and treatment may be justified for these patients.

Elevated homocysteine is treated with 12.5 mg vitamin B_6, 0.5 mg B_{12}, and 1 mg folic acid orally per day. Measurement of pretreatment vitamin levels may be interesting, but is not required to start therapy.

Drugs

Statins—In addition to lowering LDL cholesterol, it is now well accepted that statin therapy stabilizes plaque. Cholesterol lowering accounts for some of this, as the cholesterol content of plaque is reduced, and cholesterol-rich plaque is more prone to rupture. But statins appear to have direct actions that are unrelated to cholesterol levels: they augment endothelial synthesis of nitric oxide, inhibit inflammation (C-reactive protein [CRP] decreases), and are antithrombotic, blocking expression of plasminogen activator inhibitor-1 by the endothelium.[24]

One reason for the success of statin therapy is a relative absence of side effects when compared with other agents. After 1 year of treatment, more than 95% of patients on statins remain on therapy, compared with less than half of those taking niacin, gemfibrozil, or resins.[25] That may surprise you, because there is such concern about liver toxicity and myositis with statins. Liver dysfunction is dose-related. Serial liver function testing is more important at high dose therapy, although a threefold increase in liver enzymes is still rare, developing in less than 1% of patients. Serial liver function testing is generally not recommended for those on low dose treatment (you should check the *Physician's Desk Reference* [PDR] guidelines for monitoring therapy, whatever you prescribe).

Myositis also occurs at higher doses. It may develop out of the blue, and serial testing of muscle enzymes is not useful. Statins are metabolized by the liver's cytochrome (CYP) enzyme system. Other drugs that share this metabolic route may inhibit degradation of the statin, leading to increased concentrations and adverse effects. These include gemfibrozil, amiodarone, cyclosporine, erythromycin (and other antibiotics), HIV protease inhibitors, and large quantities (>1 quart/day) of grapefruit juice. Another important drug interaction is warfarin—the International Normalized Ratio increases with statin therapy as protein-bound warfarin is displaced by the statin.

Fibrates—This is the drug class of choice for lowering triglyceride, with a modest (5% to 15%) increase in HDL as a bonus. Fibrates increase the oxidation of free fatty acids in the liver, blocking synthesis of VLDL triglyceride.

The side effect of gemfibrozil of greatest concern is myositis. The risk is higher in patients with renal failure. It is substantially increased when gemfibrozil is combined with high dose statin therapy. Many of the statins have a recommended maximum dose if they are used with gemfibrozil. An exception to this is atorvastatin. Note that the package insert (and PDR) states that the simvastatin dose should not exceed 20 mg per day when combined with gemfibrozil. A problem is that general physicians often do not know this (how much minutiae can anyone retain?), and I commonly see patients on high-dose simvastatin plus gemfibrozil.

Myositis can be a big problem: in the last year I consulted on two patients on combination therapy who had creatine kinase levels above 40,000. Azotemia developed in both along with their rhabdomyolysis, but both patients recovered with hydration and sodium bicarbonate therapy. While the combination of gemfibrozil and statins is not a violation of the standard of care, I try not to use it, because there are effective alternatives.

Fenofibrate (Tricor) is a third-generation fibrate that is slightly more potent than gemfibrozil. With experience to date, it appears that the risk of myositis is much lower with fenofibrate than with gemfibrozil. Fenofibrate is safer than gemfibrozil when used with statins, and most lipid clinics use it rather than the gemfibrozil-statin combination. On the other hand, it is much more expensive. Gemfibrozil is no longer on patent (lowering its costs) and would be a reasonable choice for use alone.

Another side effect of fibrates that may be missed is erectile dysfunction. Like other drugs that bind to protein, fibrates may displace warfarin from protein, requiring an approximate 30% reduction in the warfarin dose.

Niacin—In many ways it is the ideal drug, substantially raising HDL while lowering LDL cholesterol. It works by preventing mobilization of free fatty acids from the periphery (adipose), which leads to reduced hepatic production of triglycerides and secretion of VLDL. In addition, it inhibits conversion of VLDL to LDL.

At high doses, it can raise HDL concentrations by 30%, more than can be achieved with gemfibrozil. We tend to limit therapy to 1.5–2 g of nicotinic acid per day, and this raises HDL slightly, while lowering triglycerides substantially.

Use of the short-acting preparation is difficult, because most patients experience flushing. Aspirin given 30 minutes before taking niacin may block this prostaglandin-mediated side effect. The extended release formulation of niacin (Niaspan) causes less flushing and fewer gastrointestinal side effects. Other, potentially serious side effects tend to occur when the dose exceeds 3 g/day, including hyperuricemia and gout (blocked tubular excretion of uric acid), a modest worsening of glycemic control in diabetes, and hepatotoxicity.

Combination drug therapy—Problems with the combination of statins and gemfibrozil have been discussed. It is a particular problem with simvastatin (the dose should not be above 20 mg), but less so with atorvastatin (to date there has been no limit placed on the atorvastatin dose). Fenofibrate (Tricor) is probably safer with statins (although the PDR continues to list this combination in its warnings section).

Another effective combination is niacin plus a statin. The HATS trial was a serial angiographic study with 3-year follow-up.[28] Patients were treated with niacin, 2 g/day, plus simvastatin titrated to lower LDL to the mid-70s. Those treated with placebo or with antioxidants alone had progression of atherosclerosis, but simvastatin plus niacin led to regression of plaque. This translated to clinical benefit. The placebo group had a 24% event rate (death, MI, stroke or revascularization), compared with 3% in the treatment group.[28]

Other agents may be added to statins, especially when the patient does not tolerate niacin. The resins (cholestyramine, colestipol, and colesevelam) bind bile acids in the intestine, blocking their enterohepatic circulation. They may also bind with and block absorption of drugs such as warfarin, digoxin, thiazides, statins, and thyroxine; these agents should be given 1 hour before or 4 hours after a resin. Colesevelam (Welchol), the newest of the resins, causes fewer gastrointestinal side effects.

Ezetimibe (Zetia) is the first of a new class of agents that blocks both dietary and biliary cholesterol absorption.[28] With less delivery of cholesterol to the liver, LDL receptor density increases, and LDL is removed from the circulation. The usual dosage, 10 mg/day, reduces dietary absorption by 50%. It may be used in combination with statins to achieve the LDL target. There are no unfavorable interactions with statins or gemfibrozil; it is not metabolized by the CYP enzyme system.

Antioxidants—Oxidized LDL is cytotoxic, leading to endothelial injury and dysfunction, and enhancing recruitment of monocytes and their transformation to macrophages. There was hope that inhibiting the modification of LDL with antioxidant vitamins would block progression of ASCVD. The results of clinical trials of monotherapy with antioxidants have been mixed. Synthetic vitamin E, beta-carotene, or vitamin cocktails showed no benefit, while natural vitamin E reduced event rates in two trials.[29] One of these favorable studies involved patients with renal failure on dialysis, and oxidation of LDL may be especially important in this population (dialysis membranes with an antioxidant coating are being tested). As an element of combination therapy, antioxidants have added little, and in one trial, a vitamin cocktail added to simvastatin plus niacin appeared detrimental.[28]

The role of oxidation in genesis of plaque is complicated. For example, it is uncertain where, in vivo, oxidation takes place, and pharmacokinetics may determine where and whether a drug blocks LDL oxidation. Further research based on the oxidation hypothesis is warranted. But at this stage, the clinical use of antioxidants is not.

Fish oil—The polyunsaturated fatty acids (PUFAs) found in fish oil are known to raise HDL and lower LDL cholesterol and triglycerides. Fish oil supplements are especially helpful for hypertriglyceridemia. Endothelial function improves, and there is a reduction in inflammation. Multiple studies have documented a reduction in ASCVD clinical endpoints.[30]

The hottest news is a reduction in the risk of sudden cardiac death (SCD). An increase in dietary PUFA content has been found to increase the PUFA level in the myocardial cell membrane.[31] This alters the action potential and has an antiarrhythmic effect. Lowering the vulnerability to ventricular fibrillation may be more important than the effect on atherosclerosis. The current American Heart Association (AHA) recommendation is that everyone should have two oily fish meals per week (burp), and others have suggested additional supplements for those at high risk for SCD.

Hormone replacement therapy—This is an odd story that underscores the importance of the modern clinical trial. A series of observational studies, beginning in the 1960s, suggested that hormone replacement therapy (HRT) could lower the risk of ASCVD by as much as 50% in postmenopausal women.[32,33] Many effects of estrogen are consistent with cardioprotection. It raises HDL, and lowers LDL, Lp(a), and fibrinogen. It also inhibits oxidation of LDL and improves endothelial function. On the negative side, it raises triglycerides and CRP and promotes thrombosis. Adding progestin blocks the HDL benefit.

Most were surprised by a negative result from the first randomized trial of HRT, the Heart and Estrogen Replacement Study (HERS). There was no long-term benefit, and there was an unexpected increase in ASCVD risk during the first year after starting HRT.[32] Since then, multiple randomized trials have confirmed the HERS result, finding no clinical or anatomic benefit from HRT for those with established CAD, and an increased risk soon after starting HRT.

More recently, *primary prevention* trials have indicated potential harm with HRT. The estrogen plus progestin arm of the Women's Health Initiative trial was stopped early because of adverse effects. This study of healthy, normal women found that

HRT caused a 29% increase in MI, a 41% increase in stroke, a twofold increase in venous thromboembolic disease, and a 26% increase in breast cancer.[32]

One explanation for the discrepancy between the observational studies and clinical trials is the tendency of complications to develop soon after starting HRT.[32] Most observational studies are weighted with subjects who have been on treatment for some time. Those with early complications, especially if they are fatal, have dropped out before the observational study has begun. Reexamination of the observational data, focusing on patients on HRT for less than 1 year, eliminated previously described benefits.[32,33]

Possible explanations for the higher risk of vascular events soon after starting HRT include the prothrombotic and pro-inflammatory effects of estrogen. It is also possible that a subgroup of women genetically predisposed to adverse effects of HRT develop them promptly after starting treatment. The early clustering of adverse effects provided a rationale for the recommendation that a woman who is not on HRT should not start it, but that another who has been on it for some time need not stop it. This recommendation, however, does not appear in clinical guidelines, and HRT is not indicated for the primary or secondary prevention of ASCVD.

At present, HRT is indicated just for the control of menopausal symptoms, including sleeplessness and hot flashes. The safest approach is low-dose HRT and a short duration of therapy.[34] HRT is also approved for prevention of osteoporosis for those with early disease or falling bone density. The issue of ASCVD prevention is not entirely settled; different hormone combinations may be safer. For example, the unopposed estrogen wing of the WHI study is ongoing.

Diet therapy—The prevalence of obesity in the United States has doubled in the past 20 years; roughly 45% of women and 30% of men are dieting at any given time.

Two extreme approaches to dieting have been promoted. One is the vegetarian, high carbohydrate, high fiber and extremely low fat diet; the Pritikin and Ornish diets are examples. On this diet patients lose weight, often in an eponymous summer camp setting. But this diet of roots, unprocessed grains and herbs is not palatable, and once away from supervision few are able to stick with it. Increasingly popular—perhaps because it is palatable and is often effective—is the opposite extreme, a low carbohydrate, high fat, high protein diet. The Atkins diet is the most notable example. (As a general rule, palatability is determined by fat content.) Between these two extremes is the Mediterranean diet, currently recommended by the Heart Association. It is low in calories, saturated fats, trans fats and cholesterol, but includes animal protein, and is rich in fruits, vegetables, and fiber.

Small trials that randomized less than 200 patients have compared the Atkins with a higher carbohydrate diet and found greater weight loss at 6 months with the Atkins diet, but no difference at 12 months.[35]

There are some potential benefits with the Atkins diet. Those with diabetes and the metabolic syndrome who lose weight also have an increase in HDL, a decrease in triglycerides and increased insulin sensitivity. It may be attractive to a person used to eating a lot, as the diet does not aggressively restrict caloric intake, and with high fat content, it tastes good. Ketosis is thought to help limit intake.

But there are substantial arguments against the Atkins diet.[35] First, there is no evidence that it has any beneficial effect on ASCVD, while clinical studies have shown that the Mediterranean diet reduces risk. The long-term effect of high fat intake is uncertain and worrisome, and Atkins is supposed to be a lifelong diet. The Atkins diet does not lower LDL, although there is an increase in HDL. It may lack important vitamins and fiber. Side effects of high protein intake induce calciuria (a potential problem with stones and bone mass), and aggravation of liver or kidney disease.

Weight loss is so important that any diet approach that achieves it is hard to proscribe, and many of our patients have success with the Atkins diet. Nevertheless, long-term clinical effects of the Atkins must be understood before we can recommend it for those with or at high risk for developing ASCVD. We may expect further study, but for now the NCEP and other practice guidelines recommend the Mediterranean diet for weight loss and lowering ASCVD risk.[18,36,37]

Another diet issue is the function of additives. B vitamins prevent oxidation of LDL, and observational studies have found less ASCVD with a vitamin rich diet. As noted above, trials of vitamin (antioxidant) supplementation have shown no benefit.

Flavonoids may be beneficial, as epidemiologic studies have found an inverse relation between dietary intake and the incidence of ASCVD. These compounds may help explain the "French paradox," a reduced incidence of ASCVD despite a high fat diet that has been attributed to red wine consumption. Flavonoids are a component of red wine, dark beer, other dark spirits and the skins, seeds, and stems of purple grapes and other fruits. The mechanism of benefit may be improved endothelial function. Of particular interest, flavonoids block the endothelial dysfunction that follows consumption of a high fat meal.

Alcohol, used moderately, is another dietary supplement associated with a lower incidence of ASCVD in observational studies.[38] It is known to raise HDL, reduce platelet aggregation and promote fibrinolysis. Up to 2 ounces of spirits a day may prove beneficial, but the evidence is not compelling enough to recommend that nondrinkers take it up.

Atherosclerosis

Response to Injury Hypothesis of Atherogenesis

The intimal surface of arteries is lined with endothelial cells that form a barrier between elements of the blood and the arterial wall. Injury of the endothelium appears to be the first step in atherogenesis. The nature of early vascular injury is uncertain, and multiple factors may interact. Increased turbulence at branch points and shear stress may be responsible for this common location of plaque. Infection has been proposed, as viral elements and Chlamydia have been isolated from plaque (though small trials of antibiotic therapy have shown no benefit). Oxidized LDL cholesterol is cytotoxic and appears to have a role in endothelial injury.

Table 3.7 Substances Released by Endothelial Cells		
System	Anti-ischemic Effect	Pro-ischemic Effect
Vascular tone	Vasodilate: NO, prostacyclin, bradykinin, C-natriuretic peptide	Vasoconstrict: ET-1, A-II, thromboxane A-2
Smooth muscle proliferation	Inhibit: NO, prostacyclin (and others)	Promote: ET-1, A-II, oxidant radicals, PDGF, insulin-like growth factor, inter-leukins
Thrombosis	Anti-thrombotic: NO, prostacyclin, plasminogen activator, protein C, von Willebrand factor	Pro-thrombotic: ET-1, oxidant radicals, PAI-1, thromboxane A-2, fibrinogen, tissue factor
Inflammation		Pro-inflammatory: CAMs that promote migration of leukocytes to the subintima. Note that CRP may increase production of CAMs.

NO, nitric oxide; ET-1, endothelin-1; A-II, angiotensin-II; PDGF, platelet derived growth factor; PAI-1, plasminogen-activator inhibitor-1; CAMs, cellular adhesion molecules; CRP, C-reactive protein.

After disruption of the endothelium, the next step is the complex interaction of a number of different cell types, which leads to propagation of endothelial injury and infiltration of lipids and other blood elements into deeper layers of the arterial wall (Table 3.7). Circulating, oxidized LDL binds to monocytes and facilitates their migration into the endothelium where they become macrophages. These cells scavenge more lipid, particularly oxidized LDL, become foam cells, and form the fatty streak. Activated macrophages produce cytotoxic substances that promote further endothelial injury. They also produce growth factors that stimulate proliferation and migration of smooth muscle cells into the early plaque. In turn, smooth muscle cells secrete growth factors and cytokines and produce connective tissue. As the plaque matures, this fibroproliferative process dominates, with the replication of smooth muscle cells, attraction of fibroblasts, and production of connective tissue. The core of the mature plaque is rich in lipid.

Platelets have an important role. They adhere to injured endothelium, particularly at branch points where there is turbulence and stasis. Like other cellular elements, they produce growth factors and vasoactive substances. Platelets are critical in the genesis of unstable syndromes. Advanced lesions commonly develop surface cracks and fissures, and platelets are activated by exposed collagen, forming mural thrombi that are incorporated into the plaque. This is one mechanism of rapid disease progression. Arterial occlusion by mural thrombus is a common mechanism for MI. Blocking platelet function is more effective than other forms of anticoagulation for the prevention of unstable coronary syndromes.

Angiotensin II also works at the endothelial level, promoting endothelial dysfunction and vasoconstriction. It promotes generation of superoxide radicals by macrophages by aiding uptake of oxidized LDL by the macrophage. ACE inhibition has been shown to have direct vascular protective actions apart from its effect on blood pressure.

Inflammation and Infection

Atherosclerosis is now considered a chronic inflammatory process that begins with vascular injury. Like autoimmune disorders there is activation of macrophages, B and T cells and endothelial cells, and there is elevation of cytokines. Circulating immune cells are recruited to the injured and inflamed vessel.

C-reactive protein is a marker of inflammation that has been found to predict MI, SCD, stroke, and peripheral arterial disease.[39] It has been found to be a stronger predictor than LDL cholesterol, and adds additional prognostic information when considered with other risk factors for ASCVD. A level of 1–3 mg/L corresponds to moderate risk, and greater than 3 mg/dL, to high risk. Note that these are low levels; with bacterial infection, the CRP may approach 100 mg/dL. A highly sensitive CRP assay is required for accurate measurement of these low levels. When the CRP is above 10 mg/L the test should be repeated and other processes excluded (low-grade infection, malignancy).

Among patients with the metabolic syndrome, the CRP level correlates with the level of insulin resistance, endothelial dysfunction, and impaired fibrinolysis (features of the metabolic syndrome that are not easily measured). Thus, CRP helps differentiate high- from low-risk patients with the metabolic syndrome. The relationship between inflammation, atherothrombosis, and diabetes suggests a common etiology related to the immune system, and influenced by diet and exercise.

CRP levels tend to be stable in an individual, have no circadian variation, and are not influenced by eating; fasting blood sampling is unnecessary. It is not age- or gender-dependent, but it is higher during HRT. The molecule has a long half-life, and is stable during storage; this has made it possible to return to earlier clinical trials and measure CRP using stored serum. There are other biomarkers of inflammation that predict ASCVD events (interleukin-6, cytokines, cellular adhesion molecules, CD40 ligand, and others), but they are no more sensitive or specific than CRP and are difficult to measure. The erythrocyte sedimentation rate and white blood cell count have not proven useful.

CRP is a predictor of acute clinical events, as well as a marker of atherosclerosis. Inflammatory cells are concentrated in the culprit lesions of patients dying with acute coronary syndromes.[40]

Suppression of inflammation may help. Among men in the Physicians' Health Study, aspirin for primary prevention was most effective in those with high CRP. Statins are the most potent vascular anti-inflammatory agents, suppressing the CRP levels. This action is independent of the lipid-lowering effects of statins.[24] The anti-inflammatory effect is prompt, leading to a reduction in ischemic event rates within a week of beginning statin therapy.[41]

On the other hand *nonsteroidal anti-inflammatory drugs* (NSAIDs) do not influence coronary event rates.[42] Apparently, the action of statins is specific for vascular inflammation, and NSAIDs do not have it. Furthermore, NSAIDs do not have the cardioprotective action of aspirin, even though they inhibit platelet aggregation; they should not be substituted for aspirin (note further discussion of aspirin and COX-2 inhibitors in Chapter 4).

Trials of antibiotic therapy have demonstrated no effect on the natural history of CAD.[42]

Endothelial Function

The endothelium was originally considered a passive interface between blood and the vascular wall. We now recognize this single-cell layer as an active paracrine organ that releases vasoactive substances in response to hemodynamic forces and other blood-borne signals.[43] It produces both vasodilators (nitric oxide [NO]) and constrictors (endothelin-1 [ET-1], and angiotensin-II), and the balance between them determines vascular tone. In addition, these substances may promote or retard atherosclerosis through their effects on platelet function, thrombosis, vascular smooth muscle proliferation and inflammation (Table 3.7).

Endothelial dysfunction—a predominance of the pro-ischemic substances in Table 3.7—is a probable link between risk factors and atherosclerosis. It has been described with cigarette smoking, hyperlipidemia, obesity, renal failure, high CRP, hypertension, left ventricular hypertrophy, immunosuppression after transplantation, aging, and multiple other clinical states. Endothelial dysfunction is well described at the molecular level. For example, high insulin levels in the metabolic syndrome decrease the bioavailability of NO and increase the production of ET-1.

In addition to the impact of endothelial dysfunction on atherogenesis, it has a key role once atherosclerosis is established. Vasoconstriction of the arterial bed distal to a stenosis—which contributes to increased resistance and reduces flow—may initiate ischemia. This may explain the *warm-up phenomenon*, the patient who develops angina with minimal exertion early in the day, but does not have it with similar exertion later (suggesting better endothelial function later in the day). Unstable coronary syndromes, including MI, are clearly influenced by endothelial-mediated changes in platelet function, coagulation, and plaque architecture.

Endothelial dysfunction may be measured noninvasively in the peripheral circulation. The peripheral arterial changes correlate with coronary artery dilatation that is endothelium-dependent, but requires quantitative coronary angiography for measurement. Normally, upper arm occlusion with a blood pressure cuff for 5 minutes is followed by reactive hyperemia—vasodilatation—that is mediated by an increase in NO production. Absent or blunted vasodilatation after cuff release indicates endothelial dysfunction and subnormal NO production.

Endothelial dysfunction can be treated. The first step is modification of risk factors. Lowering LDL cholesterol improves endothelium-mediated vasodilatation. In addition, the statin class of drugs has cholesterol-independent, direct beneficial actions on endothelial function.

ACE inhibitors also have an effect on endothelial function, and the benefit is apparent after short-term treatment.[43] ACE inhibition promotes fibrinolysis, reduces angiotensin II, has an antioxidant action, and increases bradykinin. While not proven, improved endothelial function—a direct arterial effect—probably explains the efficacy of ACE inhibitors in the HOPE trial (see Chapter 4). This study showed that ramipril reduced stroke, MI, and death, independent of blood pressure lowering.

Screening for Pre-clinical Atherosclerosis

The following chapters will discuss the evaluation of angina pectoris, other chest pain syndromes, and MI. How do we evaluate the patient who is asymptomatic, with no history of CAD? There is an obvious benefit to identifying pre-clinical disease, as this would shift the patient from a primary prevention to a secondary prevention treatment strategy. We do that now. An occasional patient having angiography is found to have *luminal irregularity* or nonstenosing plaque unrelated to symptoms. This calls for more aggressive LDL lowering therapy aspirin, and ACE inhibitor therapy (Chapter 4).

Risk factor evaluation is a first step in screening, and there are guidelines for cholesterol management (Table 3.4). But with the exception of diabetes, risk factors do not serve as *surrogates* for established disease. The incidence of CAD is high enough with diabetes to warrant more aggressive statin therapy, and ACE inhibitor therapy is indicated for the prevention of renal as well as heart disease. It is possible that future study will identify combinations of risk factors that may be considered surrogates. Elevation of both CRP and LDL cholesterol comes to mind, but there are currently no data to support secondary prevention for patients who have this combination.

Another surrogate for CAD is arterial disease elsewhere. The rationale is the diffuse nature of ASCVD. Those with peripheral or carotid artery disease usually have coronary artery plaque as well, and the selection criterion for the HOPE trial was any arterial disease. Thus, patients with carotid bruit and abnormal Doppler studies, or others with noninvasive evidence for peripheral vascular disease qualify for a secondary prevention approach to ASCVD.

Fast CT scanning for coronary artery calcium—Plaque contains calcium, and there are increasingly accurate CT methods for detecting calcium. Electron-beam CT was the earliest of these, but newer techniques include spiral CT and multi-detector CT. Early studies have shown that a high coronary artery calcium (CAC) score predicts future ischemic events including death, MI, and a need for revascularization.[44,45]

Attractive features of this technique include low cost (now $350 in our hospital, bring your charge card), speed (it takes less than a minute to do), and safety (no catheter, no intravenous line, no dye). A normal study predicts an excellent prognosis.

An advantage of CAC imaging is that it detects preclinical plaque, a lesion that narrows the vessel by less than 50%. Many of our middle-aged patients want to be screened with stress testing, often requesting perfusion imaging (retail cost, $3500). But these provocative tests for ischemia are positive only when there is flow-restricting stenosis, with narrowing of the arterial diameter greater than 70%. Asymptomatic patients[46] are more likely to have early rather than flow restricting plaque, and CAC imaging makes more sense for them. I usually recommend it for the person with no history of heart disease, who has risk factors for ASCVD, and *who wants a screening test.*

Nevertheless, at this stage there are inadequate data for us (or the AHA) to promote this new technique as a routine screening method. As with any screening technique, its use for low risk individuals who do not have risk factors for ASCVD will produce false-positive results.[44–47] Having said that, I will admit that I—and most of my colleagues—have had it done. I expect that further experience will show that a high CAC score is a surrogate for established ASCVD, and an indication for a secondary prevention strategy. Of course, I may be wrong, and there is no substitute for clinical trials.

Treatment of Atherosclerosis

Subsequent chapters will review the management of CAD in detail. Based on clinical trials, there are three treatments that are indicated for all who have ASCVD. The indication for treatment is any atherosclerotic disorder, including CAD, cerebrovascular and peripheral arterial disease. If your patient is not on each of these drugs, you should document the reason it is contraindicated. They are:

• Aspirin

• LDL lowering therapy

• ACE inhibitor therapy

References

1. American Heart Association. 2002 Heart and Stroke Statistical Update. Dallas, TX: American Heart Association; 2001.

2. Dawber TR, Meadors GF, Moore FE Jr. Epidemiological approaches to heart disease: the Framingham Study. Am J Public Health 1951;41:279–281.

3. Assmann G, Cullen P, Schulte H. Simple scoring scheme for calculating the risk of acute coronary events based on the 10–year follow-up of the prospective cardiovascular Munster (PROCAM) study. Circulation 2002;105:310–315.

4. Prevention of stroke by antihypertensive drug treatment in older persons with isolated systolic hypertension: final results of the Systolic Hypertension in the Elderly Program (SHEP). SHEP Cooperative Research Group. JAMA 1991;265:3255–3264.

5. Collins R, Peto R, MacMahon S, et al. Blood pressure, stroke, and coronary heart disease. Short-term reductions in blood pressure: overview of randomized drug trials in their epidemiological context. Lancet 1990;335:827–838.

6. Leon AS, Connett J. Physical activity and 10.5 year mortality in the multiple Risk Factor Intervention Trial (MRFIT). Int J Epidemiol 1991;20:690–697.

7. Carney RM. Psychological risk factors for cardiac events: could there be just one. Circulation 1998;97:128–129.

8. Braunwald E. Cardiovascular medicine at the turn of the millennium: triumphs, concerns and opportunities. N Engl J Med 1997;337:1360–1369.

9. Bonow RO. Primary prevention of cardiovascular disease: a call to action. Circulation 2002;106:3140–3141.

10. Stampfer MJ, Hu FB, Manson JE, et al. Primary prevention of coronary heart disease in women through diet and lifestyle. N Engl J Med 2000;343:16–22.

11. Kottke TE. Managing nicotine dependence. J Am Coll Cardiol 1997;30:131–132.

12. Dwyer JH. Exposure to environmental tobacco smoke and coronary risk. Circulation 1997;96:1367–1369.

13. Kannel WB, Higgins M. Smoking and hypertension as predictors of cardiovascular risk in population studies. J Hypertens Suppl 1990;8:3–8.

14. Negri E, Franzosi MG, La Vecchia C, et al. Tar yield of cigarettes and risk of acute myocardial infarction. BMJ 1993; 306:1567–1570.

15. Bolinder G, Alfredsson L, Englund A, de Faire U. Smokeless tobacco use and increased cardiovascular mortality among Swedish construction workers. Am J Public Health 1994;84:399–404.

16. Reaven G, Tsao PS. Insulin resistance and compensatory hyperinsulinemia: the key player between cigarette smoking and cardiovascular disease. J Am Coll Cardiol 2003;41:1044–1047.

17. Sobel BE, Frye R, Detre KM. Burgeoning dilemmas in the management of diabetes and cardiovascular disease; rationale for the Bypass Angioplasty Revascularization Investigation 2 Diabetes (BARI 2) Trial. Circulation 2003;107:636–642.

18. Wilson PW, Grundy SM. The metabolic syndrome: a practical guide to origins and treatment. Part I, Circulation 2003.108:1422–1424. Part II, Circulation 2003.108:1537–1540.

19. Gerich JE. Contributions of insulin-resistance and insulin-secretory defects to the pathogenesis of type 2 diabetes mellitus. Mayo Clin Proc 2003;78:447–456.

20. Opie LH, Parving HH. Diabetic nephropathy; can renoprotection be extrapolated to cardiovascular protection. Circulation 2002;106:643–645.

21. Yanovski SZ, Yanovski JA. Obesity. N Engl J Med 2002;346:591–602.

22. Weinstock RS. Treating type 2 diabetes mellitus: a growing epidemic. Mayo Clin Proc 2003;78:411–413.

23. Marso SP. Optimizing the diabetic formulary: beyond aspirin and insulin. J Am Coll Cardiol 2002;40:652–661.

24. Libby P, Aikawa M. Mechanisms of plaque stabilization with statins. Am J Cardiol 2003;91(suppl):4B–8B.

25. Grundy SM, Cleeman JI, Bairey Merz CN, et al. Implications of recent clinical trials for the National Cholesterol Education Program Adult Treatment Panel III Guidelines. Circulation 2004;110:227–239.

26. Nissen SE, Tuzcu EM, Schoenhagen P, et al. Effect of intensive compared with moderate lipid-lowering therapy on progression of coronary athesosclerosis. JAMA 2004;291:1071–1080. Also, Cannon CP, Braunwald E, McCabe CH, et al. Intensive versus moderate lipid lowering with statins after acute coronary syndromes. N Engl J Med 2004;350:1495–1504. Also, Rader DJ. Therapy to reduce the risk of coronary heart disease. Clin Cardiol 2003;26:2–8.

27. Homocysteine Studies Collaboration. Homocysteine and risk of ischemic heart disease and stroke: a meta-analysis. JAMA 2002;288:2015–2022. Also, Gauthier GM, Keevil JG, McBride PE. The association of homocysteine and coronary artery disease. Clin Cardiol 2003;26:563–568.

28. Brown BG, Zhao XQ, Chait A, et al. Simvastatin and niacin, antioxidant vitamins, or the combination for the prevention of coronary disease. N Engl J Med 2001;345:1583–1592. Also, Bruckert E, Giral P, Tellier P. Perspectives in cholesterol-lowering therapy; the role of ezetimibe, a new selective inhibitor of intestinal cholesterol absorption. Circulation 2003;107:3124–3128.

29. Gotto AM. Antioxidants, statins, and atherosclerosis. J Am Coll Cardiol 2003;41:1205–1210.

30. Siscovick DS, Lemaitre RN, Mozaffarian D. The fish story: a diet-heart hypothesis with clinical implications: n-3 polyunsaturated fatty acids, myocardial vulnerability and sudden death. Circulation 2003;107:2632–2634.

31. Leaf A, Kang JX, Xiao YF, Billman GE. Clinical prevention of sudden cardiac death by n-3 polyunsaturated fatty acids and mechanism of prevention of arrhythmias by n-3 fish oils. Circulation 2003;107:2646–2652.

32. Herrington DM. Hormone replacement therapy and heart disease: replacing dogma with data. Circulation 2003;107:2–4.

33. Michels KB, Manson AE. Postmenopausal hormone therapy: a reversal of fortune. Circulation 2003;107:1830–1833.

34. Hulley SB. Hormone therapy after menopause: An update. Cardiol Rev 2003;20:11–15.

35. Freedman JE. High-fat diets and cardiovascular disease: are nutritional supplements useful. J Am Coll Cardiol 2003:41:1750–1752.

36. Yancy WS, Westman EC, French PA, Califf RM. Diets and clinical coronary events: the truth is out there. Circulation 2003;107:10–16.

37. Trichopoulou A. Adherence to a Mediterranean diet and survival in a Greek population. N Engl J Med 2003;348:2599–2608.

38. Goldberg IJ. To drink or not to drink. N Engl J Med 2003;348:163–164.

39. Ridker PM. Clinical application of C-reactive protein for cardiovascular disease detection and prevention. Circulation 2003:107:363–369.

40. Kinlay S, Selwyn AP. Effects of statins on inflammation in patients with acute and chronic coronary syndromes. Am J Cardiol 2003;91(suppl):9B–13B.

41. Lefer DJ. Statins as potent antiinflammatory drugs. Circulation 2002;106:2041–2042.

42. Ray WA, Stein CM, Hall K, et al. Non-steroidal anti-inflammatory drugs and risk of serious coronary heart disease: an observational cohort study. Lancet

2002;359:118–123. Also note, O'Connor CM, Dunne MW, Pfeffer MA, et al. Azithromycin for the secondary prevention of coronary heart disease events: the WIZARD Study: a randomized controlled trial. JAMA 2003;290:1459–1466. (*7747 patients with stable CAD and high titers to* C. pneumoniae *randomized to three months of antibiotic therapy. No cardiac benefit.*)

43. Verma S, Anderson TJ. Fundamentals of endothelial function for the clinical cardiologist. Circulation 2002;105:546–549.

44. Hecht HS. Atherosclerotic risk factors revisited. Am J Cardiol 2003;93:73–75.

45. Wong ND. Detection of subclinical atherosclerosis: Implications for evaluating cardiovascular risk. ACC Curr J Rev 2004;13:30–35.

46. Greenland P, Gaziano JM. Clinical practice. Selecting asymptomatic patients for coronary computed tomography or electrocardiographic exercise testing. N Engl J Med 2003;349:465–473.

CHAPTER 4

ANGINA PECTORIS: EVALUATION OF CHEST PAIN AND THE MANAGEMENT OF ANGINA PECTORIS AND ACUTE CORONARY SYNDROMES

Abbreviations

ACS	acute coronary syndrome	ECG	electrocardiogram
AHA	American Heart Association	ED	emergency department
ASCVD	atherosclerotic cardiovascular disease	H2	histamine-2
		LAD	left anterior descending (coronary artery)
AV	atrio-ventricular		
CABS	coronary artery bypass surgery	LDL	low density lipoprotein (cholesterol)
CAD	coronary artery disease	LV	left ventricle (ventricular)
CHF	congestive heart failure	LVEF	LV ejection fraction
CK	creatine kinase	MET	metabolic unit
COX	cyclooxygenase	MI	myocardial infarction
CPUE	chest pain of uncertain etiology	MVO$_2$	myocardial oxygen demand
		NSTEMI	non-ST elevation MI
CRP	C-reactive protein	USAP	unstable angina pectoris

Scientific medicine in the 20th century evolved in a series of steps. The first was the recognition of pathoanatomy and physiology of a disease. Next was the development of mechanical solutions (when possible), followed by their replacement with pharmacologic therapy. Take the case of peptic ulcer disease: the recognition of gastric acid as a cause was followed by surgical procedures to resect the ulcer and block acid secretion. The Billroth procedure was the general surgeon's bread-and-butter when I was a medical student in the 1960s. Then development of H2 blocker and proton pump inhibitors eliminated the need for surgery.

We are watching a similar story unfold with the treatment of coronary artery disease (CAD). My early years in practice witnessed the evolution of mechanical treatment. Coronary artery bypass surgery (CABS) was new when I trained, and had its golden era in the 1980 to 1990s. Its turf has been steadily eroded by angioplasty over the past 20 years.

However, the hot news of the past decade has been the rapid development of pharmacologic therapy. While there is still a bias to fix the blockage, a succession of clinical trials are demonstrating less need for that as medical therapy becomes more and more effective. I tell students that 1980 to 2000 was a great time to be in the catheterization laboratory, but now the action is in the clinic. Coronary artery disease will become a medical illness.

Chest Pain of Uncertain Etiology

There is no diagnostic code for chest pain of uncertain etiology (CPUE), but I think of it as a clinical entity because its evaluation is such a common clinical exercise. I am not referring to the evaluation of a patient with known CAD and typical angina pectoris. Instead, I refer to the patient in the emergency department (ED) or clinic with somewhat vague, atypical pain and no ECG changes.

It may or may not be cardiac. After a careful history and physical examination, I know that my best guess about the etiology of chest pain will be wrong at least one third of the time. We are used to being fooled, and understand that our job is often about managing uncertainty.

Nevertheless, because chest pain is so common (3 million ED visits a year, and I took an antacid last night), most who practice general medicine become adept with the differential diagnosis (Table 4.1). The first goal is recognition of cardiac pain and dissection of the aorta, because they may be fatal while most other causes of chest pain are not.

Table 4.1 describes a number of noncardiac causes of chest pain. The most common are gastroesophageal reflux and chest wall syndromes. In these cases, the history, alone, may allow a diagnosis. A patient with pain at night when recumbent that is relieved by sitting, is associated with a sour taste, and is provoked by a late meal has reflux. And discomfort that occurs with movement—reaching, twisting, or use of the arms—or is reproduced with pressure on the chest wall is musculoskeletal. When the bedside evaluation indicates one of these conditions, and the ECG is normal, I may not pursue further cardiac workup.

Esophageal diagnostic studies, in my experience, are seldom helpful. If you suspect uncomplicated gastroesophageal reflux, try a therapeutic trial of antacids (a proton pump inhibitor in the morning and ranitidine at night are effective), elevation of the head of the bed, avoidance of late meals, and so forth. If the symptoms do not resolve, then consider gastrointestinal evaluation. The therapeutic trial should be evaluated with a follow-up visit.

Laboratory Evaluation of Chest Pain

The need for blood work varies. Most benefit from a complete blood count. Anemia alone does not cause angina, but it lowers the angina threshold in the presence of CAD. Inflammatory conditions that may affect the heart do not usually raise the white blood cell count. A normal erythrocyte sedimentation rate excludes pericarditis. A more sensitive marker of inflammation, the C-reactive protein (CRP), is frequently elevated in chronic CAD, and more so with acute coronary

Table 4.1 The Differential Diagnosis of Chest Pain			
Syndrome	Associated Conditions	Physical Examination	Laboratory Evaluation
Angina pectoris	Risk factors for CAD	Usually normal. During pain, an S_4 gallop or soft systolic murmur (papillary muscle dysfunction)	ST segment changes on the ECG during pain (may be normal without pain); abnormal stress study (see text)
Aortic dissection (see Chapter 8)	Young patients: Marfan's syndrome. Older patients: hypertension and ASCVD risk factors	Unequal or missing pulses. Murmur of aortic regurgitation with proximal dissection.	Wide mediastinum on chest x-ray. Diagnosis requires CT scan or transesophageal echocardiogram.
Esophageal spasm	Middle to older age. Often smoking and obesity.	Normal	Endoscopy, pH monitoring, motility studies.
Esophageal rupture	Follows severe vomiting.	Subcutaneous emphysema	Chest x-ray shows air in the mediastinum
Pancreatitis	Alcoholism, gall bladder disease	Epigastric tenderness	Elevated amylase, lipase, and white count
Peptic ulcer disease	Possibly smoking	Usually normal, epigastric tenderness is possible	Endoscopy
Chest wall pain	Osteoarthritis, chronic neck or back pain.	Pain with deep palpitation, breathing, reaching or changing position	None; the diagnosis is confirmed by physical findings. Often a diagnosis of exclusion.
Herpes zoster	Old age, immuno-compromised host, history of shingles	Pain may precede the rash by 2–3 days.	Tzanck smear of a lesion, rise in antibody titer (although the diagnosis is usually made on clinical grounds)
Pericarditis	Young patient, may follow a flu-like illness	Friction rub, often fever	High sedimentation rate. ST elevation on ECG. White count usually normal. Small pericardial effusion on echo.

ASCVD, atherosclerotic cardiovascular disease; CT, computed tomography; ECG, electrocardiogram.

syndromes (ACS). In most hospitals, the assay is not immediately available, so the CRP may not be useful when evaluating a patient in the ED.

None of the chest pain syndromes alters electrolytes, but it is always worth checking serum potassium and magnesium in a patient who is taking diuretics. I do not order the Chem-20 unless there is a specific reason (e.g., a new patient, one who is being admitted to the hospital, other medical problems that should be monitored, suspicion of gallbladder disease). If the differential diagnosis includes angina, a lipid panel will be useful, although it is not a part of the ED evaluation.

Cardiac enzymes, troponin or CK, are frequently measured as part of the ED evaluation of chest pain. The indication for drawing enzymes is to rule out myocardial infarction (MI). If there is no clinical suspicion of MI, there is no need to measure them. Cardiac enzymes are drawn frequently when they are not indicated, and elevated levels that are false-positive results lead to unnecessary further workup. Chapter 5 discusses cardiac enzymes in some detail.

The resting ECG is essential when evaluating a patient with chest pain.[1] It is cheap, safe, easy to do, and always available. It is hard to justify not doing an ECG when the diagnosis might be cardiac, and malpractice cases often hinge on the misuse of the ECG. If there are ST segment or T wave changes that could be from ischemia, and they are not known to be old, the patient may need admission to the hospital for more evaluation.

On the other hand, the ECG may be normal between episodes of angina. During angina there usually is ST segment depression, and an absence of ECG changes during pain is evidence against ischemia. Unfortunately, it is not absolute proof, because there are some myocardial regions that are electrocardiographically silent. In particular, ischemia involving the lateral wall of the left ventricle (LV) supplied by the circumflex artery may not cause ST segment alteration.

If no previous ECG is available for comparison, the ECG on presentation or during pain is less useful. Establishing a baseline is another reason for obtaining an ECG for any patient with chest discomfort.

The chest x-ray is a crude screen for thoracic aneurysm; mediastinal widening is present in 80% who have aortic dissection. A normal study does not exclude dissection, and the workup for aortic dissection requires a transesophageal echocardiogram or CT scan.

Deciding to Admit or not Admit

Unstable angina is the criterion for admission. An initial diagnosis of unstable angina could be wrong, and the patient may be having noncardiac chest pain. Nevertheless, a clinical impression of unstable angina justifies admission. A minority of patients with unstable angina are at low risk for MI in the near future, and they may be safely evaluated as outpatients (vide infra). But when in doubt, admit.

Stable Angina Pectoris

The clinical definition of chronic stable angina is *exercise-induced discomfort that is relieved in minutes by rest or nitroglycerin, with symptoms that have been stable for more than 2 months with no change in frequency or severity* (Table 4.2). In the absence of left main coronary artery stenosis, the mortality rate is less than 3% per year.

Table 4.2 Classification of Angina Pectoris		
Parameter	Chronic Stable Angina	Unstable Angina
Clinical syndrome	Angina at a predictable level of exertion (the angina threshold). Relief with rest or nitroglycerin. No change in the angina pattern for ≥2 months.	Angina with any of the following: 1. New onset (<2months) 2. Accelerating pattern 3. Angina at rest 4. Nocturnal angina 5. Longer episodes of pain 6. New ST-T changes on the ECG
Prognosis	Annual mortality <3% if LV function is normal. The short term risk of MI is low.	10–40% chance of MI or death within 3–4 months (depending on clinical presentation, Table 4.5)
Coronary artery lesion (angiographic appearance)	Flow-restricting stenosis (>70 reduction in lumen diameter), but smooth plaque surface.	The stenosis may not be tight. Ragged plaque surface with ulceration, exposed collagen and thrombus.

ECG, electrocardiogram; LV, left ventricular; MI, myocardial infarction.

The number of angina episodes per week is not related to prognosis, as long as the spells are exercise-induced and brief.

Pathophysiology

Myocardial ischemia occurs when oxygen supply falls below myocardial oxygen demand (MVO_2). Variables in the supply-demand equation are illustrated in Figure 4.1. The typical coronary stenosis causing chronic, stable, effort angina is fairly tight, reducing the vessel diameter by more than 70%. The lesion tends to be calcified, rigid, and have smooth plaque surface. It is not a dynamic lesion; that is to say, the percent stenosis changes little, and there is no spasm or thrombus at the site of the lesion.

The hydraulics of coronary blood flow thus approximates those of fuel lines in machines (this is a good way to describe it to patients). A car with a fuel line stenosis runs normally when idling. Opening the throttle increases the workload of the engine, but fuel flow is limited and the engine misses. Because of the fixed nature of the fuel line stenosis, you would expect the engine to begin missing at the same workload—speed—every time. That speed is the angina threshold.

The same holds true for stable, exercise-induced angina. Myocardial oxygen demand is proportional to heart rate and systolic blood pressure at any level of physical work. The heart rate–blood pressure product at which angina occurs defines the *angina threshold*. Serial exercise testing shows that the angina threshold, the heart rate-blood pressure product that elicits angina, is consistent from day to day. Patients usually can identify the level of physical work that provokes angina, and try to avoid it.

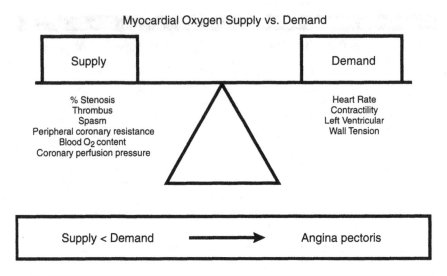

Figure 4.1 Ischemia occurs when myocardial oxygen demand exceeds supply, and most patients experience angina pectoris. There are two clinical syndromes. *Chronic stable angina*: the stable coronary artery stenosis reduces the vessel diameter >70%, placing a ceiling on blood flow. With an increase in cardiac work, the increased demand for oxygen exceeds this ceiling, causing ischemia. *Unstable angina*: the severity of stenosis is variable, usually because of thrombus on the plaque surface (spasm has a role in a minority of patients). The initiating event leading to ischemia is reduced supply, rather than increased demand. Inadequate supply may be aggravated by reduced oxygen-carrying capacity of blood (anemia), failure of peripheral coronary vasodilatation, or low coronary perfusion pressure. Increased demand may result from conditions that increase heart rate, myocardial contractility, or ventricular wall tension. (Reprinted with permission from Taylor GJ. The Cardiology Rotation. Malden, MA: Blackwell Science, 2001:105.)

A change in the angina threshold usually means a change in the plaque. Developing angina at a lower workload—a worsening of the angina pattern—is one of the clinical definitions of unstable angina, and it signifies a higher risk of MI.

Variable threshold angina: a qualification of the fixed plaque model—The fixed lesion, supply–demand model works most of the time to explain how angina develops. But some patients have variation in the angina threshold. For example, they may describe good days, with no angina despite much exercise, or bad days when angina develops with little exertion. Another common example of this is the *warm-up phenomenon*: angina with minimal exertion early in the day, with improvement later and no angina despite vigorous activity.

A possible explanation is variability of the coronary artery lumen at the site of plaque. Although uncommon, this may occur when the plaque is eccentric, and does not cover the entire circumference of the arterial wall. The uninvolved arterial segment may relax or contract, and thus change luminal diameter and flow.

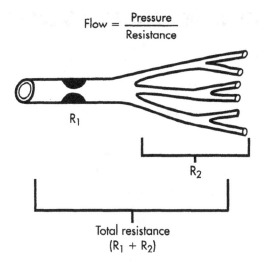

$$\text{Flow} = \frac{\text{Pressure}}{\text{Resistance}}$$

R_1

R_2

Total resistance
$(R_1 + R_2)$

Figure 4.2 Blood flow is proportional to perfusion pressure and inversely proportional to vascular resistance. We are used to thinking that resistance to flow is from the fixed coronary stenosis in the patient with effort angina (R_1). However, the total resistance to flow comes from the combined resistances at the stenosis (R_1) and downstream (R_2). R_1 probably does not change with vasodilator therapy, but R_2 may (this has been shown with calcium channel blockade). In addition, the angina threshold may fall when R_2 is high, explaining why a patient with fixed coronary stenosis can have variation in symptoms (e.g., good vs. bad days, the warm-up phenomenon). (Reprinted with permission from Taylor GJ. Primary Care Management of Heart Disease. St. Louis: Mosby, 2000:141.)

More common is a change in vascular resistance distal to the stenosis (Figure 4.2). Coronary blood flow is governed by resistance in the entire vascular bed, not just at the site of stenosis. Lowering downstream resistance can improve overall blood flow, raising the angina threshold.

Blood flow in distal coronary artery branches is autoregulated, controlled largely by local factors. Vasodilatation occurs with increased tissue CO_2 tension and endothelial nitric oxide. The major vasoconstrictor influence is alpha-adrenergic stimulation. When there is a tight proximal stenosis that limits flow and creates persistent low-level ischemia, autoregulation of the distal vessel is maxed out. There is no vasodilator reserve to counter an alpha-adrenergic, vasoconstrictor stimulus.

This was initially worked out in catheterization laboratory experiments using the cold pressor test, which provokes alpha-adrenergic discharge. Placing the patient's hand in ice water lowered the angina threshold by causing peripheral coronary vasoconstriction. A change in alpha tone affecting distal coronary resistance may be the link between angina and emotional stress, the warm-up phenomenon, or walking into a cold wind. Calcium channel blockers appear to contribute to distal coronary vasodilator reserve; nifedipine blocked the changes seen during the cold pressor test.

Table 4.3 Indicators of Poor Prognosis with Coronary Artery Disease	
Clinical Predictors	Congestive heart failure or low LVEF Prior MI (indicates increased risk of death with subsequent MI) Complex ventricular arrhythmias (a marker of low LVEF) Resting tachycardia (a marker of low LVEF) Diabetes Left ventricular hypertrophy (a risk factor for sudden cardiac death) Advanced age
Resting ECG	New T wave inversion, or resting ST-T wave changes ST segment depression during angina ST segment elevation during angina New bundle branch block Long QT interval Q waves indicating prior MI
Stress ECG	>2 mm ST segment depression ST depression in exercise stage I ST depression in multiple leads ST depression persisting for >5 minutes during recovery Poor exercise tolerance (<4 METS or <6 minutes using the Bruce protocol) Symptoms and ST depression at heart rate <120 (off beta-blockers) Angina during exercise A drop in blood pressure >10 mm Hg with exercise (may indicate left main CAD) Exercise-induced PVCs or ventricular tachycardia Delayed recovery of heart rate (it should fall >12 beats/min in the first minute)
Perfusion Imaging	Defects in multiple vascular distributions (indicates multivessel CAD) Anterior plus lateral defects (possible left main CAD) Increase lung uptake of thallium (marker of poor LV function) Post exercise LV dilatation Anterior perfusion defect (left anterior descending CAD)
LV Function Imaging (Echocardiography or Radionuclide Angiography)	Poor LV function at rest Fall in LVEF with exercise (≥10 percentage points) LV dilatation with exercise Wall motion abnormalities involving multiple vascular regions
Coronary and LV Angiography	Left main CAD*—always an indication for CABS Three-vessel CAD—usually an indication for revascularization Proximal left anterior descending CAD (when present, it upgrades the risk, e.g., moves two-vessel disease into a higher risk category) Ragged plaque surface and associated filling defects (thrombus)—indicators of unstable plaque Depressed LV function—when present increases the need for revascularization for those with active ischemia; a graded effect: the worse the LV, the greater the need for revascularization

MI, myocardial infarction; LVEF, left ventricular ejection fraction; CAD, coronary artery disease; METS, metabolic unit (1 MET is the energy used sitting at rest, 5 METS is the equivalent of walking up stairs, or doing housework); PVC, premature ventricular contraction; CABS, coronary artery bypass surgery.

*Stenosis and disease indicate luminal diameter reduced ≥70%.

I have found calcium channel blocker therapy especially effective for the patient who describes a variable angina threshold.

Evaluation of the Patient with Angina

Stable angina tends to be stable, and a patient who has had it for years does not require frequent cardiac reevaluation. Lipid-lowering therapy (as well as other medical therapy) should be monitored, and an updated ECG in the record is useful for comparison if symptoms change. Repeated stress testing with or without imaging is of little use unless there is a change in the angina pattern. The stress test is usually positive, as the patient does, after all, have angina. Most important, it does not help to predict the future; a yearly stress test does not predict when the patient will become unstable or have an MI.

On the other hand, a patient who first presents with angina needs evaluation to exclude a risk for early MI or death, even if it is effort angina. There are a few clinical principles that influence management (Table 4.3):

1. *More extensive CAD indicates a worse prognosis.* Natural history studies in the 1970s found annual mortality rates of 2% to 3% with single-vessel CAD, 4% to 6% with two-vessel CAD, and 7% to 10% with three-vessel disease. The mortality risk is much lower with modern medical therapy (vide infra). Tight (≥70%) left main coronary artery stenosis is especially dangerous (Figure 4.3), with an annual mortality more than 50%. Infarction of this vessel means the simultaneous loss of two of the three vascular regions, the anterior and lateral walls. Early evaluation must screen for left main and/or multivessel CAD.

2. *Exercise tolerance during treadmill testing correlates with survival.* Patients who have to stop the exercise test before completing stage 2 in the Bruce protocol (Table 4.4) have 6% to 10% annual mortality, compared with 1% for those who reach stage 4. Thus, a patient with poor exercise tolerance plus ischemia during an exercise test would be a candidate for angiography, while good exercise tolerance would make us more comfortable with a trial of medical therapy. Using the Bruce protocol, an ability to exercise more than 7 minutes establishes a good prognosis, independent of ECG changes (e.g., those with a positive test still have a good prognosis if exercise tolerance is good).

3. *Poor LV function indicates a bad prognosis.* This is true for most adults with heart disease, and especially with CAD. Defining LV function is an important part of the initial evaluation. LV dysfunction is suggested by a history of MI, Q waves on the ECG, or symptoms of congestive heart failure (CHF) including easy fatigue. These clinical factors or poor LV function identified by noninvasive testing weigh in favor of angiography, even when the angina pattern is stable.

Noninvasive Screening for Coronary Artery Disease

Stress testing—The resting ECG tends to be normal, but during angina, there is ST segment depression. As noted, an absence of ST segment changes weighs against angina. *Be sure to note—on the tracing—that the ECG was obtained during pain.* If you do not, you will have difficulty identifying the chest pain ECG later.

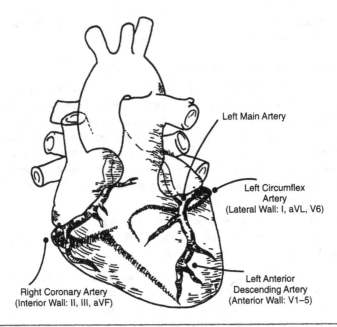

Left Main Artery

Left Circumflex
Artery
(Lateral Wall: I, aVL, V6)

Left Anterior
Descending Artery
(Anterior Wall: V1–5)

Right Coronary Artery
(Interior Wall: II, III, aVF)

Figure 4.3 Coronary artery anatomy. The circumflex and right coronary arteries circle the heart in the atrioventricular groove; branches of the circumflex leave the groove to supply the lateral wall of the left ventricle. The major right coronary branch, the posterior descending artery, supplies the inferior wall. The anterior descending artery is located over the interventricular septum and sends branches into the septum and over the anterior wall of the left ventricle. The spatial orientation of the ECG allows groups of leads to be particularly sensitive to events in a given region of the heart. This patient has a right dominant circulation, with the posterior descending branch originating from the right coronary. A small number of patients (15%) have left dominance. In this case the right coronary is tiny, and the posterior descending comes off a large circumflex vessel that reaches the base of the heart. (Reprinted with permission from Taylor GJ. The Cardiology Rotation. Malden, MA: Blackwell Science, 2001:113.)

The coronary arteries are on the epicardial surface of the heart, and they send perforating branches into the myocardium (Figure 4.3). Exercise-induced ischemia first affects the muscle farthest from the epicardial source, the subendocardium. Thus, angina usually produces the ECG pattern of subendocardial ischemia, ST segment depression (Figure 4.4). ST depression more reliably indicates ischemia (is more specific) when the patient also experiences angina.

The treadmill ECG (a.k.a., stress test, graded exercise test) is straightforward. The goal is to provoke ischemia in a controlled setting so that both symptoms and the ECG may be evaluated (Table 4.4). The test is positive when the coronary stenosis is tight enough to limit flow, reducing luminal diameter more than 70%. That is usually the case with exercise-induced angina, and stress testing has good sensitivity in chronic stable angina.

Table 4.4 Bruce Exercise Test Protocol (The patient walks in each stage for 3 minutes)				
	Treadmill Setting			
Stage	Speed	Grade	METS	Exercise Equivalent
1	1.7 mph	10%	5*	The average peak cost of activities of daily living (walking up stairs, sex with a spouse). It is the exercise level recommended after discharge after MI.
2	2.5 mph	12%	7	
3	3.4 mph	14%	9.5	An ability to walk 7 minutes indicates good prognosis, even in those with known CAD and stable angina.
4	4.2 mph	16%	13	The average exercise capacity for moderately active young men.

1 MET (metabolic equivalent) is the energy used sitting quietly at rest; at this baseline the average oxygen consumption is 3.5 mL/kg/min (thus, 5 METS assumes an oxygen consumption of 17.5 ml/kg/min); MI, myocardial infarction; CAD, coronary artery disease.

*Achieving 5 METS assumes completion of stage I, or at least being able to exercise comfortably at that level. Walking slowly on level ground requires about 3 METS.

While it is a useful screening study, the stress ECG has limits. It does not identify the artery responsible for ischemia. For example, inferior wall ischemia does not cause changes in just the inferior ECG leads (Figure 4.3). Most positive stress tests have ST segment depression in V5, regardless of the location of the culprit lesion. ST segment depression in multiple leads and a failure of the ST segments to return to baseline with 6 minutes of recovery indicate worse prognosis. A drop in blood pressure during exercise suggests left main coronary stenosis; there usually is ST depression as well. Blood pressure normally increases with exercise, even during ischemia involving smaller coronary branches, but left main ischemia affects a large portion of the LV, causing transient pump failure and hypotension.

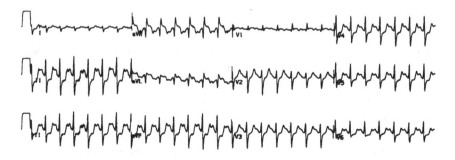

Figure 4.4 Positive stress ECG showing ST segment depression in inferior and lateral leads, the pattern of subendocardial ischemia. (Reprinted with permission from Taylor, GJ. The Cardiology Rotation. Malden, MA: Blackwell Science, 2001:108.)

The stress ECG is less sensitive with unstable angina where the lesion may be dynamic (vide infra). The person with a normal stress test who has an MI the next day or week probably had a 30% to 50% stenosis, not tight enough to cause ischemia during exercise. But such non-critical lesions can have unstable plaque surface leading to thrombosis (a frequent mechanism of unstable angina). Clot may reduce luminal diameter and cause angina at rest, or it may occlude the artery and cause MI. For this reason, I usually tell patients that a normal stress test indicates low risk for MI, "but not zero risk."

Despite this limitation, the stress ECG is still an effective tool for evaluating CPUE, particularly when it is exertional. False positives are common, and are more likely in women, in patients taking digoxin, and when there are baseline ST-T wave changes. A false positive test can be identified as such by repeating it with an imaging study.

Perfusion scanning—Thallium enters the myocyte via the Na^+-K^+ ATPase pump. Think of thallium as a potassium analog, an intracellular cation. Most is extracted by muscle with the first pass, and myocardial accumulation is proportional to myocardial blood flow. A normal scan shows homogenous uptake by all LV segments. With ischemia there is a cold spot on the scan, less uptake in the vascular distribution of the stenosed or occluded coronary artery.

An anterior defect indicates left anterior descending (LAD) disease, a lateral defect indicates circumflex disease, and inferior defect, right coronary disease (in 85% of patients, the other 15% have a dominant circumflex that supplies the inferior wall). Defects involving more than one region indicate multivessel CAD, and a worse prognosis. A defect in both the lateral and anterior walls suggests left main CAD (Figure 4.3).

Two scans are obtained, the first with stress. Ischemic muscle does not accumulate thallium and there is a cold spot. However, over the next couple hours, after recovering from ischemia, viable muscle accumulates thallium from the circulation. The second, resting scan shows redistribution of thallium into the area, indicating that it is viable. A perfusion defect on both the stress scan and the delayed scan indicates scar (prior MI).

An occasional patient with severe ischemia has a resting defect that fails to normalize in a couple hours, giving the appearance of scar. With more time this stunned or hibernating myocardium can accumulate thallium from the circulation. The *viability study* is a delayed scan, 24 hours after injection of thallium. A cold spot that fills in indicates viable muscle, not scar. The viability study is usually done when LV function is poor, hoping to find viable muscle that can recover after bypass surgery.

Sestamibi is another perfusion imaging agent. It is a technetium-99m compound that binds to mitochondria and is not transported by the Na^+-K^+ ATPase pump. There is rapid initial uptake, but no late redistribution into the ischemic region. The advantage of this for the stress study is that there is no rush to do the scan after sestamibi is injected; with stress thallium, the scan must be done immediately because of redistribution. Because there is no redistribution, sestamibi cannot be used for viability studies. Some laboratories use dual isotope imaging, with thallium for the resting scan, and sestamibi for the stress study.

Perfusion imaging improves both the sensitivity and specificity of stress testing. A negative study is especially valuable, with less than 1% risk of cardiac events (MI or cardiac death) in the next year. The risk is slightly higher at older age, among women with diabetes, and when there has been previous CAD.[2]

A question that comes up in the clinic is how long the patient remains low-risk—what is the warranty period of a normal scan? A history of CAD and advanced age are associated with a higher coronary event rate in the second year after the scan, but it is still low. Here are data from a study of 7376 patients followed for 2 years after a scan showing no active ischemia:[2] a 50-year-old man without previous CAD has a 0.1% event rate (MI or death) the first and second years after the exercise perfusion scan. With known CAD a 50-year-old man has a 0.9% event rate the first year, and a 1.5% rate the second year. For an 80-year-old man with known CAD, the event rates in the first and second year are 1.4% and 2.4%. One message from this study is that myocardial perfusion imaging is quite good, but the history still adds to the assessment of prognosis.

Pharmacologic stress testing—Exercise testing should be done when possible. It allows assessment of exercise tolerance, which is related to prognosis. An ability to complete an exercise stress test is another predictor of better outcome when the perfusion scan is normal.[2] However, many of our patients cannot walk on the treadmill.

There are two approaches to pharmacologic stress. The first really is a stress test. Dobutamine is infused at progressively higher doses to raise heart rate and blood pressure, attempting to induce ischemia. The perfusion scan, or echocardiogram, is first done at rest and then during maximum dobutamine infusion.

The second non-exercise approach is the coronary vasodilator scan, using adenosine or dipyridamole (which blocks the uptake and removal of adenosine). Adenosine is a powerful coronary vasodilator, raising coronary blood flow twofold or more. Adenosine does not cause an increase in cardiac work, and it usually does not provoke ischemia. Instead there is differential dilatation, with the normal coronary artery dilating more than a stenosed vessel. Flow thus increases to the normal area, but much less in the stenosed region. This heterogeneous flow pattern creates the illusion of ischemia and a positive scan—or you may argue that there is relative ischemia. But most patients to not have chest pain with ST segment depression.

An occasional patient does have angina and ST changes; this usually indicates an occluded artery supplied by collaterals. Dilating the vessel that is the source of the collateral reduces flow through the collateral vessels—the *coronary steal syndrome*. Another group of patients have chest pain but no objective evidence for ischemia (ST changes or a perfusion abnormality). Adenosine is the neurotransmitter at cardiac sensory nerve endings, and stimulation of pain receptors may be the mechanism (note the discussion of silent ischemia and syndrome X near the end of this chapter).

Adenosine (and thus, dipyridamole) can provoke bronchospasm or AV nodal block and bradyarrhythmias. Both effects are reversed by theophylline.

The vasodilator scan has been found superior to exercise scanning in patients with left bundle branch block (a fact that has found its way to the medicine boards).

Stress echocardiogram and radionuclide angiogram—Like perfusion imaging, LV function and wall motion studies raise the sensitivity and specificity of stress testing, and they are able to identify the ischemic region. There is prompt cessation of contractility when muscle becomes ischemic. The stress test report will describe a new wall motion abnormality or region of akinesis. Both the echocardiogram and radionuclide angiogram (also called the *MUGA scan*) can be used to assess wall motion before and during exercise. A large ischemic region indicates a worse prognosis. Anterior wall ischemia tends to be more dangerous than inferior or lateral wall disease, as the LAD artery supplies a larger amount of myocardium. Likewise, a substantial fall in LV ejection fraction (LVEF) during exercise and ischemia indicates higher risk.

Choosing a noninvasive imaging technique—The sensitivity and specificity of stress perfusion imaging and stress echo are close. Studies of these tests are from centers with medical and technical personnel who work full time on either nuclear imaging or echocardiography. Although self evident, this is worth mentioning, as both techniques are operator-dependent. The average cardiologist reading echocardiograms—me for example—is not capable of interpreting the stress echo. That requires further training for the cardiologist and echo technician, then a relatively high practice volume to maintain skill. The same holds true for nuclear stress testing. If your scans are being read by a radiologist who has no cardiac training and minimal experience, and who reads an occasional perfusion scan while doing other nuclear studies, you will see a lot of false-positive results. Day in and day out, use the technique favored by your center.

Left bundle branch block affects wall motion. The septum contracts late, and this reduces stroke volume (note the discussion of resynchronization therapy in Chapter 1). Vasodilator perfusion imaging is the most accurate noninvasive technique in this setting.

Cost may influence choice. In our hospital, the retail cost of a stress perfusion scan is $3500, compared with $1200 for stress echocardiography. Isotopes are expensive.

Coronary Angiography

The indication for cardiac catheterization is suspicion of high risk based on the history and results of noninvasive studies (Tables 4.2 and 4.3). Remember that myocardial injury is cumulative, and the chance of a patient with MI dying is much higher when there is a history of MI. Thus, a history of MI and known depression of LV function are both clinical indicators of high-risk CAD. The most frequent indication for angiography in a patient who has had chronic stable angina is a change in the frequency or severity of the angina. When this happens, the patient has essentially developed unstable angina (Table 4.2). Unstable angina is probably the most common diagnostic code used as an indication for catheterization.

Angiography is considered a low risk, although invasive procedure. The chance of a major complication—death, MI, stroke, or another embolic event—is about 1 in 700. The risk is higher for those with peripheral artery disease or diabetes, yet it is remarkable how well critically ill patients with advanced disease tolerate the procedure.

A pulsatile *psuedoaneurysm* may develop in the groin. This infrequent complication occurs with failure of the arterial puncture site to close. There is persistent communication between the arterial lumen and the surrounding hematoma. It may be unstable, leading to rupture or to bleeding into the retroperitoneal space. When evaluating a large hematoma, the key finding is pulsation, which suggests pseudoaneurysm. It requires either surgical repair or correction using special catheterization laboratory techniques. On the other hand, hematomas are common after catheterization, as most of our patients are on antiplatelet therapy. The hematoma may be large, then forms a hard knot and resolves with time. There is no need for surgical intervention.

Contrast nephropathy—Most studies define contrast nephropathy as a rise in creatinine of 0.3 mg/dL or more over baseline. It usually occurs in those with elevated creatinine or diabetes. Use of lower osmolar contrast agents, good hydration before catheterization, and acetylcysteine (Mucomyst; 600 mg the night before and twice daily the day of catheterization) have been shown to lower the risk of nephropathy. For those with near-normal renal function, spontaneous recovery during the week after angiography is the rule. However, with advanced renal disease, contrast exposure may be the final insult leading to dialysis. When on the fence about the need for catheterization, severe renal dysfunction weighs against it.

Nephropathy begins with vasoconstriction. When the kidney is exposed to a high osmotic load, adenosine is released, which leads to vasoconstriction and glomerular ischemia. Pretreatment with theophylline, an adenosine receptor blocker, prevents vasoconstriction and moderates the fall in creatinine clearance that follows contrast exposure. It has no effect on renal adenosine release (measured as the urine adenosine level). Studies of theophylline prophylaxis measured pre and post catheterization creatinine clearance in patients with normal renal function or mild azotemia who were at low risk for nephropathy (defined as a rise in serum creatinine). I assume that theophylline's beneficial effect on creatinine clearance would translate to prevention of contrast nephropathy in higher risk patients, but this has not been proved. The regimen used in most studies has been long-acting theophylline (Theo-Dur) 200 mg the night before and twice daily the day of catheterization; at this dose, the risk of use is minimal.

Acetylcysteine, a free radical scavenger, also protects the kidneys. Oxygen free radicals are produced by glomerular ischemia. An additional source of free radicals is the breakdown of adenosine to xanthine. The xanthine oxidase inhibitor, allopurinol, has been shown to prevent a drop in creatinine clearance after angiography, but it is a potentially toxic drug. Acetylcysteine, however, is quite safe at the effective dose. Note that theophylline blocks the adenosine receptor, and not the release of adenosine following hyperosmolar challenge. Thus, there is an argument for using both agents: theophylline to block ischemia, and acetylcysteine to remove free radicals produced by the degradation of adenosine. While the renoprotective effects of these drugs have been documented in randomized trials—and both are quite safe at the low, recommended doses—there has been no study of combination therapy.

Treatment of Stable Angina

It is useful to think about what you will accomplish with any therapy. In particular, you should know what treatments prolong life, and distinguish them from others that just relieve symptoms. Both goals are important, but highest on the list would be the life-prolonging therapies. In fact, if you are not providing a life-prolonging treatment, you would be wise to document the reasons for avoiding it in the medical record.

Survival with CAD is better with aggressive lipid lowering, aspirin, and angiotensin-converting enzyme (ACE) inhibitors. Those with a history of MI live longer on beta-blocker therapy.[3]

Low-Density Lipoprotein–Lowering Drugs

Serial angiographic trials showed that pushing the low-density lipoprotein (LDL) cholesterol below 70 mg/dL halts the progression of CAD for many patients and leads to regression of disease for some. Furthermore, statins stabilize the artery independent of their effects on cholesterol levels (see Chapter 3). We now understand that therapy should be started soon after establishing the diagnosis of atherosclerotic cardiovascular disease (ASCVD), because there is a survival benefit within the first weeks of treatment. Practice guidelines call for lowering the LDL below 70 mg/dL, regardless of the pretreatment level (see Chapter 3).

The NCEP target LDL has been lowered because of new clinical trials (Table 3.4). The AVERT trial compared medical therapy with angioplasty in patients with one- or two-vessel CAD and stable angina.[4] The medical group received atorvastatin 80 mg/day, which lowered LDL cholesterol 46%, to a mean of 77 mg/dL; 71% in the angioplasty group also had statin therapy but at a lower dose, resulting in an 18% reduction in LDL to about 120 mg/dL. During 18 months follow-up, mortality was similar in the two groups. However, high-dose atorvastatin resulted in 36% fewer ischemic events than angioplasty (including MI, revascularization, and hospitalization for angina).

I describe the AVERT trial in some detail for a couple reasons. 1) It supports my claim at the beginning of this chapter: the trend is for CAD to become a medical illness. 2) It is a reason that the NCEP has lowered its LDL targets for both primary and secondary prevention (see Chapter 3).

Antiplatelet Therapy

Aspirin prevents MI and lowers the risk of death in patients with established ASCVD—including CAD—as well as those with risk factors for ASCVD.[5] Clopidogrel is a good substitute for those who do not tolerate aspirin. The CAPRI trial compared aspirin 325 mg/day with clopidogrel 75 mg/day in 19,000 patients with stable vascular disease.[6] The risk of MI, stroke, or vascular death was 8.7% lower in the clopidogrel group (5.3% vs. 5.8%). That difference is not great enough to justify its use for all patients, especially considering the low cost of aspirin. Perhaps more important, CAPRI documented the safety of clopidogrel.

Nonsteroidal anti-inflammatory drugs(NSAIDs)—The issue of other COX inhibitors is more complicated. Stimulated platelets release arachidonic acid, which is converted to thromboxane A_2, a platelet agonist and vasoconstrictor.[7] Aspirin, a nonselective COX inhibitor, blocks the generation of thromboxane A_2, and is thus antithrombotic. Naproxen also blocks this reaction. However, clinical trials have not consistently found protective cardiac effects with naproxen or other NSAIDs, and they should not be considered substitutes for aspirin.[7,8] More recently there is concern that NSAIDs may counteract the effects of low-dose aspirin.

Keep in mind that platelets function in the neighborhood of the endothelium. Endothelial cells generate prostacyclin, nitric oxide, and carbon monoxide, which counteract platelet activity and vasodilate. The selective COX-2 inhibitors block the synthesis of prostacyclin, and have less effect on thromboxane A_2 than aspirin.[7] In fact, there is concern that patients on both drugs may have aspirin's beneficial action on thromboxane A_2 canceled by the COX-2 inhibitor effect on prostacyclin. Highlighting this possibility was the VIGOR trial, which compared rofecoxib (Vioxx) and naproxen in patients rheumatoid arthritis, and it described an increased risk of MI with rofecoxib although no increase in the risk of death.[9] This has been all attributed to cardioprotective effects of naproxen, rather than to rofecoxib toxicity.[7] (Author note: While in press, Vioxx has been withdrawn from the market. There is continued discussion about the safety of other COX-2 inhibitors.)

Furthermore, these results in patients with rheumatoid arthritis may not apply to the general population.[7] Evaluation of a 67,000 patient Canadian database found no increase in the short-term risk of MI with COX-2 inhibitors compared with naproxen or other NSAIDs.[10] More recently, the huge TennCare database assessed the risk of death or nonfatal MI in users of rofecoxib and other NSAIDs. The incidence of death or nonfatal MI was increased with high-dose rofecoxib (more than 25 mg/day), but not at the usual dose of 25 mg/day.[11] In this study, naproxen and ibuprofen did not influence the risk of coronary events.

Angiotensin converting enzyme inhibitors—ACE inhibition has direct vascular effects. It is interesting how this understanding developed. Early studies of hypertension discovered the renoprotective effect of ACE inhibition in patients who also had diabetes. Assuming this was a vascular effect, the next step was to test benefits in patients without diabetes.

The HOPE trial randomly treated 9297 patients younger than 55 years old with a history of CAD, stroke, peripheral vascular disease or diabetes, plus one additional risk factor for ASCVD with ramipril 10 mg/day or placebo.[12] During 5 years follow-up, ramapril lowered death from MI 20%, death from stroke 32%, and death from any cause 16%. Before treatment, 37% of the patients had diabetes, and in this group ramapril reduced diabetic complications (a composite of nephropathy, need for dialysis, or need for laser treatment for retinopathy). Most interesting, ramapril also prevented the development of diabetes; the explanation for this is uncertain. The benefit of ramapril was considered a direct vascular effect, independent of the trivial lowering of blood pressure noted in the study.

A smaller clinical trial of enalapril supports the vascular benefits of ACE inhibitors. Angiography was done initially and after 4 years.[13] Enalapril had no effect on degree of stenosis, but it lowered incidence of a combined endpoint of death, MI, or stroke. The vascular benefit probably involves endothelial function (see Chapter 3).

Based on these early studies, ACE inhibitor therapy is recommended for all with ASCVD, with or without diabetes. There are clinical trials in progress testing the effects of other ACE inhibitors in populations that do not include patients with diabetes.

Beta blockade—A survival benefit has been demonstrated with beta-blocker therapy after MI. The treatment of stable angina has not been well studied, but most clinicians extrapolate the post-MI data to the treatment of chronic CAD. Indeed, the AHA practice guidelines recommend beta-blockers as the initial therapy to control angina symptoms, citing the "consensus opinion of experts."

The efficacy of available beta-blockers is comparable. Bronchospasm is a relative contraindication, and would be an indication for a cardioselective, beta-1 agent, metoprolol or atenolol. At low doses, they do not provoke bronchospasm in those with mild-moderate reactive airway disease.[14] At higher doses all beta-blockers tend to lose their selective effects; when treating a patient with lung disease start with a low dose and slowly raise it (as we do with beta-blockers for CHF).

Vasospasm is another problem with beta blockade that is often overlooked. Beta-adrenergic stimulation causes both coronary and peripheral artery dilatation. Blocking this leaves alpha vasoconstriction unopposed. An increase in claudication is fairly common after starting beta-blockers. A rare patient has worsening angina with beta blockade. The mechanism is vasospastic, variant angina (vide infra). The first case of Prinzmetal's angina I encountered developed after the patient started beta-blockers for hypertension.

We usually avoid beta-blocker therapy when there is bradycardia. However, pindolol (Visken) and acebutalol (Sectral) have intrinsic sympathomimetic activity, and may be considered. They have little effect on resting heart rate, but limit the rise in heart rate with activity.

Nitrates—Nitroglycerin relaxes vascular smooth muscle, predominantly in the venous system. With vasodilatation, there is less blood return to the heart. Lower preload reduces ventricular size, lowering wall tension and MVO_2 (note the discussion of the Laplace relationship in Chapter 1). Because its effect depends on pooling of blood in the lower body, nitroglycerin is less effective when the patient is recumbent. Conversely, the Trendelenberg position reverses any hypotensive effect. Advise your patients to sit, but not to lie down when they have angina and take nitroglycerin.

Both beta blockade and nitroglycerin reduce the heart's mechanical activity. The patient is able to perform more total body work before reaching the angina threshold. The time on the treadmill is longer, but the heart rate–blood pressure product that causes angina is not changed. This is another way of saying that nitrates and beta-blockers do not increase coronary blood flow, rather they reduce oxygen demand.

At the cellular level, nitroglycerin does not work on the endothelium, but goes directly into the smooth muscle cell where it is converted to nitric oxide (NO). Nitroglycerin is thus an NO donor. The endothelium is a separate source of NO, but nitroglycerin remains active when the endothelium is not intact.

Continuous therapy leads to *nitrate tolerance*. This may occur with all of the long-acting nitrate preparations, with evidence of tolerance apparent after 24 hours of a constant blood level of the drug. A brief, nitrate-free interval restores responsiveness.

Limiting nitrate exposure to 12 to 14 hours per day prevents tolerance. That requires the patient remembering to take the nitroglycerin patch off before retiring. I have found that most patients would prefer taking a pill to the use of patches. Eccentric dosing of isosorbide dinitrate (Isordil), given at 8 AM, 1 PM, and 6 PM means that the nitrate effect is gone by midnight. The duration of action of the third dose is diminished by the tolerance effect. More convenient is the sustained release form of isosorbide mononitrate (Imdur); it works for 12 hours and can given once a day (30–240 mg). The timing of the single dose is tailored to the patient's needs; nocturnal symptoms may be controlled by giving it in the evening rather than morning.

Patients are often reluctant to use sublingual nitroglycerin because they think of it as a pain pill. Explain that it works to change blood flow when prescribing it, and recommend taking it as soon as angina begins. The duration of action is approximately 20 minutes, and it can be used prophylactically just before angina-provoking activity.

Headache is the most common side effect of nitrate therapy. I am struck by how often I see patients who have been kept on a long-acting nitrate despite headache. Long-acting nitrates do not prolong survival or prevent MI, and there are good alternatives. There is no reason to continue therapy when it causes headache.

Calcium channel blockers—Because there is no survival benefit, calcium blockers tend to be used infrequently for control of angina. I suggest that you consider them for symptom relief, because they are effective and well tolerated, especially by elderly patients. Serial treadmill testing has shown an increase in the angina threshold with calcium blockers. Thus, unlike beta-blockers and nitrates, they appear to improve coronary blood flow. They do not dilate the coronary artery at the site of stenosis, but instead dilate the downstream vessel, lowering overall resistance in the system and improving flow (Figure 4.2). A fall in peripheral vascular resistance (LV afterload), and mild depression of contractility with some agents adds to the antianginal effect by lowering cardiac work.

Diltiazem is a reasonable substitute for beta-blockers in the patient with severe bronchospasm, because it lowers heart rate. Verapamil has a greater effect on heart rate, but is a relatively weak vasodilator; it has the greatest negative inotropic effect and should be avoided when LV function is severely depressed. I have seen patients with poor LV function develop pulmonary edema with verapamil, but not with diltiazem. Nevertheless, diltiazem should be avoided when there is CHF or LVEF below 30%. The dihydropyridines are pure vasodilators, and reflex tachycardia may be an issue. They would be a good choice when there is bradycardia. This effect can be avoided by giving them with beta-blockers.

Summary—An Approach to Medical Therapy for Chronic Stable Angina:

1. Correct associated problems that may aggravate angina (anemia, hyperthyroidism, uncontrolled hypertension, valvular heart disease, etc.).

2. Modify risk factors.

3. Initiate LDL lowering therapy, with the target LDL 70 mg/dL.

4. Treat all patients with aspirin (or clopidogrel) and an ACE inhibitor.

5. Initiate symptom control using beta-blockers and sublingual nitroglycerin.

6. If symptoms are not controlled, add either a calcium blocker or a long-acting nitrate.

Revascularization

Generally, there are three indications for angiography and revascularization for chronic stable angina:

1. There is high risk for MI or cardiac death based on clinical and laboratory evaluation (Table 4.3).

2. Medical therapy fails to control symptoms.

3. There is a change in symptoms (with acceleration of symptoms, the patient has developed unstable angina).

Accepted anatomic indications for revascularization include left main coronary disease, three-vessel CAD, and multivessel CAD with poor LV function.

Intolerable angina despite medical therapy is a common indication for revascularization. Intolerable for some may be an inability to play competitive sports. On the other hand, elderly or sedentary patients may prefer to live with exertional angina, adjusting activities to avoid symptoms (and invasive therapy). Angina at low workloads, after just a couple minutes on the treadmill, is a relative indication for angiography, because it indicates poor prognosis. In practice, the indications for revascularization often overlap.

Percutaneous coronary revascularization—Angioplasty and stenting have developed rapidly. The usual criticism of newly published studies is that the technology is already outmoded. For example, comparative trials of balloon angioplasty and coronary bypass surgery were out-of-date within a year of completion because of the introduction of coronary stents.

Coronary stenting has been a breakthrough technology. Before stents were available, abrupt occlusion of the coronary artery at the time of angioplasty or during the next 12 hours was common. In fact, the logistics of balloon dilatation included cardiac surgery back up. With stenting, abrupt closure is rare. Emergency surgery is so infrequent that scheduled back up is unnecessary. This has become an argument for performing angioplasty/stenting in hospitals that do not have heart surgery programs, although that does not presently meet the standard of care. (Perhaps the best argument against it is volume. Freestanding programs—without surgery—are more likely to be low-volume, which means higher risk for these operator-dependent techniques.)

Restenosis with recurrent angina develops in approximately 20% of patients after balloon angioplasty. Angiographic follow-up detects another 10% with recurrent stenosis without angina (so that a total of 30% have angiographic restenosis). The mechanism of restenosis has been the subject of intense investigation. While a bit simplistic, think of it as hyperactive scarring at the site of vascular injury.

Every method for enlarging the arterial lumen damages the endothelium and arterial wall. It apparently makes no difference how the plaque and artery are altered; with mashing, cutting, or burning, there is a damaged surface that must heal by scarring. Removing or debulking plaque with cutting devices (atherectomy or rotoblator techniques) or laser has no special benefit. The size of the vessel is the best predictor of restenosis. A large caliber artery has more room for the inevitable lump of scar, so there is less stenosis when healing is complete. Stenting of large caliber vessels further lowers the chance of restenosis, yet with multivessel stenting almost 20% need a repeat procedure.[15]

When it occurs, restenosis happens within 7 months of the procedure. A patient who has recurrence of angina during that time should have repeat catheterization, with plans to restent the vessel. It is interesting that restenosis has no adverse effect on survival, while abrupt closure of the vessel does.[16] As long as the patient returns promptly with recurrence of angina, restenosis is a clinical problem with a good outcome. With present techniques, surgery is infrequently needed.

One approach to in-stent restenosis is intracoronary radiation. Deploying a radioactive stent has been shown to lower the subsequent restenosis rate, but the technique is cumbersome. Our hospital requires a radiation oncologist's presence in the catheterization laboratory! (As an interventional cardiologist I had a short attention span, and wanted to be able to pull a tool off the shelf and fix the problem.)

Drug-eluting stents may change everything.[16] The polymer coating of the stent contains an anitproliferative drug that leaches out over about 30 days and inhibits scarring. The initial study comparing the sirolimus-eluting stent with the standard stent for de novo lesions showed 0% and 27% angiographic restenosis, respectively.[16] Survival at 1 year without MI or another revascularization proceedure was 94% versus 71%. The results from this manufacturer-sponsored trial may seem too good to be true. Nevertheless, other clinical experience with the drug-coated stents suggests a restenosis rate below 5%. We currently use it for patients who have had restenosis with standard stents, and I suspect the coated stent will become the device of choice for de novo lesions that are high risk for restenosis (e.g., long lesions or those in small caliber vessels). There is hope it will improve the results of stenting for diabetic patients.

Follow-up after angioplasty is straightforward. The patient still has CAD and should be on the medicines that promote survival: aggressive LDL lowering, antiplatelet and ACE inhibitor therapy. Those who have had MI should be taking a beta-blocker.

Practice guidelines allow noninvasive screening for restenosis, but do not require it. I do not think that routine screening is the standard of care, and few of my colleagues have patients return for expensive follow-up studies. Most patients with restenosis have a recurrence of angina. An exception may be the patient who initially presented with silent ischemia or an angina equivalent, such as dyspnea on exertion or exercise-induced, episodic fatigue. In such cases, consider a follow-up perfusion scan or stress echo, not another angiogram. If you are going to screen for restenosis, wait until the restenosis period has expired: 7 months with the standard stent, 8 to 9 months with the drug-coated stent (that number may change with experience). A screening study done earlier does not exclude the possibility of restenosis.

Coronary artery bypass surgery—It is common to see an elderly patient with new angina who had CABS many years earlier. When dealing with these often-difficult cases, it helps to remember that CABS is probably responsible for the patient reaching old age—it is a therapeutic triumph. There is general agreement that revascularization surgery has contributed to improved longevity with CAD.[17]

A number of technical advances have improved outcomes with CABS. These include the routine use of the left internal mammary artery for grafting the anterior descending artery, better myocardial protection during surgery, and minimally invasive, off-bypass surgery. Endoscopic surgical techniques are being developed that will allow some patients to avoid thoracotomy.

The risk of surgery is largely determined by patient selection. Major determinants of risk are age, cardiac function and general health ("how brightly does the fire of life burn?"). It is noteworthy that the average age of patients having CABS has steadily risen, as younger patients with less extensive CAD have angioplasty. A 78-year-old woman with low LVEF having a second bypass operation would have a mortality risk as much as 15 times that of a 55-year-old man having a first, elective operation. Ejection fraction does not tell the entire story. Patients with depressed LVEF but no history of heart failure tend to do well. When there has been clinical heart failure, the risk is much higher. Viability studies occasionally help sort this out, but my experience is that the surgeon usually asks for this study hoping for an excuse to avoid surgery—a scan showing viable but stunned muscle rarely generates enthusiasm for the operation.

Other comorbidities that increase the risk of surgery include recent MI, CABS in emergency circumstances, ventricular arrhythmias, diabetes, cerebral vascular disease, obstructive lung disease, and elevated creatinine. Related, life-altering (or ending) complications of CABS include stroke, deep wound infection, MI, and renal or pulmonary failure. Surgeons discuss these possibilities with the patient and family before surgery, and the decision to operate involves balancing risk and benefit.

Follow-up after coronary artery bypass surgery—Although fixed, the patient still has CAD and should be on the usual life-prolonging therapy (an LDL-lowering drug, aspirin, an ACE inhibitor, and a beta-blocker when there has been MI). During the first couple months after surgery, most complain of easy fatigue and poor exercise tolerance. They may be alarmed because they have been told they will be ready to return to work after 6 weeks. In reality, it is a small minority that is able to return to normal activity this quickly. Those who do physical work require more time before they are able to resume working. Older patients commonly take 6 months to recover. Cardiac rehabilitation programs speed the recovery process, and help with risk factor modification.

With better coronary blood flow, the cardiac risk of exercise is lower after surgery than it was before. There are few activities that must be avoided, and walking and other aerobic exercise are key elements in the recovery process. Chest wall soreness will limit upper body exertion, and symptoms are a reasonable guide. The chest wall is stable after surgery, and nothing will fall apart if the patient over-exerts and is sore. Most who are walking regularly can resume driving 3 to 4 weeks after surgery, avoiding prolonged sitting and long trips at first. There is no reason to delay resumption of sexual activity; the usual recommendation is "if you can walk up the stairs to the bedroom, you can have sex."

Patients are now being discharged just a few days after uncomplicated CABS. There are a few complications of CABS you may encounter in a primary care practice:

Atrial fibrillation (AF) occurs in 15% to 20% during the week after CABS. There are no risk factors for postoperative AF, and it is not related to the severity of heart disease. Nor does it injure the heart, and you should reassure your patient that while AF is aggravating, it has few serious consequences (stroke may occur but it is rare in this setting). The usual treatment principles apply (see Chapter 7). Cardioversion with ibutelide or countershock is effective and safe. If it persists for longer than 48 hours, warfarin is indicated. Late recurrence is rare, and warfarin can be stopped a couple months after cardioversion.

Note that low magnesium or potassium is a common cause of AF after any surgery, and electrolyte replacement may correct the arrhythmia. Small studies have found that prophylactic beta blockade and aggressive magnesium replacement may prevent perioperative AF. It is common to see patients on amiodarone after CABS—AF is the usual reason it was started, and it should be stopped 1 month after surgery.

Postpericardiotomy syndrome is another complication of heart surgery that brings patients to their family doctor. It is an autoimmune illness with fever and pleuropericarditis that develops 1 to 6 weeks after surgery. Any mechanical manipulation of the pericardium can cause it, including cardiac trauma or perforation of the heart by a pacemaker wire. The serositis is like that of Dressler's syndrome. The incidence is approximately 10% with heart surgery, with mild cases unrecognized.

It is easy to diagnose when you are aware of it. The usual clinical picture is fever, cough and pleuritic chest discomfort, plus flu-like symptoms. The patient usually feels poorly out of proportion to physical findings. Patchy pneumonitis is common, and it may be mistaken for pneumonia. There may be a pericardial friction rub, and ECG and echocardiography may suggest pericarditis. Granulocytosis is uncommon, but there may be mild lymphocytosis. All patients have a *high sedimentation rate*—above 100 mm/hr—and that is the key test for making or excluding the diagnosis.

Mild cases respond to NSAIDs. A short course of steroids (e.g., a methylprednisolone [Medrol] dose-pack) is frequently needed. Most patients have a single episode, but some have intermittent recurrence, with episodes as late as 1 year after surgery. Recurrence is easily identified by symptoms and re-elevation of the sedimentation rate. Postcardiotomy tends to burn out with flare-ups becoming farther apart and less severe with time. Although possible, pericardial fibrosis and constriction are rare. We reassure patients that the inflammatory process does not hurt the heart and that they may expect to do well long term.

Neurocognitive dysfunction is a long suspected but just recently described complication of CABS.[17] It may appear to be transient, with some improvement in the months after surgery, but this is often followed by later decline. Predictors of late cognitive dysfunction are advanced age, dysfunction before or early after surgery, and low educational level. The severity of the heart disease and the duration of cardiopulmonary bypass have not been identified as risk factors for cognitive dysfunction. On the other hand, many suspect that the heart-lung bypass machine plays a role, and suggest that cognitive decline may be avoided with off-pump surgery.

Choosing between coronary stenting and coronary artery bypass surgery— Approximately 60% of the patients with multivessel CAD treated with CABS or angioplasty could have been treated with either procedure. After reading the above descriptions, you can see that arguments can be made for or against either procedure. Early and more recent comparison studies have shown that survival is similar with each technique.[15]

There is a basic trade-off: With angioplasty and stenting, the patient avoids major surgery but has chance of restenosis leading to repeat angiography, re-stenting and rarely, CABS. With CABS, the patient probably will not need follow-up procedures. In practice, most patients are willing to go through a lot to avoid a major operation, and choose angioplasty/stenting. A rare patient wants to know he is fixed for good and chooses CABS. Measured 1 year after surgery, stenting is less expensive than CABS, despite more procedures during follow-up.[15] The effect of drug-eluting stents on this calculus is uncertain.

Diabetes is a special situation. Long-term survival with diabetes and multivessel CAD has been better with CABS than angioplasty. On the other hand, this datum comes from an older study where not all patients were stented, and none with drug-coated stents.[18]

Acute Coronary Syndromes

Pathophysiology

The ACS include unstable angina pectoris (USAP) and non-ST elevation MI (NSTEMI). The two conditions represent a continuum of the same process, and distinguishing between them is often an exercise in semantics. For example, some studies of USAP include patients with elevation of troponin and CK. You could argue that any patient with elevated enzymes has had an MI. Semantics aside, large clinical trials now lump USAP and NSTEMI in studies of ACS.

The initiating event in stable angina is exercise leading to an increase in MVO_2. With ACS, there is no increase in cardiac work, and ischemia begins with a drop in oxygen supply. This was initially described using ambulatory 12-lead ECG and blood pressure monitoring. A rise in heart rate and blood pressure preceded ST depression with chronic stable angina. But with USAP, ST segment changes (ischemia) occurred before any change in heart rate or blood pressure. The coronary lesion in USAP is dynamic. By some mechanism the lesion tightens and causes ischemia.

Atherosclerotic plaque morphology is different with stable and unstable coronary disease. Paradoxically, those with stable angina often have tighter stenosis. This fits the demand-outweighing-supply physiology of stable angina (Figure 4.1). In contrast, the culprit lesions of ACS and MI may not be stenotic. Something happens to disrupt this nonstenotic but vulnerable plaque, leading to plaque rupture, platelet activation, thrombosis, and ischemia. Some triggers of instability are local. Unstable atheroma tends to have a large, necrotic lipid core with a thin fibrous cap. The site of plaque rupture is often the shoulder of the cap, where it meets normal arterial wall, and this site appears susceptible to shear forces.

Multiple lines of evidence implicate inflammation in plaque instability and rupture:[20,21] Post-mortem examination indicates a concentration of inflammatory cells in ruptured plaques. The degree of instability with ACS is proportional to the degree of elevation of CRP; all patients with MI preceded by USAP had elevated CRP, compared with less than 50% of patients who had MI without USAP.[20] Intracoronary angioscopy and ultrasound indicate that ACS tends to involve multiple sites in the coronary tree in addition to the culprit lesion, suggesting a more systemic process—perhaps widespread acute coronary endothelial inflammation. The inflammatory activation of metalloproteases can weaken the fibrous cap of lipid-rich plaque, leading to rupture. Inflammation may be local, at the plaque, or systemic. ACS can result from unstable plaque or unstable blood that is thrombogenic or proinflammatory.

The bottom line is a complex interaction among (1) plaque anatomy (thin cap and lipid core), (2) plaque inflammation, and (3) exogenous factors (vasomotor tone, mechanical stress related to plaque location, systemic inflammation, possibly from infection, and coagulability). The relative contribution of these factors varies from patient to patient, and possibly from plaque to plaque.

Rupture of a vulnerable plaque exposes the necrotic lipid core to the circulation, and these tissue factors activate platelets and initiate the clotting cascade. If the resulting thrombus occludes the artery, it causes ST segment elevation MI. If the thrombus does not occlude, but rather causes stenosis, unstable angina or NSTEMI is the result. A balance between endogenous thrombolysis and the thrombotic process moderates this process.

The treatment of ACS is based upon interrupting thrombosis, with emphasis on antiplatelet therapy, and stabilizing the coronary artery. Anti-inflammatory therapy is the most recent addition to these principles of treatment. Many of the drugs currently used to treat CAD and ACS have been found to suppress vascular inflammation: statins, fibrates, ACE inhibitors, clopidogrel, low-molecular-weight heparin, and platelet IIb/IIIa inhibitors.[21]

The Clinical Syndrome and Risk Stratification

The term *unstable* is more than descriptive. USAP is a well-defined clinical syndrome that is associated with a 10% to 40% risk of death or MI within 4 months (Table 4.5A). The clinical definition of unstable angina includes angina at rest, prolonged episodes of pain (longer than 10 to 15 minutes), worsening of the angina pattern, or recent onset of symptoms (less than 2 months). The prognosis varies with the severity of symptoms, and risk stratification is largely based on the history (Table 4.5 A). Findings that indicate the highest risk for MI or early death are prolonged and ongoing chest pain, angina within the last day, new ST segment or T wave changes on the resting ECG, angina plus heart failure or hypotension, angina with a new or worsening mitral regurgitation murmur, and elevation of cardiac enzymes. A common presentation is the patient with prolonged pain and new T wave inversion—changes that look like those of non-Q wave MI—but no rise in cardiac enzymes. Conversely, another patient may have minimal or no ECG changes, but a small rise in troponin or CK-MB. Both patients fall in the high-risk category and should be admitted to hospital for early angiography.

Management of Acute Coronary Syndrome

The first step is stabilization using medical therapy, with emphasis on anticoagulation (vide infra). Subsequent treatment is related to the risk of near-term MI (Tables 4.5A and B):

1. Low-risk patients. Most stabilize with medical therapy, and further risk stratification using noninvasive studies (e.g., stress imaging studies) is reasonable. The workup may be done as an outpatient. This group is largely comprised of patients with exertional angina with onset of symptoms less than 2 months earlier, and with no angina during the 2 days before your evaluation. In a sense,

Table 4.5 Risk Stratification for Patients with Acute Coronary Syndromes (Unstable angina or non-ST elevation MI)

A. Risk stratification and treatment based upon Braunwald's classification[19]

Level	Clinical Presentation	Treatment
Low risk	No previous angina; no ongoing angina; little previous use of anti-ischemic therapy; normal or unchanged ECG; young; normal cardiac enzymes	Initial medical therapy, risk stratifying tests, possibly as an outpatient
Intermediate risk	New-onset or accelerating angina; angina at rest or ongoing angina; no ST segment changes; normal cardiac enzymes	Initial medical therapy; admit to hospital. With recurrent ischemia (angina) or a positive noninvasive study, angiography.
High risk	1. Angina at rest or prolonged angina 2. Ongoing angina 3. Angina after MI 4. Previous use of anti-angina therapy 5. Older age 6. New ST changes or ST changes during angina 7. Elevated cardiac enzymes 8. Hemodynamic instability (including heart failure)	Initial medical therapy, add a IIb/IIIa inhibitor with elevated enzymes, early angiography and revascularization

B. The TIMI Risk Score for ACS, and treatment decisions.[22]

Characteristic	Points
1. Age >65 years	1
2. >3 risk factors for CAD	1
3. Known CAD (stenosis >50%)	1
4. Aspirin use in previous 7 days	1
5. Angina within last 24 hours	1
6. ST segment deviation >0.5 mm	1
7. Increased cardiac enzymes	1
Total	0–7

MI, myocardial infarction.

Table 4.5 B: Risk of death, MI or need for urgent revascularization in the next 2 weeks is proportional to the point total: 0–1 point, 4.7% risk; 3 points, 13.2%; 4 points, 20%; 5 points, 26%; 6–7 points, 41%.

Treatment recommendation: patients with an enzyme rise, prior revascularization, heart failure, or with a risk score >3 should have early angiography. Lower risk patients may have noninvasive testing.

they have stable angina that is not yet chronic. A low-risk patient who has a positive noninvasive study should have angiography, especially if the study suggests high risk CAD (Table 4.3).

2. Intermediate-risk patients. The practice guidelines allow risk-stratifying tests (stress imaging studies). However, a number of trials support early angiography, especially when there are new ST segment or T wave changes, or any rise in cardiac enzymes.[2]

3. High-risk patients. Early angiography is advisable.

More recently, multivariable analysis of almost 2000 patients in the TIMI 11 trail has allowed development of a simple risk stratification tool that probably will replace the Braunwald classification (Table 4.5). Seven clinical variables were identified as independent predictors of risk, and appeared of equal importance.[22] Hence, the scoring system assigns each variable 1 point, and the point total predicts the risk of death, MI, or a need for urgent revascularization within the next 2 weeks (Table 4.5).

The two risk stratifying systems in Table 4.5 A and B have considerable overlap. A problem with any scoring system is remembering it, especially if you do not use it often. At least remember that an increase in cardiac enzymes, recent prolonged or ongoing pain, and ST segment changes require hospital admission and early angiography.

Medical Therapy

Antithrombotic therapy—This is the critical, initial therapy.[23] Unstable angina and non-ST-elevation MI is about platelets and thrombosis. Initial treatment with aspirin reduces adverse outcomes by 50% to 70%, and aspirin should be started if there is *any suspicion* the patient may have CAD and an ACS. Heparin provides an additional benefit, and should be added if ACS is *likely*. Comparative trials have found enoxaparin superior to unfractionated heparin, and the 2002 practice guidelines indicate that it is the preferred agent. This is especially true if troponin is elevated.

The addition of clopidogrel to aspirin and heparin reduces cardiac death or MI another 20% *in both low- and high-risk patients* with ACS. A benefit with early clopidogrel therapy was apparent at 24 hours and persisted during the next year, even for those who had revascularization. Clopidogrel has thus been added to the practice guidelines for the initial treatment of ACS.

Clopidogrel should be started at least 6 hours before angiography and angioplasty/ stenting, as there is a substantial lowering of post-procedure complications. A loading dose of 300 mg may be given. When the drug was new, the usual practice was to continue it for 1 month after stenting. However, the CREDO trial compared 1 month with 1 year of treatment with clopidogrel plus aspirin, and found a 27% reduction in death, MI, or stroke with prolonged therapy.[23] We now recommend aspirin plus clopidogrel for a year. (I expect that future studies will support lifelong treatment.)

On the other hand, clopidogrel within 5 days of CABS increases the risk of serious perioperative bleeding at least 50%. If it appears likely that CABS will be needed, delay starting clopidogrel until angiography has been done.

Finally, patients with elevation of troponin or CK-MB should receive a glyco-protein IIb/IIIa antagonist soon after admission, before going to the catheteriza-tion laboratory. Both tirofiban and eptifibatide are effective, but abciximab is of no benefit in a setting of ACS (this drug is used primarily in the catheterization labo-ratory, at the time of stenting).

It seems like a lot. Quadruple antithrombotic therapy—aspirin + clopidogrel + enoxaparin + IIb/IIIa inhibition—has not been tested for ACS alone, but it has been found beneficial as adjunctive therapy during angioplasty. A majority of patients in the angioplasty trials had ACS, and most patients with ACS are headed for angioplasty. It thus seems reasonable to extend these results to the treatment of ACS, and the practice guidelines now recommend this four-drug combination. Studies that added clopidogrel to the other three drugs found little increase in bleeding.[23] Nevertheless, bleeding is the most common compli-cation with this aggressive anticoagulation regimen. Patients at high risk for bleeding, or with a recent history of bleeding should not be given the four-drug combination.

Beta blockade—Meta-analysis of studies of USAP indicates that beta-blockers reduce the risk of MI by 13% (not much and far less affective than antithrombotic therapy).[19,23] Various preparations have similar efficacy, and intravenous beta block-ade is not necessary. The dose should be titrated to bring the heart rate between 50 and 60 beats/minute.

Nitrates—Intravenous nitroglycerin is prescribed for ongoing ischemic pain. Although it helps with pain control, there are no data showing that nitroglycerin prevents MI or death in patients with ACS. Nitrate tolerance develops after about 24 hours of intravenous treatment. This is managed by increasing the dose, or by switching to non-parenteral treatment with an appropriate nitrate free interval. As they are not cardio-protective, oral nitrates can be stopped after successful revascu-larization.

Calcium channel blockers—Short-acting nifedipine is a pure vasodilator, and this effect provokes reflex tachycardia. In the absence of beta blockade, short-acting nifedipine increases the risk of MI. Adding metoprolol to nifedipine prevents tachycardia, and the dihydropyridine–beta-blocker combination is safe and effec-tive for relieving angina. Long acting nifedipine and the newer dihydropyridines have less effect on heart rate, but have not been studied as therapy for ACS. Consider them if the patient remains symptomatic despite effective beta blockade (e.g., the heart rate is below 60 beats per minute). I have been impressed with how often symptoms improve on calcium channel blockers, possibly because of their coronary vasodilating effects or increased flow through collateral vessels (note the earlier discussion of calcium blocker therapy in stable angina).

Diltiazem is the most useful calcium blocker in the setting of ACS. A random-ized trial compared diltiazem 360 mg/day with placebo in patients with NSTEMI, and found a 30% reduction in mortality or reinfarction after mean follow-up of 2 years.[19] In this study, patients with CHF or LVEF below 30% were excluded. An earlier trial showed that diltiazem lowered the risk of MI during the first 2 weeks of treatment by 50%. These studies are overlooked, and there is a common misconception that calcium channel blockade just relieves symptoms.

As a general rule, medicines that lower the heart rate help patients with CAD. Beta blockade is the first choice, but many of our patients cannot tolerate it, especially those with obstructive lung disease. Diltiazem is a useful alternative; start with 240 mg/day, and raise the dose if the heart rate remains above 60 beats per minute. Diltiazem depresses contractility, but the effect is minor. I have not seen it cause heart failure in the absence of prior symptomatic CHF. However, clinical trials found that benefits were limited to patients with LVEF over 50%, so CHF and low LVEF are relative contraindications.

Other drugs—As noted, generalized vascular inflammation may contribute to plaque instability. A number of the drugs recommended for treatment of ACS have anti-inflammatory effects: clopidogrel, low-molecular-weight heparin, and glycoprotein IIb/IIIa inhibitors. Because of their anti-inflammatory properties, both statins and ACE inhibitors may be helpful during the acute phase of the illness. There have been no trials that tested this possibility, and practice guidelines do not call for early anti-inflammatory therapy. On the other hand, if it is certain that the patient will eventually be treated with either drug, and there is no contraindication to early treatment (i.e. hypotension in the case of ACE inhibition), consider starting them soon after admission.

A possible infectious etiology of atherosclerosis and vascular inflammation has led to a handful of antibiotic trials.[23] None has shown a favorable effect.

Revascularization

The benefit of angiography and revascularization for intermediate or high-risk patients with ACS is well established (Table 4.5). The relative merits of CABS and angioplasty/stenting have been reviewed. There may be concern about sending a patient to the catheterization laboratory with four-drug antithrombotic therapy on board. While there is a risk of bleeding and hematoma, clinical trials have shown a better outcome with aggressive anticoagulation.

Better understanding of plaque anatomy and physiology will influence interventional therapy. At present, stenting is a "one shoe fits all" business. But our current tools may not be good for every patient. For example, deployment of metallic stents on a plaque that has a large lipid core—identified by intravascular ultrasound—has been associated with poor distal flow after stenting. It is thought that oozing of plaque contents through the stent wire and microembolism are responsible for the poor result. Perhaps a rigid metallic stent deployed by a high-pressure balloon is not necessary for the soft, noncalcific and noncritical stenosis typical of ACS. A biodegradable stent that releases anti-inflammatory and antithrombotic medicine may be better. In the future we may have devices better suited for a specific plaque type and clinical circumstances.

Outcomes have been slightly better with early angiography. There is no benefit from a cooling off period with medical therapy. On the other hand, angiography is not an emergency procedure (unlike the case with ST segment elevation MI). Rather, the patient with USAP may be scheduled for the next available slot in the catheterization laboratory.

Other Clinical Syndromes, and Special Issues

Prinzmetal's Variant Angina

This variant of angina pectoris occurs at rest and is not provoked by exercise. During pain there is ST segment elevation, and angiography confirms coronary artery spasm as the cause. Spasm may occur at the site of atherosclerotic plaque, as with Dr. Prinzmetal's initial cases, but also may occur in normal-appearing arteries. It may be a facet of generalized vasospasm; there is occasional association with Raynaud's phenomenon or migraine headache.

There is no apparent etiology for most patients. The most common identifiable cause is cocaine. It blocks the presynaptic uptake of norepinephrine and dopamine, increasing alpha-adrenergic tone. Similarly, beta-adrenergic blockers may aggravate coronary spasm by leaving alpha stimulation unopposed. Prinzmetal's angina develops in an occasional patient after starting beta-blocker therapy for hypertension. There are reports of coronary spasm after treatment with 5-fluorouracil or cyclophosphamide.

The attack frequency may wax or wane, with occasional symptom-free intervals. The quality of angina discomfort is typical. Pain usually occurs at rest, and it tends to occur at the same time and commonly at night. Continuous ST segment monitoring has shown that many ischemic episodes are painless, especially when they are brief. Exercise tolerance is usually normal.

Another presentation is syncope. Ischemia may be severe enough to provoke ventricular tachycardia. Heart block may occur with right coronary spasm and ischemia of the AV node.

Laboratory evaluation—The diagnosis of coronary spasm is confirmed when an ECG during chest pain shows ST segment elevation. A patient with no ST changes during typical pain probably does not have spasm, and would not benefit from angiography. Exercise stress testing may be considered to screen for fixed coronary stenosis, but is of no use for the diagnosis of spasm.

Angina at rest is, by definition, unstable angina, so many of these patients have coronary angiography. It is justified when there is ST segment elevation with pain, and when there is uncertainty about the diagnosis. In addition to identifying spasm, an angiogram determines the extent of atherosclerotic CAD.

Provocative testing with ergonovine maleate during angiography is the standard test for spasm. After identifying normal appearing coronary arteries, the patient is given increasing doses of ergonovine. With spasm, a repeat angiogram shows occlusion or near-occlusion of a segment of coronary artery, and there is ST elevation plus pain. Spasm is focal. An overall reduction in the caliber of the vessel is a normal response to ergonovine, and does not cause pain or ST elevation.

We used to do a lot of provocative testing to exclude spasm in the catheterization laboratory in patients with chest pain and normal coronary arteries. However, the yield was low. Patients with atypical chest pain syndromes seldom have coronary spasm. The ergonovine stress is now reserved for those with normal arteries and chest pain at rest that sounds like angina.

Ergonovine testing is sensitive and specific, and it is safe. Angina and ST segment elevation are usually relieved by sublingual nitroglycerin, but some require intracoronary nitroglycerin. For this reason, provocative testing has been a catheterization laboratory procedure. There are reports of using ergonovine stress with noninvasive imaging, but this approach has not been validated by large studies.

Therapy—Calcium channel blockade is the mainstay of therapy. These agents are so effective that I think of spasm as an illness of the calcium channel (realizing that the basic mechanism has not been identified with certainty). All of the long-acting preparations work, and may need to be given at high dose. An occasional patient who does not respond to one of them may respond to another. A rare patient needs treatment with two different calcium blockers, from different drug classes.

There may be rebound of symptoms when calcium blockers are stopped, such as perioperatively. Intravenous diltiazem may be used if symptoms have been frequent.

Angina attacks are relieved by nitroglycerin, and long-acting nitrates may be used with calcium blockers. As the mechanism of action is different with the two drug classes, combination therapy makes sense. One reason it is important to recognize spasm as the mechanism of angina is that two of the standard therapies for CAD and angina may cause worsening of symptoms. Beta-blockers leave alpha adrenergic stimuli unopposed. Consider coronary spasm if your patient with hypertension develops angina after starting a beta-blocker. Aspirin inhibits synthesis of prostacyclin, a coronary vasodilator, and may thus aggravate spasm. Avoiding aspirin may help the patient with variant angina and no underlying ASCVD. With coronary artery plaque plus spasm, benefits of aspirin may exceed risks—but monitor symptoms.

Hypomagnesemia may cause spasm. Serum magnesium often falls after major surgery, and spasm is a rare complication. It responds to magnesium replacement.

Pure vasospasm with no underlying atherosclerosis is a medical condition, not a surgical one. A failure to recognize that a stenosis is from spasm rather than plaque may lead to a surgical/interventional disaster. Spastic arteries are touchy, and often develop spasm at the site of manipulation or graft insertion. Postoperative ST segment elevation, arrhythmias and infarction may follow. (Remember magnesium replacement!) On the other hand, when spasm develops at the site of a tight plaque, stenting or CABS are effective.

Natural history—As noted, symptoms may wax and wane. Many patients are better 4 to 6 months after initial presentation. When symptoms resolve, it is reasonable to slowly taper therapy, and possibly to stop it. If symptoms recur, they respond to the same medicines.

The risk of MI and death is highest for those with spasm plus underlying atherosclerosis. Those with angiographically normal coronary arteries have a good prognosis, with 5-year survival about 95% and MI risk less than 10%. If cocaine use is the cause of spasm, continued use confers higher risk.

Silent Ischemia

About 20% to 60% of heart attacks are unrecognized by the patient, and about half of these are truly painless.[24] There are some patients who have a defective angina warning system, and are at risk for MI and death. Others have angina with longer episodes of ischemia, but also have shorter asymptomatic spells. Ischemia is bad, regardless of the presence or absence of symptoms. Exercise-induced ST segment depression without angina indicates a four to five times increase in cardiac mortality compared with those having a normal stress test.

Pathophysiology—Pain-sensing nerves, the C fibers, accompany cardiac sympathetic afferent fibers.[25] They follow the path of the coronary arteries, originating at the base of the heart and moving to the apex, and are primarily subepicardial. The sensory nerves pass through ganglia in the heart, mediastinum and thorax, then to the nucleus of the solitary tract, and finally with other visceral and somatic afferents in the spinothalamic tract. After passing through the hypothalamus and thalamus they are projected bilaterally to the frontal cortex.

At the myocardial end, adenosine is the neurotransmitter. Chest pain without ischemia (e.g., there is no ST segment change or perfusion abnormality) is common during adenosine or dipyridamole infusion; it may be a neurotransmitter effect.

Silent ischemia may develop from peripheral neuropathy. This is the probable cause with diabetes, where asymptomatic ischemia is common. Those with autonomic neuropathy are more likely to have silent ischemia. Neuropathy has also been described after reperfusion therapy for acute MI; prolonged ischemia apparently damages cardiac nerves, and subsequent infarct-zone ischemia is more likely to be silent (the patient is left with stunned nerves and live muscle, see Chapter 5).

Asymptomatic ischemia may also be a central phenomenon. Study of hypertensive patients with silent ischemia demonstrated a generally higher pain threshold (to tooth pulp stimulation, of all things). They may have higher endorphin levels. Positron emission tomography scans in others with painless, dobutamine-induced ischemia showed activation of the thalamus, but a failure of the impulse to project to the left frontal cortex.

The duration of ischemia often determines symptoms. Ambulatory ECG monitoring shows that a majority of patients with stable angina also have brief periods of ST segment depression without pain. They develop pain only when ischemia is present for 2 to 5 minutes.

Management—Observational studies have found that prognosis with CAD is related to the extent of disease and LV function, and not to the presence or absence of symptoms. It has been argued both ways: 1) With a defective warning system, the patient has a higher risk, or 2) the absence of symptoms may mean less severe ischemia. However, available data show that silent ischemia indicates neither lower nor higher risk.

Silent ischemia is usually diagnosed with stress testing or following an asymptomatic MI. While there is monitoring equipment designed to detect ST segment depression, ambulatory monitors used for arrhythmia detection do not provide information about ST segment changes. Following the diagnosis of silent ischemia, further testing is indicated to assess the risk of MI or cardiac death (Table 4.3).

The medical treatment of silent and symptomatic ischemia is the same. High-risk patients benefit from revascularization. The asymptomatic cardiac ischemia pilot (ACIP) study assigned patients with surgical CAD to three treatment strategies: 1) medical therapy designed to control symptoms, 2) medical therapy to prevent ischemia on serial ambulatory ST segment monitors, and 3) revascularization.[26] The 2-year mortality in the three groups was 6.6%, 4.4%, and 1.1%. Based on this and observational studies, revascularization should be considered for those with high risk CAD but no angina (Table 4.3).

Syndrome X: Microvascular Coronary Artery Disease

This syndrome has been defined as angina or angina-like chest pain with normal appearing coronary arteries. It is a mixed bag: Most are having noncardiac pain.

Some have microcirculatory disease and ischemia. The stress test is abnormal and there may be patchy thallium perfusion defects. Increased myocardial lactate production during induced angina has been demonstrated in such cases. Microvascular constriction, or inadequate vasodilator reserve are possible mechanisms, as coronary blood flow does not increase with exercise or dipyridamole infusion.

The third mechanism is abnormal cardiac pain perception. I think of this as the flip side to silent ischemia—the heart is hypersensitive.[27] In such cases, low-dose adenosine infusion may cause severe pain without objective evidence for ischemia. Some of these patients with sensitive hearts have heightened visceral pain sensitivity elsewhere (e.g., an abnormal pain response to esophageal stimulation).

The rare patient with syndrome X who has objective evidence for ischemia will respond to antianginal therapy. However, treating those with chest pain, normal coronary arteries and no objective evidence for ischemia with antianginal therapy rarely helps. It is important to reassure the patient. Most have spontaneous resolution of symptoms with time. The risk of MI and death is low, even for those with ischemia on the stress ECG or perfusion scan.

Erectile Dysfunction and Sildenafil (Viagra)

Erectile dysfunction affects almost 30 million men in the United States. Risk factors for erectile dysfunction parallel those of ASCVD. A survey of men in their late fifties with diabetes, hypertension, or both found erectile dysfunction in 62%, 46%, and 67% respectively.[28] The evaluation of a patient with heart disease before sildenafil therapy is a common cardiology consultation.

My first comment to a man beginning sildenafil is, "Congratulations, it works, and you'll be a happy guy." In addition to hearing good things from patients, I have noticed that following the introduction of sildenafil, the number of patients seeking penile implants has declined. Another constructive development is that patients are more willing to discuss ED than in the past. As part of your initial evaluation, be aware that many of the cardiovascular drugs may cause ED (diuretics, beta-blockers, statins, fibrates, and digoxin to name a few). Impotence is among the intolerable complications of medical therapy, and there are few cases where I feel compelled to continue therapy (perhaps an exception is beta blockade that has had a dramatic effect on symptoms and LVEF in a patient with heart failure).

Another bit of good news is that sildenafil is safe for men with CAD. A study of hemodynamic changes after 100-mg sildenafil in men with flow-restricting coronary artery stenoses found a trivial drop in arterial and pulmonary artery pressure, no change in cardiac output or pulmonary wedge pressure, and no change in coronary blood flow in the stenosed artery measured using intracoronary Doppler.[29] Clinical trials in men with stable CAD, CHF, or hypertension have shown no increase in cardiac risk.[30–32] While there are reports of death or MI during sex with sildenafil, a US Food and Drug Administration survey found that the number of cases is below what would be expected considering the large number of men who have received prescriptions for it.[33] The usual workload associated with sex with a spouse is 4 to 6 METs (Table 4.4). If there is uncertainty about exercise tolerance based on history, a treadmill test may be appropriate.

Mechanism of action and the interaction of sildenafil and nitroglycerin—This is worth reviewing because nitrates contraindicate the use of sildenafil.[34] Relaxation of arterial smooth muscle is promoted by cyclic guanylate monophosphate (cGMP), which through a series of steps affects an ion channel, reducing intracellular calcium. (Calcium ion in the cell stimulates muscle contraction.) Phospodiesterase (PDE) leads to the degradation of cGMP; PDE *inhibitors* thus lead to higher levels of cGMP, and to vasodilatation. Nitrates work upstream. Nitric oxide, produced by the endothelium or from a nitrate donor like nitroglycerin, stimulates the production of cGMP.

The net effect of increasing cGMP production (nitroglycerin) and impeding its breakdown (PDE inhibitor, sildenafil) is maximal vasodilatation. This combination can lead to life-threatening hypotension. Hypotension does not require simultaneous administration of the two drugs, but may be delayed. Recent guidelines suggest a 24-hour interval between administration of sildenafil and nitrates. In practice I do not prescribe sildenafil when the patient is on any nitroglycerin preparation.

There are some cardiologists who think that any patient with CAD should carry nitroglycerin, even an asymptomatic person after revascularization. Although this seems a common sense practice, it is not required by practice guidelines. If the patient wants sildenafil, he should not carry or use nitroglycerin. That would hold true for others with chronic CAD who are asymptomatic.

There are a number of isoforms of PDE. PDE 5 is concentrated in the corpus cavernosum, hence the effect of sildenafil on ED. There are early studies suggesting beneficial effects of PDE inhibition on pulmonary hypertension, and possibly on endothelial dysfunction in patients with heart failure.[34]

Palliative Care for End-Stage Coronary Artery Disease[35]

Everyone with CAD reaches a point where another revascularization procedure is not feasible. This can be distressing news for the patient and family. That certainly is the case when the doctor tells the patient, "There is nothing more we can do for you."

That is not a phrase that I use. Not only is it emotionally devastating, it is factually incorrect. Medical therapy is remarkably effective, and even patients with advanced CAD may expect to have symptoms and survival improve. It is better to tell the patient that "medical therapy is superior to revascularization," and then to emphasize what is true: the medicines we use to control symptoms also prolong life, including aspirin, clopidogrel, beta-blockers, ACE inhibitors, and in some situations, calcium blockers.

At the same time, it is unwise to withhold the truth about prognosis. I address this frankly, telling the patient with end-stage disease the condition may be fatal. But the timing of death is uncertain. With metastatic lung cancer, we know that most are dead in 6 months. With advanced CAD, some will be dead in 6 months, but it is possible to live much longer. "If I hear that you have died 3 months from now, I will be surprised, although I realize that is a possibility. On the other hand, if we are still visiting in clinic 3 or 5 years from now, I will not be surprised, as I know that is possible." This is a hopeful message. After years of following patients with advanced CAD, I also know that it is true.

In addition to usual therapy for angina, consider these treatments for the end-stage patient.

Calcium channel blockers are often overlooked when treating chronic CAD, because they are not on that list of medicines that prevent death or MI. But they are quite effective in controlling symptoms and are well tolerated by sick and/or elderly patients. They are easy to use in combination with other antianginal drugs. Dihydropyridines do not slow heart rate, so may be used when there is bradycardia. Diltiazem does slow the rate, and is the choice for the patient with tachycardia. It may depress the myocardium, so must be used with caution when there is heart failure or low LVEF. All calcium blockers may lower blood pressure.

Adding *clopidogrel* to aspirin often helps. Patients with end-stage CAD usually have some rest angina, and thus have unstable angina. This justifies more aggressive antiplatelet therapy, and it works to control symptoms.

Morphine is commonly used to treat end stage heart failure, but it also palliates angina when all else has failed. In addition to its analgesic effect, it is a venodilator, reducing blood return to the heart and therefore, cardiac work—a nitroglycerin-like action, but without the problem of nitrate tolerance.

Hospice care is appropriate by the time a patient with angina needs morphine. While hospice is not required for those on morphine, I usually recommend it. Some consider morphine an unconventional treatment for CAD, and hospice involvement obviates any medical-legal question. More important, hospice nurses are good at monitoring opiod therapy. Patients with heart disease frequently improve with the attention of a skilled hospice nurse. After a few months many are ready for discharge from hospice.

Home oxygen has not been tested in clinical studies, but an occasional patient has less angina with it. Some of this may be a placebo effect, a well-documented and important component of all therapies for angina. Oxygen is easier to justify for those with low arterial oxygen saturation on room air.

Correcting mild anemia has been shown to relieve symptoms in studies that tested effects of erythropoietin plus iron and folate. The patient with advanced illness often has the anemia of chronic disease, and boosting the hematocrit from 30% to 33% to 35% changes the angina threshold.

Smoking cessation is worth pursuing, even for the end-stage patient. There is an immediate effect on arterial oxygen-carrying capacity. Smoke contains carbon monoxide, and active smokers have elevated arterial carboxyhemoglobin levels. A person with advanced symptoms may note an improvement a few days after reduced smoking.

Spinal cord stimulation has been tested using electrodes implanted in the epidural space, and with transcutaneous stimulation (TENS). Randomized small studies have found improved exercise tolerance and decreasing frequency of angina episodes. By reducing the number of hospital admissions, this may be cost effective.

Chelation therapy does not work, and I mention it because patients still ask about it. Originally, the rationale for chelation was the removal of calcium from plaque using ethylenediaminetetraacetic acid (EDTA) infusion. This was supposed to debulk the plaque. A more recent claim is that EDTA plus vitamins have an anti-oxidant effect that improves endothelial function. This has been tested in a randomized trial, and endothelial function did not improve with the treatment.[36] Furthermore, randomized trials have indicated no clinical benefit.[37,38] Nevertheless, chelation clinics continue to peddle this expensive technique, and there are stories of miraculous cures. The placebo effect of any treatment for CAD can be remarkable.

Rest therapy is a final step in palliation. One of my mentors, Dr. Julian Beckwith, taught me that a sensible treatment option for uncontrolled symptoms is reduced activity, a bed-to-chair lifestyle. This was a common approach before the1960s, and at times is still appropriate. There is no doubt about the efficacy of aerobic activity for patients with heart disease, both CAD and heart failure. But there comes a time when it no longer works, and reduced activity offers palliation.

References

1. Lee TH, Goldman L. Evaluation of the patient with acute chest pain. N Engl J Med 2000;342:1187–1195.

2. Hachamovitch R, Hayes S, Friedman JD, et al. Determinants of risk and its temporal variation in patients with normal stress myocardial perfusion scans: what is the warranty period of a normal scan? J Am Coll Cardiol 2003;41:1329–1340.

3. Gibbons RJ, Abrams J, Chatterjee K, et al. ACC/AHA 2002 guideline update for the management of patients with chronic stable angina—summary article. Circulation 2003;107:149–158.

4. O'Keefe JH, Cordain L, Harris WH, et al. Optimal low-density lipoprotein is 50 to 70 mg/dl: lower is better and physiologically normal. J Am Coll Cardiol 2004; 43:2142–2146. Also, Pitt B, Waters D, Brown WV, et al. Aggressive lipid-lowering therapy compared with angioplasty in stable coronary artery disease. Atorvastatin versus Revascularization Trial (AVERT). N Engl J Med 1999;341:70–76. Also note, Henderson RA, Pocock SJ, Clayton TC, et al. Seven-year outcome in the RITA-2 trial: coronary angioplasty versus medical therapy. J Am Coll Cardiol 2003;42:1161–1170. (7-year follow-up showed no difference in mortality, but better symptom control with angioplasty. Like the AVERT trial, just a small percentage of patients had stenting.)

5. Antiplatelet Trialists' Collaboration. Collaborative overview of randomized trials of antiplatelet therapy. Prevention of death, MI and stroke by prolonged antiplatelet therapy in various categories of patients. Br Med J 1994;308:81–106.

6. A randomized, blinded trial of clopidogrel versus aspirin in patients at risk of ischaemic events (CAPRIE). CAPRIE Steering Committee. Lancet 1996;348: 1329–1339.

7. Howard PA, Delafontaine P. Nonsteroidal anti-inflammatory drugs and cardio-vascular risk. J Am Coll Cardiol 2004;43:519–525.

8. Ray WA, Stein CM, Hall K, et al. Non-steroidal anti-inflammatory drugs and risk of serious coronary heart disease: an observational cohort study. Lancet 2002;359:118–123.

9. Bombardier C, Laine L, Reicin A, et al. Comparison of upper gastrointestinal toxicity of rofecoxib and naproxen in patients with rheumatoid arthritis. VIGOR Study Group. N Engl J Med 2000;343:1520–1528.

10. Mamdani M, Rochon P, Juurlink DM, et al. Effect of selective cyclooxygenase 2 inhibitors and naproxen on short-term risk of acute myocardial infarction in the elderly. Arch Intern Med 2003;163:481–486.

11. Ray WA, Stein CM, Daugherty JR, et al. COX-2 selective non-steroidal anti-inflammatory drugs and risk of serious coronary heart disease. Lancet 2002;360:1071–1073. Also note, Verma S, Szmitko PE. Coxibs and the endothelium. J Am Coll Cardiol 2003;42:1754–1757. (Review of studies of endothelial function which found no effect of COX-2 therapy on endothelial function or inflammation.)

12. Yusuf S, Sleight P, Pogue J, et al. Effects of an angiotensin-converting-enzyme inhibitor, ramipril, on cardiovascular events in high-risk patients. The Heart Outcomes Prevention Evaluation Study Investigators. N Engl J Med 2000;342: 145–153.

13. Teo KK, Burton JR, Buller CE, et al. Long-term effects of cholesterol lowering and angiotensin-converting enzyme inhibition on coronary atherosclerosis: The Simvastatin/Enalapril Coronary Atherosclerosis Trial (SCAT). Circulation 2000; 102:1748–1754.

14. Salpeter SR, Ormiston TM, Salpeter EE. Cardioselective beta-blockers in patients with reactive airway disease: a meta-analysis. Ann Intern Med 2002;137: 715–725.

15. Serruys PW, Unger F, Sousa JE, et al. Comparison of coronary artery bypass surgery and stenting for the treatment of multivessel disease. N Engl J Med 2001;344:1117–1124. Also note, Hueb W, Soares PR, Gersh BJ, et al. The medicine, angioplasty, or surgery study (MASS-II): a randomized, controlled clinical trial of three therapeutic strategies for multivessel coronary artery disease:one-year results. J Am Coll Cardiol 2004;43:1743–1751.

16. King SB. Restenosis: the mouse that roared. Circulation 2003;108;248–249. Also note, Morice MC, Serruys PW, Sousa JE, et al. A randomized comparison of a sirolimus-eluting stent with a standard stent for coronary revascularization. N Engl J Med 2002;346:1773–1780.

17. Newman MF, Kirchner JL, Phillips-Bute B, et al. Longitudinal assessment of neurocognitive function after coronary-artery bypass surgery. N Engl J Med 2001;344:395–402.

18. Comparison of coronary bypass surgery with angioplasty in patients with multivessel disease. The Bypass Angioplasty Revascularization Investigation (BARI) Investigators. N Engl M Med 1996;335:217–225.

19. Yeghiazarians Y, Braunstein JB, Askari A, Stone PH. Unstable angina pectoris. N Engl J Med 2000;342:101–114. *Note these two clinical trials:* Gibson RS, Boden WE, Theroux P. Diltiazem and reinfarction in patients with non-Q-wave myocardial infarction. N Engl J Med 1986;315:423–429. And, The effect of diltiazem on mortality and reinfarction after myocardial infarction. The Multicenter Diltiazem Postinfarction Trial Research Group. N Engl J Med 1988;319:385–392.

20. Maseri A, Fuster V. Is there a vulnerable plaque? Circulation 2003:107:2068–2071.

21. Kereiakes DJ. The emperor's clothes: in search of the vulnerable plaque. Circulation 2003:107:2076–2077.

22. Sabatine MS, Antman EM. The thrombolysis in myocardial infarction risk score in unstable angina/non-ST-segment elevation myocardial infarction. J Am Coll Cardiol 2003;41(suppl):89S–95S. (*The following is a good description of the use of the risk score:* Cannon CP. Evidence-based risk stratification to target therapies in acute coronary syndromes. Circulation 2002;106:1588–1591).

23. Boden WE. Practical approach to incorporating new studies and guidelines for antiplatelet therapy in the management of patients with non-ST-segment elevation acute coronary syndrome. Am J Cardiol 2003;93:69–72. Also note, Brieger D. Optimizing adjunctive antithrombotic therapy in the treatment of acute myocardial infarction: a role for low molecular weight heparin. Clin Cardiol 2004;27:3–8.

24. Stern S. Angina pectoris without chest pain: clinical implications of silent ischemia. Circulation 2002;106:1906–1908.

25. Crea F. New look to an old symptom: angina pectoris. Circulation 1997;96:3766–3773.

26. Davies RF, Goldberg AD, Forman S, et al. Asymptomatic Cardiac Ischemia Pilot (ACIP) study two-year follow-up: outcomes of patients randomized to initial strategies of medical therapy versus revascularization. Circulation 1997;95:2037–2043.

27. Cannon RO. The sensitive heart. A syndrome of abnormal cardiac pain perception. JAMA 1995;273;883–887.

28. Roth A, Kalter-Leibovici O, Kerbis Y, et al. Prevalence and risk factors for erectile dysfunction in men with diabetes, hypertension, or both diseases: a community survey among 1,412 Israeli men. Clin Cardiol 2003;26:25–30.

29. Herrmann HC, Chang G, Klugherz BD, Mahoney PD. Hemodynamic effects of sildenafil in men with severe coronary artery disease. N Engl J Med 2000;342:1622–1626.

30. Kloner RA. Cardiovascular risk and sildenafil. Am J Cardiol 2000;86:57F–61F.

31. Arruda-Olson AM, Mahoney DW, Nehra A, et al. Cardiovascular effects of sildenafil during exercise in men with know or probable coronary artery disease: a randomized crossover trial. JAMA 2002;287:719–725.

32. Bocchi Ea, Guimaraes G, Mocelin A, et al. Sildenafil effects on exercise, neurohormonal activation, and erectile dysfunction in CHF: double-blind, placebo-controlled, randomized study followed by a prospective treatment for erectile dysfunction. Circulation 2002;106:1097–1103.

33. Wysowski DK, Farinas E, Swartz L. Comparison of reported and expected deaths in sildenafil users. Am J Cardiol 2002;89:1331–1334.

34. Reffelmann T, Kloner RA. Therapeutic potential of phosphodiesterase 5 inhibition for cardiovascular disease. Circulation 2003;108:239–244.

35. Taylor GJ, Kurent JE. A Clinician's Guide to Palliative Care. Malden: Blackwell Publishing, 2003.

36. Anderson TJ, Hubacek J, Wyse DG, Knudtson ML. Effect of chelation therapy on endothelial function in patients with coronary artery disease: PATCH substudy. J AM Coll Cardiol 2003;41:420–425.

37. Lamas GA, Ackermann A. Clinical evaluation of chelation therapy: is there any wheat amidst the chaff? Am Heart J 2000;140:4–5.

38. Knudtson M, Galbraith PD. Chelation therapy for ischemic heart disease: a randomized controlled trial. JAMA 2002;287:481–486.

CHAPTER 5

MYOCARDIAL INFARCTION

Abbreviations			
ACE	angiotensin-converting enzyme	LVEF	LV ejection fraction
ACS	acute coronary syndromes	MI	myocardial infarction
AICD	automatic implantable cardioverter-defibrillator	MR	mitral regurgitation
		NSTEMI	non–ST-segment elevation MI
AIVR	accelerated idioventricular rhythm	PVC	premature ventricular contraction
AV	atrio-ventricular	RCA	right coronary artery
CAD	coronary artery disease	rt-PA	recombinant tissue plasminogen activator
CK	creatine kinase		
CPR	cardiopulmonary resuscitation	RV	right ventricle (ventricular)
ED	emergency department	S3	third heart sound
EMS	emergency medical services	S4	fourth heart sound
EP	electrophysiology	SCD	sudden cardiac death
LAD	left anterior descending (coronary artery)	STEMI	ST-segment elevation MI
		VF	ventricular fibrillation
LV	left ventricle (ventricular)	VT	ventricular tachycardia

Over the past two decades, the incidence of myocardial infarction (MI) has declined, while that of unstable angina has increased. Patients are coming to the emergency department (ED) earlier with warning symptoms rather than later with infarction. Nevertheless, more than 1 million Americans have MI each year, and about one third of them die. Roughly one third of the deaths occur within an hour of the onset of symptoms, before the patient reaches the hospital.

Pathophysiology

When blood flow to the heart muscle is interrupted, contractile activity stops within a few heartbeats. Energy is then devoted to maintaining cellular viability. During the subsequent minutes to hours, cell death occurs. Cell membrane deteriorates, and cellular contents, including the contractile proteins we call cardiac enzymes, leach out of the infarct zone and into the circulation.

The underlying illness is atherosclerosis. With stable angina, the atherosclerotic plaque that causes ischemia during exercise is tight, reducing the cross-sectional

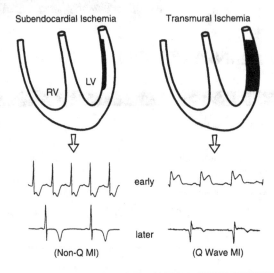

Figure 5.1 Patterns of myocardial infarction (MI). Tight stenosis of a coronary artery with some antegrade flow causes subendocardial ischemia and ST segment depression. If ischemia persists long enough to cause necrosis, there may be T wave inversion the next day. This has been called non-Q MI, or at its outset, non–ST-segment elevation MI (NSTEMI). Total occlusion of the coronary artery affects the full thickness of the myocardium, causing ST-segment elevation (STEMI). With necrosis, Q waves develop. (Reproduced by permission from Taylor GJ. The Cardiology Rotation. Malden, MA: Blackwell Science, 2001:136.)

diameter of the coronary artery more than 70%. The pathophysiology of acute coronary syndromes (ACS), including unstable angina and non–ST-segment elevation MI (NSTEMI), has been reviewed in Chapter 4. With these illnesses, the culprit lesion often is not flow restricting. Instead, a vulnerable plaque with a soft lipid core covered by a thin cap of endothelium ruptures, exposing the lipid core to the circulation. This activates platelets and the clotting cascade, and the abrupt accumulation of thrombus is responsible for rapid progression of symptoms, angina at rest, or ischemia that is severe enough to cause minor injury and an enzyme leak. A more detailed account of this process is in Chapter 4.

Think of acute MI with ST-segment elevation as the most unstable of the ACS. The process of coronary thrombosis is the same, but the clot totally occludes the artery, leading to the ECG pattern of transmural ischemia (Figure 5.1).

Prognosis, Infarct Size, and Cumulative Injury

I tell students that the measurement most useful for predicting the future of an adult with heart disease is LV ejection fraction (LVEF). There are a few exceptions, but this is generally true, and it certainly is for those with coronary artery disease (CAD). EF is a simple measurement with normal above 50% to 55%, depending on the technique used to measure it (Box 5.1). An LVEF of 50% simply means that the ventricle ejects 50% of its content with each heartbeat.

Infarct size is proportional to the rise in cardiac enzymes and to the loss of EF points. The size of the infarct is related to the size of the artery that occludes. The vascular distribution of the left anterior descending (LAD) artery is big, including the anterior wall of the LV and the interventricular septum. Thus, anterior MI is usually the largest: peak creatine kinase (CK) may be 3500 IU, and LVEF after recovery is often less than 30%. Both the right and circumflex arteries supply smaller LV regions, and inferior or lateral infarction pushes the CK to the 1000 IU range, with minimal effect on LVEF. On the other hand, there is considerable anatomic variation. An occasional patient has an especially large right coronary artery (RCA) supplying a large portion of the lateral as well as the inferior walls of the LV; occlusion causes a large inferolateral MI.

Cardiac injury is cumulative. Following infarction, dead muscle cannot regenerate. I tell patients that losing heart muscle with an MI is like losing a toe; neither can grow back. Thus, a patient who loses 10 EF points with a first MI, and loses another 10 with a subsequent MI must then live with an LVEF in the 35% range. When a large anterior MI, or multiple smaller MIs have pushed the LVEF below 30%, there usually is a loss of exercise tolerance or heart failure. In fact, one of the Social Security Administration's criteria for disability benefits with heart failure is LVEF less than 30%.

Since damage is cumulative, a major goal after MI is the prevention of future ischemic injury. The mortality risk with a second MI is much higher than that of the first. You may tell your patient with MI, "You have lost all the muscle you can afford to lose."

ST-segment Elevation versus Non–ST-segment Elevation Myocardial Infarction

This is now the preferred nomenclature, replacing non-Q and Q-wave MI. As noted, ST-segment elevation indicates ischemia of the full thickness of the LV. MI with ST depression or T wave inversion—also called non-Q or subendocardial MI—has ischemia largely of the subendocardial region (Figure 5.1). It's a nice model, but pathologic studies have found that the two ECG and clinical presentations may look identical at autopsy. Nontransmural infarction has been shown to generate Q waves about half the time.[1]

Angiography during infarction has taught us a lot. With ST-segment elevation, the infarct artery is totally occluded in most cases. When the artery is opened in the catheterization lab, the ST segments move down, toward the isoelectric baseline. If the artery is not opened, and infarction runs its course, and Q waves develop the next day (Figure 5.1). It is useful to think of this as a *completed MI*. That is to say, there is completed injury of all of the muscle supplied by the infarct artery, and the infarct zone will become a scar.

A completed infarct tends to be stable—scar tissue is not subject to further ischemic injury. We have always thought there is no need to open or bypass the totally occluded artery, as it is not possible to turn scar back into muscle. Furthermore, totally occluded vessels have been considered more stable than tightly stenosed ones. After all, whatever can happen has already happened to a closed artery. But who knows what will happen to the patient with a tightly stenosed coronary artery when that vessel finally closes?

These long-accepted concepts about clinical stability with coronary occlusion and completed infarction are now being questioned, but I am not yet convinced by the data. A pilot trial has claimed better LV function and exercise tolerance with angioplasty of a persistently occluded LAD artery a month after MI.[2] Presumably, restoration of flow salvages stunned and non-functioning muscle that is still viable in the infarct and peri-infarct zones. A large prospective study of late intervention, the Open Artery Trial (OAT) is in progress.

One of the surprises with early reperfusion therapy was the rapid appearance of Q waves with restoration of flow. It can happen within minutes of opening an infarct artery that has been occluded 3 to 6 hours. In such cases, the infarct zone may have viable muscle, and the infarction has not been completed. This is another problem with the Q wave as the indicator of transmural injury or scar. During the course of infarction, the artery may spontaneously open and close. If it is closed long enough, and then opens, a Q wave can develop.

This is the probable pathophysiology of *infarct extension*. A patient with coronary occlusion has spontaneous thrombolysis and resolution of pain after a few hours, and Q-waves develop. A couple days later there is recurrent chest pain and ST segment elevation. Apparently, this transmural infarct was not completed. Early thrombolysis interrupted the infarction. Viable muscle in the infarct zone remained at risk for reinfarction with reocclusion of the unstable vessel days later.

Angiography during a NSTEMI usually documents a stenosed vessel with antegrade flow. The surface of the stenotic plaque appears ragged and hazy, possibly with a filling defect in the contrast shadow, all characteristics of thrombus on the plaque surface (see Chapter 4). It does not have the concentric shape with smooth endothelial borders seen with stable angina.

Persistent flow in the vessel means there is less injury. Non-ST-segment elevation MI causes a smaller rise in cardiac enzymes and leaves the patient with a near-normal LVEF. On the other hand, the patient is left with an incomplete MI, and the unstable vessel may occlude, causing ST-elevation infarction. Formerly, NSTEMIs were considered mild heart attacks, but follow-up studies found that the 1-year mortality equaled that of ST-segment elevation MI (STEMI). Within weeks to months, reocclusion of the infarct artery led to completion of the MI, exposing the patient to the possible complications of acute infarction. We now recognize the small, incomplete MI as the most unstable of the ACS.

Noninvasive imaging studies may help determine whether an infarct is complete or incomplete. Scar does not contract, and the infarct zone is akinetic on the echocardiogram. The wall motion abnormality is regional, involving the vascular distribution of the occluded coronary branch. (An echo report that describes global rather than regional hypokinesis is less consistent with CAD as the cause of LV dysfunction.) On the other hand, partially injured myocardium or muscle that is persistently ischemic may not contract. Distinguishing this stunned myocardium from scar is possible with a viability study, a thallium perfusion scan with late images looking for delayed uptake of thallium (see Chapter 4).

Clinical Presentation

The chest discomfort of MI is like that of angina pectoris, though it becomes more severe. With both, the discomfort is mild at first, and then worsens with a crescendo pattern ("like a balloon blowing up in my chest"). This is different than chest pain with dissection of the thoracic aorta, where the pain is at maximum intensity at its onset. This may be the best clinical feature that distinguishes the two illnesses (and has figured into board questions).

The quality or location of pain does not point to the location of MI. Those with inferior infarction may have more vagal symptoms, including nausea, but nausea is a common enough feature of anterior and lateral infarction as well. While severe, the pain of MI does not knock the patient down, leaving him writhing in agony. Usually, a person with MI sits quietly and appears anxious. There is a sense of impending doom, even though the pain is not as severe as that of some other illnesses (i.e., pancreatitis, or migraine headache). But there is a connection between the heart and brain that tells the patient that something is profoundly wrong.

The peak incidence of MI is between 6 AM and noon, a pattern that coincides with an elevation of plasma catecholamines and cortisol, and an increase in platelet aggregability during the morning hours. Patients who are taking beta-blockers and aspirin do not exhibit this circadian variation in the timing of MI.

There are a number of well-recognized triggers of MI: heavy physical work, particularly when fatigued or exposed to temperature extremes (heat and cold); stress (MI is more common on Monday mornings!), anger, and upsetting life-events; hypoxemia from any cause, including anemia; drugs that may provoke coronary spasm (cocaine, ergot preparations, beta-blockers, rarely, 5-fluorouricil or cyclophosphamide); and rarely the abrupt withdrawal of beta blockade or nitrate therapy. Sexual activity can trigger the onset of MI but this is uncommon, occurring in less than 1% of cases.[3] MI is especially rare when sex is with a spouse or regular partner. On the other hand, a syndrome of sudden motel death has long been recognized.

At least one third of patients with acute MI describe a symptom during the days or weeks before admission that, in retrospect, was unstable angina. On the other hand, MI develops in less than 10% of patients admitted with unstable angina. Actually, 10% is an old number, and using the aggressive management described in Chapter 4, it is the rare patient with unstable angina who has an MI in the hospital.

Painless, silent MI accounts for at least 10% of cases. It is more common in those with diabetes or hypertension, and in patients with no history of angina before MI. Silent MI is more commonly followed by silent ischemia, a positive stress ECG without angina. The prognosis of silent MI is similar to that of MI with symptoms.

Physical Examination

Everyone is in a hurry when a fresh MI rolls into the ED. But a methodical examination is still important. As antithrombotic and possibly thrombolytic therapy will be important, take a careful stroke and bleeding history and look for signs of bleeding or trauma. The most common cardiac finding is an S_4 gallop. A soft systolic murmur indicating papillary muscle dysfunction is more common with inferior or lateral MI. A loud friction rub suggests pericarditis as a cause of chest pain. Soft and transient friction rubs are common during the 3 days after large transmural MI.

It is important to note the presence or absence of rales. The Killip classification relates the severity of heart failure during acute MI to the risk of death during hospitalization. The following mortality figures in Table 5.1 are from Dr. Killip's 1967 report. Although the risk is lower with modern therapy, the Killip class still provides a rough guide.

Table 5.1 Killip Class and Mortality Risk During Acute Myocardial Infarction		
Killip Class	Criterion	Mortality Risk*
I	no rales	6%
II	rales	17%
III	pulmonary edema	38%
IV	cardiogenic shock	81%

*Mortality based on Dr. Killip's study in the 1960s. With current therapy, risk is lower (see text).

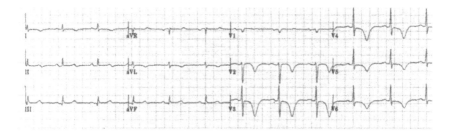

Figure 5.2 Anterior NSTEMI (or non-Q wave MI). There is symmetric T wave inversion in anterior leads. (Reproduced by permission from Taylo, GJ. The Cardiology Rotation. Malden, MA: Blackwell Science, 2001:142.)

Sinus tachycardia during the week after MI is frequently overlooked, and when present it may be the most important physical finding. In fact, resting tachycardia in a patient no longer having pain indicates a worse long-term prognosis than does successfully treated ventricular fibrillation (VF) during the acute phase of MI. That is because sinus tachycardia at rest is a marker of poor LV function; VF *during the early hours* of MI is an electrical event that may occur with a small MI, and does not indicate LV dysfunction. (At any other time, complex ventricular ectopy *is* an indicator of low LVEF.)

Electrocardiogram

ST segment depression is the pattern of subendocardial ischemia, and is the earliest change with NSTEMI. This is followed by symmetrical T wave inversion (Figures 5.1 and 5.2). Occluding a coronary artery with a balloon catheter causes ST segment elevation after a few heartbeats, and that is the pattern of transmural ischemia and STEMI (Figures 5.1 and 5.3).

With persistent occlusion of the coronary artery—in the absence of reperfusion therapy—the ST segments usually remain elevated for a day, and T wave inversion occurs. By the next day, ST elevation tends to resolve, and Q waves have developed. This process is accelerated with reperfusion.

Anterior Myocardial Infarction—Anterior infarction follows occlusion of the LAD artery (see Figure 4.3). It tends to be a large MI because of the size of the vessel and a vascular distribution that includes both the free anterior wall and much of the interventricular septum. Occlusion of the proximal LAD is the worst, because it means loss of largest diagonal branches (supplying the antero-lateral wall of the LV) and septal branches. Most with heart failure after a first MI have had proximal LAD occlusion.[4] Occlusion distally is less devastating, because some of the diagonal and septal branches are spared.

Occlusion of the LAD causes ST segment elevation in the V leads (the so-called precordial or anterior leads). It is possible to estimate the size of an anterior MI from the initial ECG: the number of leads with ST segment elevation is proportional to

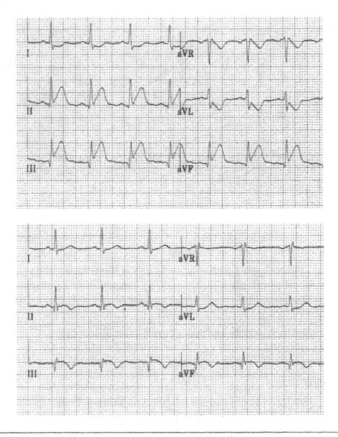

Figure 5.3 Evolution of inferior transmural MI (just six limb leads). *Top ECG:* During the acute phase of infarction there is ST-segment elevation in the inferior leads (II, III, and aVF). Reciprocal ST-segment depression is seen in leads I and a VL. *Bottom ECG:* The next day there is less ST-segment elevation, and the reciprocal ST-segment depression has resolved. The T waves have inverted and deeper Q waves have evolved. (Reproduced by permission from Taylor, GJ. The Cardiology Rotation. Malden, MA: Blackwell Science, 2001:143.)

infarct size (Figure 5.4). Thus, ST elevation in leads V_{1-4} plus aVL usually means occlusion proximal to the first diagonal branch. ST elevation of just a couple V leads is more consistent with mid-LAD occlusion.

Inferior myocardial infarction—Most (85%) are caused by occlusion of the RCA (see Figure 4.3). The RCA is dominant and supplies the inferior wall. The remaining 15% have a left dominant circulation, with the circumflex coronary artery (CCA) supplying the inferior wall. Both the RCA and CCA encircle the heart in the AV groove. The "dominant" vessel is the one that reaches the crux of the heart—where the AV and interventricular grooves intersect at the base—and is the source of the large posterior descending (PDA) that moves toward the apex in

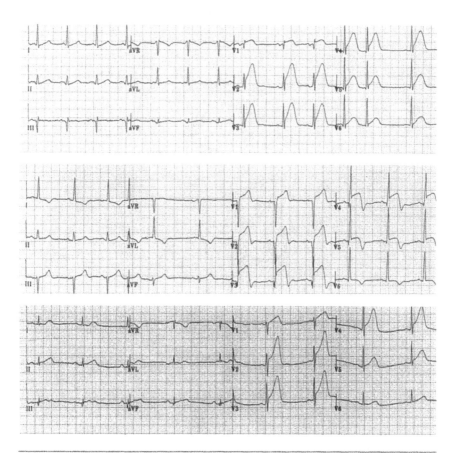

Figure 5.4 Three patients with acute anterior MI and ST elevation. Patient A has upwardly convex ST segments. Patient B has similarly shaped ST segments in V_3 through V_5, but still has some upward concavity in V_1 and V_2. This patient has T inversion in addition to ST elevation. Patient C has ST elevation plus tall, peaked T waves. These *hyperacute T wave changes* would indicate ischemia in the absence of ST elevation. The size of anterior MI is proportional to the number of leads with ST elevation. Each of these patients has ST elevation in five different leads and is having large infarction. (Reproduced by permission from Taylor GJ. 150 Practice ECGs, 2nd ed. Malden, MA: Blackwell Science, 2002:60.)

the interventricular groove (see Figure 4.3). Occlusion of the PDA causes inferior MI, regardless of whether it originates from the RCA or CCA.

RCA occlusion causes ST segment elevation in limb leads, II, III, and aVF (the inferior leads). It is also possible to estimate the size of inferior MI from the initial ECG, but in a manner different from that for anterior MI. Rather than the number of leads with ST elevation, the sum total of ST elevation in the inferior leads (II, III and aVF) is proportional to infarct size (Figure 5.5). Thus, a patient with 3- to 5-mm ST segment elevation in each of the inferior leads is having a much bigger infarct than another with 1- to 2-mm ST elevation. Another marker of large inferior MI

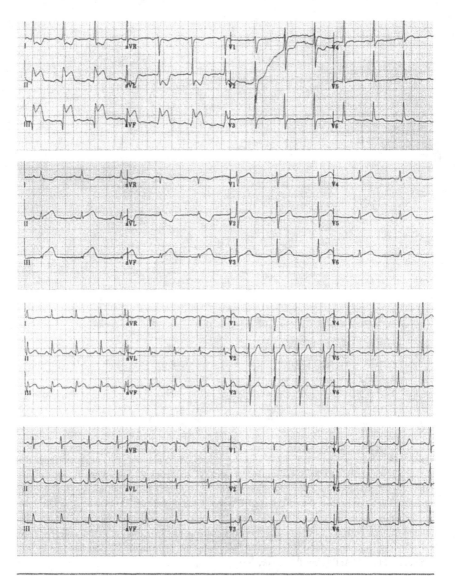

Figure 5.5 Four patients with acute inferior MI. The size of inferior MI is proportional to the sum of ST elevation in the three inferior leads. In addition, those with reciprocal ST depression in anterior or lateral leads tend to have larger infarctions. Using these criteria, patient A was having the largest MI, patients B and C, moderate-sized MIs, and patient D, a small infarct. Patient B also had ST elevation in V_5 and V_6; this may be called inferolateral MI. In this case, the distal right coronary artery in the AV groove was large, and it terminated in a branch to the lateral wall (see Figure 4.3). Patient D is an arguable case of infarction, because the ST-segment elevation is minimal. I am tempted to say that the mild J-point depression in V_2 through V_4 represents reciprocal ST depression; typical chest pain and a subsequent rise in cardiac enzymes would be needed to make the diagnosis of MI with certainty in this case. The ECG changes of transmural infarction are usually obvious, but there are borderline cases like this one. As a rule, such borderline cases involve small MIs; big ones are obvious. (Reprinted with permission from Taylor GJ. 150 Practice ECGs, 2nd ed. Malden, MA: Blackwell Science, 2002:59.)

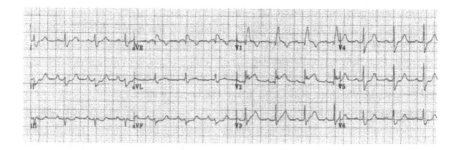

Figure 5.6 Acute anterior MI and right bundle branch block. The conduction abnormality does not obscure the ST elevation in leads V_{1-3}. (Reproduced by permission from Taylor, GJ. The Cardiology Rotation. Malden, MA: Blackwell Science, 2001:146.)

is reciprocal ST depression in anterior (V_{1-4}) or lateral (I, aVL, V_{5-6}) leads. In such cases, the infarct zone includes the postero-lateral wall, usually because the distal RCA extends beyond the PDA and supplies a postero-lateral branch.[4]

Bundle branch block—New bundle branch block occurs more commonly with anterior MI, as the LAD supplies most of the interventricular septum. Early placebo-controlled trials found improved survival with coronary thrombolysis for those with new right or left bundle branch block (RBBB, LBBB).

It is possible to diagnose acute MI with RBBB, as initial LV depolarization is unaffected (Figure 5.6). ST elevation of the early V leads plus RBBB leads indicates proximal LAD occlusion. Left bundle branch block (LBBB) obscures the ECG diagnosis of acute MI; the RV is activated first, and the initial phase of LV activation is buried in the middle of the QRS complex. In a rare case, findings that indicate ischemia with LBBB are ST segment elevation in leads where the QRS is positive (usually V_{5-6}), or ST depression where the QRS is negative (usually the inferior leads).

The usual problem with bundle branch block is deciding whether it is old or new. That is impossible without a previous ECG. With a previous ECG for comparison, and which shows LBBB, new ST segment elevation or depression may indicate acute ischemia in a patient with chest pain.

Lateral MI—The posterolateral wall of the LV tends to be electrocardiographically silent. Occlusion of a small circumflex artery may not cause ST segment elevation in lateral leads (leads I, aVL, or V_{5-6}). There may be minimal ST depression or T wave inversion in V_{5-6}, a pattern more consistent with nontransmural ischemia. Subsequent angiography proves occlusion of the lateral wall branch, with akinesis of that region, and the CK rise is higher than usual for non–ST-elevation MI.

Because there is no ST elevation or Q wave development, this technically is a nontransmural infarction. But total occlusion of the CCA and akinesis of the afflicted LV region identify completed infarction.

An occasional patient with lateral MI has no ECG changes at all. In fact, patients who are having MI without ECG changes are usually having lateral infarction. This is the rationale for observing a patient in the hospital who has convincing chest pain but no ECG changes, at least until serial cardiac enzymes exclude MI.

Anterolateral and inferolateral MI—Acute MI usually affects just one vascular distribution. It would be a remarkable coincidence for two different coronary branches to occlude simultaneously. When the distribution of infarction spills from the anterior or inferior walls into the lateral wall, it is not because a second artery has occluded. Instead, it indicates that the infarct artery—either the RCA or LAD—is unusually large, with branches to the lateral wall.

Pseudoinfarction—The ST segment elevation of *pericarditis* can mimic the changes of transmural ischemia. Usually it is diffuse, involving both anterior and inferior leads. With persistent inflammation, T wave inversion may develop. However, with pericarditis, the ST segment usually returns to baseline before the T wave flips. With ischemia, T inversion occurs while the ST segment is still elevated.

An occasional patient with *myocarditis* has ST segment elevation, then T inversion and evolution of Q waves, a pattern indistinguishable from acute MI. There may be elevation of cardiac enzymes as well. Diffuse ST elevation involving multiple vascular distributions suggests myocarditis, but angiography may be needed to sort it out.

ST segment elevation may also occur with left bundle branch block, hyperkalemia, left ventricular hypertrophy, and the Brugada syndrome (see Chapter 6). Early repolarization is a normal variant, with J point elevation in multiple leads, but with a normally shaped ST segment. With these conditions the changes in ST segments are not associated with a chest pain syndrome and usually are present on previous ECGs.

The delta wave of Wolff-Parkinson-White syndrome may appear as Q waves, usually in inferior leads. A short PR leads to the correct diagnosis, and is supported by the history (no MI) and echocardiogram (no regional wall motion abnormality). Pseudo-Qs may also occur with hypertrophic cardiomyopathy or with an infiltrative cardiomyopathy such as amyloidosis.

Cardiac Enzymes

The diagnosis of acute MI has been based on a triad of chest pain, ECG changes, and a rise in cardiac enzymes (Table 5.2). When drawn at the appropriate time, normal troponin or CK-MB would make the diagnosis of MI unlikely—the test is quite sensitive for myocardial necrosis. In fact, cardiac biomarkers—enzymes—are now so sensitive that a European Society of Cardiology/American College of Cardiology committee has suggested a standard definition MI that *begins with* the typical rise and then fall in either CK-MB or cardiac troponin, plus one of the following: (1) ischemic symptoms, (2) ECG changes (ST segment changes early, or evolution of Q waves or T inversion), and (3) coronary angiography that documents CAD.[5]

This definition of MI requires more than just an enzyme rise, because it is important to distinguish between myocardial necrosis and infarction. The cardiac troponins are more sensitive and specific than CK-MB, allowing detection of necrosis of less than 1 g of myocardium. Many of the conditions associated with a false-positive troponin elevation involve myocardial necrosis, although without ischemia (Box 5.2). For example, elevated troponin indicates a higher mortality risk

Table 5.2 Cardiac Enzymes*

	Time of Appearance (hr)		
	Earliest	Peak	Comment
Troponins	3	24	More sensitive than CK-MB. Elevation may persist for 7–14 d.
CK-MB	4	24	The area under the CK curve is proportional to infarct size. CK-MB/CK >2.5% indicates cardiac injury.
Myoglobin	1–4	6–7	Not specific for heart muscle.

CK, creatine phosphokinase; CK-MB, the myocardium specific band of CK.

*Earlier versions of this table included LDH and its isoforms and SGOT. These muscle enzymes are of little use given the better sensitivity and specificity of CK and troponin.

Box 5.2 Non-ischemic Causes of Troponin Elevation*

Cardiac trauma (contusion, pacing, ICD firing, cardioversion, biopsy, cardiac surgery)

Congestive heart failure

Hypertension

Hypotension (often with arrhythmia)

Renal failure

Postoperative (noncardiac surgery)

Critical illness (especially diabetic patients)

Drug toxicity (doxorubicin [Adriamycin], 5-fluorouracil, trastuzumab [Herceptin])

Hypothyroidism

Myocardial inflammation (myocarditis, sarcoidosis)

Sepsis

Pulmonary embolus

Burns (usually extensive)

Myocardial infiltrative disease (sarcoid, amyloid, scleroderma)

Acute neurological disease, including stroke

Rhabdomyolysis with cardiac injury

Transplant vasculopathy

in patients with advanced heart failure or pulmonary hypertension—the continued leak of troponin probably indicates ongoing myocardial injury.[6,7] Patients with end-stage renal disease often have minimally elevated troponin, and they tend to have a poor prognosis. (At this time, we do not use this as an indication for angiography.)

Troponin (molecular weight 33,000 D) tends to appear in the circulation a bit earlier than CK-MB (86,000 D), and usually is elevated 3 hours after the onset of pain. The persistent elevation of troponin 10 to 14 days after MI helps with a late diagnosis of infarction.

A marker of injury that is abnormal even sooner after the onset of MI would be useful for early diagnosis. Smaller molecules are able to leach out of the infarct zone faster. Myoglobin, weighing 18,000 D, may be elevated 1 hour after the onset of chest pain, but it is not specific for myocardium, and a reliable assay is not widely available. It is important to remember that none of the available biomarkers is elevated at the onset of MI. That is why a decision about reperfusion therapy is based on the history and ECG.

We presently draw enzymes on presentation, then 6, 12, and 24 hours later.[5]

Initial Treatment of Non–ST-Segment Elevation Myocardial Infarction

Angiography during the early phase of MI without ST segment elevation usually shows antegrade flow and a tight, ragged coronary artery lesion. The pathophysiology, presentation, and treatment of this severe variant of the ACS are reviewed in Chapter 4. Thrombolytic therapy has been tested and found no better than anticoagulation, probably because there is antegrade coronary blood flow. Four-drug antithrombotic therapy is indicated using aspirin, clopidogrel, a IIb/IIIa inhibitor, and heparin. Beta blockade has been shown to prevent recurrent ischemia and progression of the MI. Diltiazem is a reasonable substitute when beta blockade is not possible (see Chapter 4).

By the time we see these patients in hospital, the chest discomfort has usually resolved. Ongoing pain despite medical therapy is an indication for immediate angiography. In most centers, urgent, next-day angiography is scheduled for the patient without pain who is stable on antithrombotic therapy. Same-day catheterization may be advantageous (see Chapter 4), but it may not be feasible, and it is not presently the standard of care.

Initial Treatment of ST-Segment Elevation Myocardial Infarction

Reperfusion Therapy—Primary Angioplasty

Reperfusion therapy is now the standard of care of STEMI and for MI with new bundle branch block. Cell death begins within 15 minutes of coronary occlusion,

Table 5.3 Risk of Death from Myocardial Infarction and Patient Selection for Reperfusion Therapy	
Highest risk, immediate reperfusion therapy is indicated	Anterior MI Large inferior MI Inferior MI and possible RV infarction MI with new bundle branch block
Lower risk, consider emergency reperfusion based on other clinical features	NSTEMI with persistant pain Small inferior MI in a patient who is not a good candidate for reperfusion
Clinical features that increase the risk of MI, and would favor reperfusion therapy	Heart failure (Killip class II-IV) Prior MI History of heart failure RV infarction syndrome Diabetes

*MI, myocardial infarction; RV, right ventricular.

and is progressive beyond that point.[5] With each 15 minutes that passes, more heart muscle is lost. Early reperfusion saves more lives than later reperfusion. A patient in the ED does not have time to wait for a cardiologist to arrive to make a diagnosis and decision. The first doctor to see the patient in the ED should initiate treatment.

Patient selection for reperfusion therapy is influenced by the risk of the infarction. Table 5.3 suggests a hierarchy of MI risk, and identifies clinical features that would favor reperfusion therapy for the patient with a borderline ECG. Uncertainty about the diagnosis of MI—an absence of ST segment elevation—would favor immediate catheterization and stenting rather than thrombolytic therapy. In fact thrombolysis was worse than placebo for patients with chest pain and ST segment depression or no ECG changes (Figure 5.7). In such cases, the patient is exposed to the risks of lytic therapy (bleeding and stroke), without the benefit of treatment that derives from relieving total occlusion of the coronary artery.

It is now apparent that the best reperfusion technique is coronary angioplasty with stenting. I will use both terms, angioplasty and stenting, although stenting is the critical technique and is used in most cases. A meta-analysis of 23 randomized trials comparing primary angioplasty (pre-stenting) and lytic therapy showed angioplasty superior for preventing death (7% vs. 9%), nonfatal reinfarction (3% vs. 7%), stroke (1% vs. 2%), or a combination of these three outcomes at 1 month (8% vs. 14%).[8]

Furthermore, patients who are transferred from a community hospital to a tertiary referral center for interventional treatment fare better than those who are treated on site with thrombolytic therapy, as long as the time from presentation to stenting does not exceed 2 hours.[9,10] The effectiveness of thrombolysis declines with delayed therapy.

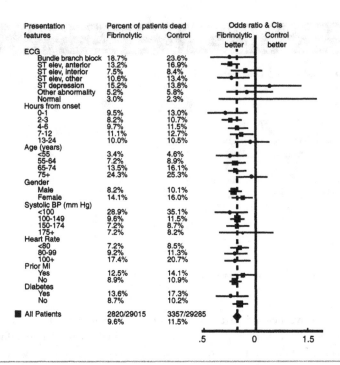

Presentation features	Percent of patients dead		Odds ratio & CIs
	Fibrinolytic	Control	Fibrinolytic better / Control better
ECG			
Bundle branch block	18.7%	23.6%	
ST elev, anterior	13.2%	16.9%	
ST elev, inferior	7.5%	8.4%	
ST elev, other	10.6%	13.4%	
ST depression	15.2%	13.8%	
Other abnormality	5.2%	5.8%	
Normal	3.0%	2.3%	
Hours from onset			
0-1	9.5%	13.0%	
2-3	8.2%	10.7%	
4-6	9.7%	11.5%	
7-12	11.1%	12.7%	
13-24	10.0%	10.5%	
Age (years)			
<55	3.4%	4.6%	
55-64	7.2%	8.9%	
65-74	13.5%	16.1%	
75+	24.3%	25.3%	
Gender			
Male	8.2%	10.1%	
Female	14.1%	16.0%	
Systolic BP (mm Hg)			
<100	28.9%	35.1%	
100-149	9.6%	11.5%	
150-174	7.2%	8.7%	
175+	7.2%	8.2%	
Heart Rate			
<80	7.2%	8.5%	
80-99	9.2%	11.3%	
100+	17.4%	20.7%	
Prior MI			
Yes	12.5%	14.1%	
No	8.9%	10.9%	
Diabetes			
Yes	13.6%	17.3%	
No	8.7%	10.2%	
■ **All Patients**	2820/29015 / 9.6%	3357/29285 / 11.5%	

.5   0   1.5

Figure 5.7 Effects of thrombolytic therapy on 1-month mortality after acute MI. Pooled data from the nine placebo controlled trials, including 58,600 patients. Most of these patients were treated with streptokinase. Newer reperfusion therapies, including rt-PA and stenting, are more efficacious than streptokinase, but will never be tested against placebo. (Reproduced by permission from Indications for fibrinolytic therapy in suspected acute myocardial infarction: collaborative overview of early mortality and major morbidity results from all randomised trials of more than 1000 patients. Fibrinolytic Therapy Trialists' (FTT) Collaborative Group. Lancet 1994;343:311–322.)

As clot becomes more organized the chance of opening the artery and achieving good flow declines. That is not the case with angioplasty. Even with late therapy more than 90% of patients have prompt restoration of excellent flow.

Nevertheless, the time of transfer is a problem. The five trials that found transfer for angioplasty superior to thrombolysis had angioplasty delayed by 43 minutes on average (compared with on site thrombolysis); 95% were treated within 2 hours of the initial presentation. I find that remarkably slick.[10] Minimizing door-to-balloon time was obviously a goal of these studies (they were as much about logistics as about the therapies). More realistic—and reflecting real world experience—are data from a large US registry that showed a door-to-balloon time averaging 185 minutes for those requiring transfer.[9] Just 3% in the registry were treated within 90 minutes.

This is a critical issue, because door-to-balloon times of 90 to 120 minutes have been associated with improved survival.[9] In one representative study of primary angioplasty that did not involve patient transfer, 565 patients had a median time from enrollment to first balloon inflation of 76 minutes. The 30-day mortality rate for those having first balloon inflation of 60 minutes or less after enrollment was 1%; 61 to 75 minutes, 3.7%; 76 to 90 minutes, 4%; and longer than 90 minutes, 6.4%.[11] The angioplasty experience is like that of early trials of coronary thrombolysis: time is still muscle.

One study found that the survival advantage of angioplasty over lytic therapy disappeared when fibrinolytic therapy was started 60 minutes or longer before angioplasty, and the composite endpoint advantage (death, stroke, or recurrent MI) was erased when the difference was 90 minutes.[9] Therefore, if the delay caused by transfer is going to be 90 minutes or longer, the patient may do as well with on-site thrombolytic therapy.[9] As the doctor providing initial treatment, it is your job to decide how long transfer for angioplasty will take (and to hustle the process along).

Another question is whether to begin thrombolytic therapy before transferring the patient for stenting, or perhaps a combination of low-dose lytic therapy plus a glycoprotein IIb/IIIa inhibitor. Early trials have shown no benefit of facilitated angioplasty with combined lytic and interventional therapy.[12] Many of these delayed stenting; more recent trials show benefits of immediate stenting, within 6 hours of thrombolytic therapy. It makes sense, because stenting stabilizes the reperfused vessel, and opens those arteries that did not reperfuse with lytic therapy.

For now, consider the approach outlined in Table 5.4, which is based upon available clinical trials.[9]

Predictors of outcome with reperfusion therapy and the no-reflow phenomenon—The time from the onset of symptoms to treatment is critical, regardless of the method used to open the artery.

Another predictor is restoration of good perfusion. The quality of flow through the coronary artery is one explanation for the superiority of angioplasty over lytic therapy. Successful angioplasty is usually accomplished shortly after arrival in the catheterization laboratory, greater than 90% have TIMI grade 3 flow in the infarct artery (e.g., there is rapid flow into the artery and rapid washout of contrast from the distal vessel). With thrombolysis, the artery may not open for 40 to 60 minutes after starting therapy, and flow often is sluggish when it is restored (TIMI grade 2). As noted, with later application, the effectiveness of lytic therapy declines.[10]

In some cases, with both angioplasty and lytic therapy, there is correction of the stenosis but poor tissue perfusion. The infarct artery looks good after initial injection of contrast, but there is delayed washout of contrast from the distal vessel. Injury of the distal microvasculature is responsible for this *no-reflow phenomenon*.[13] In addition to ischemic endothelial injury, distal capillaries and arterioles may have intraluminal platelet and fibrin thrombi. Interstitial myocellular edema may contribute to poor flow by compressing small vessels. The diagnosis of no-reflow is confirmed by the angiographic appearance of the dilated artery, and the pattern of flow.

Table 5.4 A Triage Strategy for Patients with Acute Myocardial Infarction[7]	
1	People in the community, and certainly patients with coronary artery disease, should be aware of the symptoms of MI, and should seek medical attention early. Ideally, they should arrive in the ED less than 1 hour from the onset of chest pain.
2	When possible—certainly in an urban setting—a patient with chest pain and possible MI should be taken directly to a hospital with angioplasty capability. There is no justification for stopping at a community hospital that is 15–30 minutes closer (the current practice for most ambulance services).
3 (a-c)	For patients who reach the ED <3 hours from the onset of chest pain: a. If you are in a community hospital ED, do not let the ambulance leave until you have done the initial ECG. If it shows ST segment elevation or new BBB, start an IV, begin aspirin and unfractionated heparin, and send the patient on to the tertiary center for stenting. This assumes a transfer time <60 minutes. b. While the patient is en route, notify the tertiary center so that the cath lab is ready. c. If you know that the transfer time for angioplasty will be 2 hours or longer, begin thrombolytic therapy, with the goal of starting it within 30 minutes of arrival in the ED. Follow this with transfer of the patient to the interventional cardiology center.
4	Patients who come to the ED late, >3 hours from the onset of symptoms, tend to do better with angioplasty/stenting, even with transfer delays. Likewise, those with early cardiogenic shock (including the RV infarction syndrome) should be transferred for angioplasty. In such cases, minimizing the time to angioplasty is critical.

BBB, bundle branch block; ECG, electrocardiograph; ED, emergency department; IV, intravenous; MI, myocardial infarction; RV, right ventricular.

Interestingly, the surface ECG provides an effective measure of tissue perfusion.[14,15] No-reflow is often accompanied by persistent ST segment elevation. When there is prompt and sustained resolution of ST-segment elevation with reperfusion therapy—that is, the ST segments come down by 70%—good tissue perfusion is likely. A failure of ST-segment elevation to resolve often is associated with persistent chest pain, and is an independent predictor of mortality, even for those with a successfully opened infarct artery. Thus, getting serial 12-lead ECGs is a good way to determine the success of reperfusion therapy:

The time to therapy and degree of resolution of ST elevation are the best predictors of clinical outcome.[15]

Here is why: The time to therapy reflects the amount of myocardial necrosis before treatment. Resolution of ST-segment elevation reflects the response to treatment (when the ST-segments stay up, ischemic injury is ongoing).

No-reflow may improve with coronary vasodilators, indicating an element of spasm. Intracoronary adenosine, the most potent coronary vasodilator, has been especially effective. Verapamil can be used as well, and both are better than intracoronary nitroglycerin. The IIb/IIIa inhibitors may prevent no-reflow when given before angioplasty, but intracoronary thrombolytic therapy has not proved useful in treating it. The intra-aortic balloon pump may be used to boost coronary perfusion pressure during diastole.

The response to therapy is determined by the severity of microvascular and interstitial injury. In its most severe form, there is staining of the myocardium by contrast material that leaks from injured small vessels into the interstitium. This usually is not corrected with treatment, and indicates advanced injury. The best way to avoid the no-reflow problem is early reperfusion.

Thrombolytic Therapy

The indication for coronary thrombolysis is STEMI or MI with new bundle branch block, and an inability to accomplish angioplasty within 2 hours.

You must understand your referral situation. When doctors are questioned about time of transfer, and door-to-balloon times, they uniformly claim an ability to move the patient and accomplish angioplasty in 45 to 90 minutes. However, when medical records are carefully reviewed, the reality is closer to 3 hours (note the previous discussion).

If you are sure that it will take longer than 2 hours to get your patient to angioplasty—to the initial balloon inflation in the coronary artery (not just to the hospital)—begin thrombolytic therapy immediately.

Indications and patient selection—The chance of dying with some heart attacks is higher than it is with others. The early placebo controlled trials of lytic therapy found a benefit with higher risk MI (Table 5.3, Figure 5.7). As noted, the risk of thrombolytic therapy is justified only when there is obvious coronary occlusion (e.g., ST-segment elevation). Those with suspected MI but without ST elevation are better treated with antithrombotic therapy and urgent catheterization when the chest pain does not resolve (see the discussion of ACS including NSTEMI in Chapter 4).

When the ECG does not show ST-segment elevation, but you strongly suspect MI, *repeat the ECG*. It is common for ST-segment elevation to wax and wane during the early course of MI. In addition, think of other possibilities. Severe pain and diaphoresis may be caused by aortic dissection or esophageal rupture, illnesses where thrombolysis would be a disaster.

Advanced age is not a contraindication to reperfusion. On the other hand, there is not a clear survival benefit with lytic therapy for those over 75 years old (Figure 5.7). The risk of bleeding with lytic therapy increase with age. GUSTO-I reported stroke in 0.8% of those under 65 years old, 2.1% between 65 and 74 years of age, and 3.4% over age 75. *While not zero, the risk of hemorrhagic stroke is lower with angioplasty*. Another issue with age is the patient's ability to handle aggressive and potentially stressful intervention. In community practice, most elderly patients treated with reperfusion therapy are healthy and active. Few doctors use an aggressive treatment strategy for debilitated patients from the nursing home.

Late thrombolysis is of little benefit (Figure 5.7) Lytic agents are less effective when the clot is older, and more organized. Increased fibrin cross-linking makes it harder to break up. When given 12 hours after onset of MI, less than half the patients achieve TIMI 3 flow. The LATE study addressed clinical outcomes, and found a small benefit when rt-PA was given between 6 and 12 hours after the onset of pain, but not after 12 hours. Lytic therapy greater than 12 hours from the onset of MI also introduces a new complication: the risk of *myocardial rupture* appears increased.

Stenting is a safer therapy for the late arrival with persistent pain and ST-segment elevation. It is more effective as well, as increased duration of occlusion—a more organized clot—does not influence the outcome. More than 90% have excellent restoration of flow immediately, even with late stenting.[10] Whether this translates to improved survival is uncertain, but it is preferable to late thrombolysis.

Evolution of Q waves does not mean the infarct is completed. As noted, the infarct artery may open and close. With transient reperfusion, Q waves can develop rapidly. If the ST segments are still elevated and the patient continues to have pain, Q waves are not a contraindication to reperfusion therapy.

Contraindications to thrombolytic therapy—The most important selection issue is the risk of bleeding (Table 5.5). Most bleeding is minor, occurring at vascular puncture sites. As a rule it can be controlled with local pressure, and a hematoma usually resolves without long-term sequelae.

The incidence of intracranial hemorrhage in large clinical trial is 0.75%. When the usual contraindications to lytic therapy are observed, an individual's chance of hemorrhagic stroke increases with any of four risk factors: age greater than 65 years, weight less than 70 kg, hypertension on presentation (systolic pressure ≥170 mm Hg, or diastolic pressure ≥95 mm Hg), and the use of rt-PA rather than streptokinase. With none of these risk factors, the risk of stroke is 0.26%. It is 0.96% with one, 1.32% with two, and 2.17% with three of them. Note that uncontrolled hypertension and previous stroke were contraindications to thrombolysis in the trials that produced these risk data. An even higher risk of stroke would be expected for the patient with a systolic blood pressure above 200 mm Hg.

Defibrillation and a brief period of cardiopulmonary resuscitation (CPR) are not contraindications to thrombolysis. When CPR is prolonged more than 10 minutes or there is obvious trauma with chest compression or intubation, the bleeding risk increases.

Any of the contraindications reviewed in Table 5.5 weighs in favor of primary angioplasty, even if it is delayed beyond the 2-hour limit.

Pharmacology of thrombolysis—Clot formation and dissolution are in dynamic equilibrium. Developing thrombus cannot be allowed to propagate indefinitely, and clot within blood vessels (or a ureter) must eventually be removed to restore patency. This is the role of the fibrinolytic system. As soon as clot forms, the fibrinolytic system is activated.

Plasminogen is the precursor of the active fibrinolytic enzyme, plasmin. Plasminogen is converted to plasmin by plasminogen activators. These include naturally occurring substances, tissue plasminogen activator (t-PA) and urokinase,

Table 5.5 Contraindications to Thrombolytic Therapy
Absolute contraindications
Active internal bleeding
History of cerebrovascular accident
Recent (within 2 months) intracranial or intraspinal surgery or trauma
Intracranial neoplasm, arteriovenous malformation, or aneurysm
Known bleeding diathesis
Severe uncontrolled hypertension
Relative contraindications
Recent (within 10 days) major surgery, e.g., coronary bypass graft, obstetric delivery, organ biopsy, previous puncture of noncompressible vessels
Cerebrovascular disease
Recent gastrointestinal or genitourinary bleeding (within 10 days)
Recent trauma (within 10 days)
Hypertension: systolic BP ≥180 mm Hg and/or diastolic BP ≥110 mm Hg
High likelihood of left heart thrombus, e.g., mitral stenosis with atrial fibrillation
Acute pericarditis
Subacute bacterial endocarditis
Hemostatic defects including those resulting from severe hepatic or renal disease
Significant liver dysfunction
Pregnancy
Diabetic hemorrhagic retinopathy or other hemorrhagic ophthalmic conditions
Septic thrombophlebitis or occluded atrioventricular cannula at seriously infected site
Advanced age, i.e., over 75 yr
Patients currently receiving oral anticoagulants, e.g., warfarin
Any other condition in which bleeding constitutes a significant hazard or would be particularly difficult to manage because of its location
Syndromes mimicking MI that carry a high risk of bleeding
Peptic esophagitis
Pericarditis
Aortic dissection
Intracranial bleeding with T wave changes

Reprinted with permission from Taylor GJ. The Cardiology Rotation. Malden, MA: Blackwell Science, 2001:163.

and the foreign compound, streptokinase. Plasminogen is produced by the liver and is found in the circulation. When clot forms, this free plasminogen is incorporated into the thrombus and is bound to fibrin.

The ideal thrombolytic agent would move into the thrombus and work only on fibrin-bound plasminogen. But most of the thrombolytic agents activate free, circulating plasminogen as well, producing plasmin and the so-called lytic state. Free plasmin digests circulating fibrinogen and other clotting factors, producing an hypocoagulable state.

The major difference among thrombolytic drugs is the degree to which they work on fibrin-bound plasminogen. Tissue plasminogen activator, either native (t-PA) or recombinant (rt-PA), relies on fibrin as a cofactor, and when bound to fibrin has a 500-fold increase in activity. It is not as potent when free in the circulation (and not bound to fibrin). Streptokinase works on both free and fibrin-bound plasminogen, and thus leads to a greater decline in circulating fibrinogen.

The earliest trials showing that lytic therapy is superior to placebo were performed with streptokinase—including most of those represented in Figure 5.7. Comparison studies have shown that rt-PA (alteplase) is better than streptokinase, especially when administered using a front-loading protocol. More rapid thrombolysis and earlier achievement of good flow (TIMI grade 3 flow) is the probable explanation. Newer generation rt-PA preparations, tenecteplase and reteplase, have a longer half–life so may be given as an intravenous bolus injection, rather than as a continuous infusion. These t-PA mutants have been show to produce TIMI-3 flow more rapidly than alteplase, but in comparison trials there has been no improvement in complication rates or in 30-day mortality with the newer agents.[16]

Now that angioplasty/stenting has been found superior to lytic therapy, I suspect we will see fewer research dollars spent to develop new thrombolytic agents.

Assessment of reperfusion and prognosis—Early resolution of ST-segment elevation is the best indicator of good tissue perfusion (note the earlier discussion of the no-reflow phenomenon). Improvement in chest pain is common with thrombolysis and usually accompanies improvement in ST elevation. When the artery first opens, many patients have a run of accelerated idioventricular rhythm (AIVR), and this slow-ventricular tachycardia (VT) is a reliable indicator of reperfusion. It rarely degenerates into VF, and antiarrhythmic therapy is not needed.

For many patients, ST segment elevation and chest pain do not resolve in a dramatic fashion, so there is uncertainty about the status of the infarct artery after coronary thrombolysis. Early studies found stress testing and perfusion imaging unreliable. Most of our patients have early coronary angiography.

Management after thrombolysis—Since rt-PA does not deplete fibrinogen, the patient is not anticoagulated after lytic therapy. *Heparin plus aspirin* are started with thrombolytic therapy, and the activated partial thromboplastin time should be in the therapeutic range, one and a half to two times control. Hirudin and hirulog, more potent antithrombin agents, are no more effective than heparin.

Metoprolol as an adjunct to thrombolysis has been shown to lower the rate of recurrent ischemia, but had no effect on survival or LV function. Calcium channel blocker, angiotensin converting enzyme (ACE) inhibitors, intravenous nitroglycerin, and magnesium have not been shown to augment the benefits of lytic therapy.

Coronary angiography usually shows antegrade flow in the infarct artery. It is a sign of thrombolysis, although it does not prove early and effective restoration of flow unless it is performed early. As with the ACS, the culprit lesion usually has a ragged, unstable appearance. Early reocclusion is common. Furthermore, reocclusion tends to occur without chest pain, even when there is viable myocardium in the infarct zone.[17] Prolonged ischemia stuns or damages the sensory nerves, and silent ischemia is the rule (e.g., there is nociceptive dysfunction). Pacification of the infarct artery with angioplasty and stenting is usually indicated.

A reasonable treatment strategy for the patient who cannot be transferred for primary angioplasty is 1) thrombolytic therapy using an rt-PA preparation within 30 minutes of arrival in the ED, 2) anticoagulation with aspirin and heparin, 3) angiography during the next 24 hours (the same day if possible, though I avoid middle-of-the-night transfer). If chest pain does not resolve or if there is cardiogenic shock, immediate transfer for rescue angioplasty is indicated.

Other Therapies During the Initial 12 Hours of Myocardial Infarction

Reperfusion therapy properly gets top billing, because it has the greatest potential for reducing mortality and morbidity (heart failure, serious arrhythmias, etc.).

Antithrombotic Therapy

Early in the course of coronary thrombosis there is activation of the fibrinolytic system. The infarct artery may alternate between being open and closed; aspirin increases the chance of it remaining open. One of the earliest placebo-controlled trials of thrombolytic therapy found aspirin as effective as intravenous streptokinase. Aspirin should be given upon arrival in the ED if it has not been given in the field. It is routinely administered by emergency medical services (EMS), and patients often have taken it before EMS arrives.

Clopidogrel is a good substitute for the patient with aspirin allergy. It has not been tested as an adjunct to thrombolytic therapy. On the other hand, it should be given to the patient going to the catheterization laboratory for primary angioplasty.

Patients who have had angioplasty are routinely treated with aspirin, clopidogrel, and heparin after the procedure. A number will receive IIb/IIIa inhibitor treatment as well.

Beta-adrenergic Blockade

During the acute phase of MI, patients may respond to intravenous beta blockade with prompt relief of pain and a reduction in ST-segment elevation. Randomized trials were performed before the development of reperfusion therapy, and demonstrated a reduction in mortality (by 15%), reinfarction (19%), and cardiac arrest (19%).

The greatest survival benefit was seen during the first day after MI. In contrast, thrombolytic therapy does not reduce mortality during the first 24 hours; a beneficial effect emerges over the next week. Although this suggests a complementary role for beta blockade and reperfusion therapy, synergy has not been supported by clinical trials of beta blockade as an adjunct to coronary thrombolysis. Consider beta blockade for the occasional patient with STEMI who—for whatever reason—is not to have reperfusion therapy.

Table 5.6 Beta-locker Therapy for Acute MI	
Patient selection	Acute MI, <12 hr from the onset of pain
Contraindications	1. Heart failure (diffuse rales) 2. Heart rate <60 beats/min 3. Heart block (PR interval >.24 sec) 4. Systolic blood pressure <90 mm Hg 5. Asthma or obstructive lung disease with wheezing
Dosing	**Metoprolol:** 5 mg IV at 5-min intervals for three doses if the heart rate is >60/min, and blood pressure is >100 mm Hg Then 100 mg PO qid for 48 hr Then 100 mg PO bid **Atenolol:** 5 mg IV over 5 min, repeat in 10 min (no second dose if heart rate or blood pressure decrease) Then 50 mg PO 10 min later Then 50 mg PO bid
Benefits	Blunts catecholamine effect, lowering MVO$_2$ and thus, infarct size. ST-segment elevation may resolve. Survival may also be improved by prevention of ventricular fibrillation or LV rupture.

bid, twice daily; LV, left ventricular; MI, myocardial infarction; MVO$_2$, maximal venous oxygen consumption; PO, orally; qid, four times daily.

The use of beta-blockers in the acute phase of MI is summarized in Table 5.6. If bronchospasm is a concern, use the short-acting agent, esmolol, 5–25 µg/kg per minute.

Oxygen

There is little evidence supporting oxygen therapy for a patient who does not have hypoxemia. It is not identified as a critical therapy by practice guidelines. However, patients often feel better, or describe improvement in pain with oxygen treatment. Because there is little risk with nasal oxygen, 2–4 L per minute, there is no reason to omit this traditional treatment.

A common practice has been to continue it for a couple days. In real life, it is usually overlooked, and the patient stays on oxygen until discharge (no harm done, other than the expense). It makes more sense to stop oxygen when the patient is pain-free and has normal oxygen saturation on room air, and especially when resuming ambulation.

Control of Pain

The initial treatment of chest pain with sublingual nitroglycerin is fine, even before getting the ECG. If the patient is having angina rather than MI, there may be relief. Hypotension with nitroglycerin usually resolves with recumbency. If it persists, elevate the patient's legs.

Morphine is the preferred analgesic. Meperidine is less effective, has similar side effects, and tends to raise the heart rate. Like nitroglycerin, morphine is a venodilator and thus lowers preload. A decrease in blood pressure is prevented or treated by placing the patient in a supine position or by raising the legs.

The most common error with morphine treatment is inadequate dosing. Give 4–8 mg intravenously and follow this with 2–8 mg at 5- to 15-minute intervals until there is improvement or relief of pain. There will also be improvement in anxiety and restlessness, and a blunting of autonomic output. A rare patient requires large doses of morphine for relief, as much as 2 mg/kg. This is usually tolerated, and patients with cardiac pain or pulmonary edema have a low risk of respiratory depression with morphine.

If you are concerned about morphine toxicity as a cause of hypotension, severe nausea, or respiratory depression, the effects are rapidly reversed using naloxone 0.1–0.2 mg intravenously (repeated in 5 to 15 minutes as needed).

Angiotensin-converting Enzyme Inhibition

Note the following discussion of congestive heart failure complicating MI. Early therapy with ACE inhibitors prevents infarct expansion, improving LV function and survival for those with large, anterior MI. Early treatment—started in the first 24 hours—is best (Figure 5.8 and Table 5.7). Because ACE inhibition may lower blood pressure, it must be used with caution for those already treated with nitrates or beta-blockers. Angiotensin II blockade is a suitable alternative to ACE inhibition for those with prior intolerance.

Intravenous Nitroglycerin

When used early in the course of MI, intravenous nitroglycerin decreases preload and LV wall tension, and therefore myocardial oxygen demand. This could limit infarct size. Intravenous nitroglycerin may also dilate collaterals and improve flow to the infarct zone (oral and topical nitrates probably do not have this effect).

There have been conflicting results from small clinical trials, and the routine use of intravenous nitroglycerin is not established. We do not hesitate to use it when

Table 5.7 Angiotensin-converting Enzyme Inhibition after Myocardial Infarction	
Patient selection	1. Anterior MI 2. MI complicated by heart failure 3. LVEF <30%
Contraindication	Systolic pressure <100 mm Hg, known renal artery stenosis, prior reaction to ACE inhibition.
Drugs and oral dose (begin on day 1 of MI)	Captopril (Capoten) 12.5–50 mg bid Enalapril (Vasotec) 5–20 mg bid Lisinopril (Prinivil, Zestril) 2.5–10 mg bid Ramipril (Altace) 2.5–5 mg bid

ACE, angiotensin-converting enzyme; LVEF, left ventricular ejection fraction; MI, myocardial infarction; bid, twice daily.

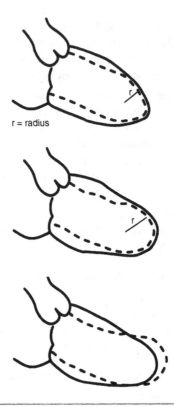

Figure 5.8 Three examples of left ventricular remodeling after MI (solid line, diastolic contour; dashed line, systolic contour). Patient A: The anterior wall is akinetic, but in diastole the left ventricle still has its ellipsoid shape (there has been no remodeling of LV shape). Patient B: In addition to anterior akinesis, the shape of the apex has changed so that it is rounded and more mushroomlike. This increases the radius (r) at the apex, and thus increases wall tension (see text). Patient C: There is an apical aneurysm. In addition to the rounded apex during diastole, there is aneurysmal bulging of the apex during systole. Not only is wall tension increased because of increased radius, but contractile energy is also absorbed by the bulging apex. This is the most extreme form of LV remodeling. (Reproduced by permission from Taylor GJ. Primary Care Management of Heart Disease. St. Louis: Mosby, 2000:198.)

there is ongoing chest pain. It is safe to use for those with large MI and/or heart failure. Nitrates to not depress heart rate or contractility, so they may be used together with beta-blockers. Both can depress blood pressure, so monitor carefully.

What Drug(s) Should You Use to Reduce Infarct Size?

Drug combinations have not been studied, and there is no algorithm. The importance of reperfusion therapy is well established. Antithrombotic therapy is the only proven adjunct to reperfusion.

An occasional patient does not have reperfusion therapy. In such cases, consider the drugs just reviewed and that are summarized in Table 5.8.

Table 5.8 A Summary of Treatment to Limit Infarct Size and/or Improve Survival When Given in the Early Phase of Myocardial Infarction

Treatment	Evidence for Efficacy	Patient Selection	Contraindication
Reperfusion therapy	Strong	STEMI or MI with new bundle branch block	Note contraindications to thrombolytic therapy (Table 5.5)
Aspirin	Strong	All with suspected MI*	Allergy or contraindication to aspirin
Intravenous beta blockade	Strong	STEMI, NSTEMI or suspected MI*; tachycardia	Hypotension, bradycardia, heart failure, bronchospasm
Oral ACE inhibitors	Strong	Anterior MI (treat on day 1)	Hypotension, known renal artery stenosis
Intravenous nitroglycerin	Equivocal	Ongoing ischemia*, anterior MI, heart failure	Hypotension, tachycardia or right ventricular infarction
Heparin, clopidogrel, IIb/IIIa inhibitor inhibitor	Strong	NSTEMI, in addition to aspirin. Add IIb/IIIa inhibitor when troponin is elevated*	Active bleeding and other contraindications to anticoagulation

STEMI, ST-segment elevation myocardial infarction; NSTEMI, non-STEMI; MI, myocardial infarction; ACE, angiotensin-converting enzyme.

*If the patient is having unstable angina rather than MI, therapy is still helpful. Beta blockade and nitroglycerin have not been shown to improve survival when given in addition to reperfusion therapy.

Complications of Acute Myocardial Infarction

Cardiogenic Shock

Before the development of reperfusion therapy, cardiogenic shock developed in approximately 20% of patients with MI, and the mortality rate was as high as 80%. With modern therapy, the incidence has been reduced to 5% to 7%, and the mortality rate to about 40%. Nevertheless, LV failure remains the leading cause of in-hospital death with MI.

Autopsy studies have shown that the pump loses its ability to maintain blood pressure when 40% of the LV is infarcted, and LV injury is responsible for 80% of cases of shock. Right ventricular infarction, acute ventricular septal defect or mitral regurgitation (MR), and LV rupture are the other causes of shock. It is important to diagnose these conditions, because the treatment is different.

When LV pump failure is the cause, there is a series of potentially harmful compensatory responses. Increased sympathetic tone and activation of the renin-angiotensin-aldosterone raise peripheral vascular resistance and ventricular afterload, further depressing LV function. A drop in arterial pressure lowers coronary perfusion pressure, aggravating ischemia. Most with cardiogenic shock have multivessel CAD. Collateral vessel flow is sensitive to a fall in perfusion pressure. It is a tough sequence of events: lower coronary perfusion pressure, further ischemic injury and depression of LV function in a stuttering, progressive fashion.

Shock usually develops during the first 3 days after MI, and is present in only 10% at the time of hospital admission. Loss of muscle at the edge of the infarct zone may have a role in the genesis of LV failure. Muscle in this watershed, peri-infarct zone is dependent on collateral flow and may be viable (and salvageable) in the early hours of infarction. With low perfusion pressure, it becomes a late casualty.

The hemodynamic definition of cardiogenic shock includes persistent hypotension with systolic blood pressure less than 80 mm Hg, low cardiac index (cardiac output corrected for body surface area < 1.8 L/min/m^2), and elevated LV filling pressure (pulmonary wedge pressure >18 mm Hg). Most with shock and elevated filling pressure also have pulmonary congestion. The bedside diagnosis is fairly certain when there is low blood pressure, pulmonary edema and clinical evidence of poor perfusion (cool clammy skin, low urine output, and altered sensorium).

Those with shock with a first MI are usually having a large anterior MI. Small infarction may cause LV failure when there has been previous LV injury; remember that LV injury is cumulative. Shock is more common in older patients and those with multivessel CAD, and both indicate a worse prognosis. The incidence of shock was reduced by about 50% in placebo-controlled studies of thrombolytic therapy. GUSTO-1 found less shock and heart failure with rt-PA, which opens arteries faster than streptokinase. Angioplasty is faster and better than rt-PA, and is thus the best therapy for preventing cardiogenic shock.

The only effective treatment for cardiogenic shock is immediate reperfusion. The SHOCK trial tested immediate angioplasty for those with early cardiogenic shock.[18] There was no survival benefit at 1 month, but the 6-month survival was better with angioplasty. The survival benefit was limited to patients less than 75 years old. The 1-month mortality of younger patients was 41% with angioplasty, compared with 57% with medical therapy (this is a bad disease). I would suspect a better outcome with present techniques including stenting and more effective treatment of the no-reflow phenomenon.

For angioplasty to work it must be applied immediately. The best results are realized by those with good reperfusion within 4 hours of the onset of MI, although minimal benefit is possible up to 12 hours.[18] Thus, a clinical diagnosis of probable cardiogenic shock is an indication for immediate cardiac catheterization and stenting. It is needed even if the patient has received thrombolytic therapy.

While moving toward the cath lab, supportive measures to maintain blood pressure and distal perfusion include catecholamine therapy. Dobutamine is the first choice; it is a pure inotropic agent with few noncardiac effects and low arrhythmogenic potential. Dobutamine may be added to dopamine. When each drug is given at rates as high as 7.5 µg/kg per minute, cardiac output and blood pressure rise without an increase in LV filling pressure. At doses above 10 μg/kg per minute, the selective actions of both drugs disappears, and they work as pure vasoconstrictors.

Intra-aortic balloon pump (IABP) counterpulsation is usually started in the catheterization laboratory. It raises cardiac output, lowers afterload while raising blood pressure, and improves coronary perfusion pressure. The 40-mL sausage-shaped balloon inflates in the descending aorta during diastole, displacing its volume into the distal circulation, including the coronary arteries (most coronary blood flow takes place during diastole). At a heart rate of 100 beats per minute, this means boosting cardiac output by almost 4 L per minute. While the IABP is an effective supportive therapy, it is useless unless there is successful reperfusion. A classic study of cardiogenic shock from the 1970s—pre angioplasty—showed a short-term hemodynamic benefit with IABP counterpulsation, but a 91% 1-year mortality.[19] Many of these patients became balloon-dependent. They were fine while the pump was working, but slipped back into shock when it was turned off.

Right Ventricular Infarct Syndrome

This usually complicates inferior MI, because the proximal RCA supplies branches to the RV (see Figure 4.3). Almost one half of patients with inferior MI have demonstrable RV dysfunction, but hemodynamically significant RV failure occurs in less than 10%. This small group has right heart failure (peripheral edema and jugular venous distension without pulmonary congestion), and when severe, can have hypotension, a form of cardiogenic shock.

LV filling pressure may be in the normal range, but this may be misleading, because LV preload may actually be low. Abrupt dilatation of the ischemic RV is limited by the rigid pericardium, and increased pressure in the pericardial space is transmitted to the LV. A common physical finding is pulsus paradoxus, falsely suggesting tamponade. With animal models of RV infarction, hemodynamics improve when the pericardium is opened, relieving pericardial crowding. Excessive fluid loading may increase pericardial pressure, further limiting diastolic filling of the heart.

Many patients with RV infarction have coexisting LV dysfunction and require an elevated LV filling pressure—above 15 to 18 mm Hg—to maintain stroke volume. LV dysfunction is severe enough in some that shock is the result of both RV and LV failure.

ST-segment elevation in both inferior leads (II, III, and aVF) and V_1 suggests RV infarction (the infero-posterior MI pattern). More specific is ST-segment elevation in lead V_{4R}, a right precordial lead in the V_4 position. Although most with this finding do not develop shock, the echocardiogram commonly shows dilatation of the right atrium and RV, and reduced RV contractility. The echocardiogram is also useful as it excludes pericardial effusion and tamponade as the cause of pulsus paradoxus. Right heart catheterization confirms the diagnosis with elevation of right atrial pressure, but minimal or no elevation of pulmonary artery diastolic pressure or pulmonary wedge pressure (e.g., LV filling pressure).

The RV infarction syndrome is prevented by early reperfusion. It is one reason that large inferior MI is an indication for reperfusion therapy. Even late angioplasty/ stenting has been recommended for patients with the RV infarction syndrome. Perhaps because wall RV wall tension is lower, late reperfusion therapy is more effective for RV than LV infarction—at least the rate of progression of injury seems less rapid.

The initial supportive treatment for hypotension is volume expansion. As long as there is no pulmonary congestion a fluid challenge is safe, giving 200 mL normal saline per hour (or more) for a couple hours. If this does not correct hypotension, the patient needs hemodynamic monitoring with a pulmonary artery catheter. It is important to keep the pulmonary wedge pressure below 20 to 22 mm Hg to avoid pulmonary congestion. A threshold level of fluid replacement is commonly reached, above which blood pressure and cardiac output no longer increase. At this point, increased pericardial pressure is limiting both RV and LV filling, and further fluid resuscitation will add little relief.

Intravenous nitroglycerin may aggravate hypotension because it reduces venous return to the heart. On the other hand, arterial vasodilators may help, as lowering left atrial and pulmonary artery pressures reduces RV afterload. When there is LV as well as RV dysfunction, dobutamine is indicated. Improved contractility of the interventricular septum boosts RV stroke volume.

Refractory hypotension often improves with the IABP, particularly for those with LV dysfunction. In addition, balloon pumping improves coronary perfusion pressure, augmenting interventricular septal performance. Spontaneous recovery of RV function is common, and there is less chance of balloon dependence than there is with cardiogenic shock caused by LV injury.

Patients with RV dysfunction do poorly with bradycardia. For this reason, the threshold for treating bradyarrhythmias with AV sequential pacing is lower.

Many with RV dysfunction have spontaneous improvement within 2 to 4 days. But it can be a serious illness, and the mortality rate with RV infarction plus shock is 40%. Without shock it is less than 10%. Chronic right heart failure with peripheral edema is rare in survivors. This favorable long-term outlook is attributed to good collateral circulation and the favorable oxygen supply-demand profile of the RV. Lower right heart diastolic pressure favors the transfer of coronary blood flow from the LV to the RV via collateral vessels.

Nevertheless, suspicion of the RV infarction syndrome, especially with hypotension, is an indication for urgent angioplasty during the early course of inferior MI.

Congestive Heart Failure

Patients with pulmonary congestion during the course of acute MI have a much higher mortality risk (note Killip's classification, Table 5.1). Early reperfusion therapy has been shown to save LV myocardium and lower the chance of subsequent heart failure.

The cause of LV dysfunction after MI is loss of contractile units. Occlusion of a large artery supplying a large myocardial region will have a greater influence on

LVEF than occlusion of a smaller side branch. In addition, ischemia increases myocardial stiffness, and diastolic dysfunction adds to elevated pulmonary wedge pressure and congestion.

Infarct expansion may contribute to LV dysfunction. During the week after STEMI, necrotic muscle softens and becomes mushy. This leads to bulging of the infarct zone, with expansion and thinning of the LV wall. It is most common with anterior infarction. The most extreme form of infarct expansion is the formation of an LV aneurysm, where there is bulging of the apex during systole.

Short of aneurysmal bulging, there is a change in the shape of the LV apex after anterior MI. It loses its normal elliptical, football shape, and becomes rounded, or mushroom-like (Figure 5.8).

As healing take place, scar is laid down in the mold provided by the altered infarct zone, resulting in a permanent alteration in shape. At that point the shape of the infarct zone is cast in scar. This change in LV geometry has a negative effect on LV function. The radius of curvature of the LV is increased. Because of the Laplace relationship (wall tension = pressure × radius), increased radius means an increase in wall tension. This has a negative effect on myocardial energetics, as wall tension is a determinant of myocardial oxygen demand (MVO_2). In addition, the bulging segment absorbs some of the contractile energy of the LV that would otherwise have gone toward ejection of blood.

Early reperfusion therapy preserves some muscle within the infarct zone and tends to prevent infarct expansion. When viewed in the operating room, the reperfused infarct zone has a marbled appearance, with patches of normal tissue mixed with injured muscle. This may explain an improvement in clinical course despite only minimal improvement in LVEF after reperfusion. Saving enough muscle to prevent infarct expansion may also prevent heart failure.

Afterload reduction therapy with ACE inhibition also prevents infarct expansion after anterior MI. It should be started early, the first day after MI if the blood pressure is stable (Table 5.7).

Ventricular Arrhythmias

It is important to distinguish between ventricular arrhythmias occurring during the early hours of infarction, and those that occur later (and are chronic). During the early hours of infarction, there is considerable electrical instability, and even a small MI can cause VT or VF. With recovery, LVEF may be normal and the long-term prognosis, good. I tell students that resting tachycardia after MI indicates a worse prognosis than VT or VF during the early phase. Resting tachycardia is a marker of low LVEF, and the early electrical storm is not.

On the other hand, complex ventricular arrhythmias in late-hospital phase of MI, days later, are limited to those with large infarction and low LVEF. These patients with ischemic cardiomyopathy have a poor prognosis. Their leading cause of death is VF (e.g., sudden cardiac death [SCD]). Studies in the 1970s found that the best predictor of complex ventricular arrhythmias was low LVEF, and the best predictor of low LVEF was complex ventricular arrhythmia 1 week after infarction.

The association is so tight that it is unnecessary to get a 24-hour monitor as a screen for SCD. An echo measurement of LVEF is enough. LVEF above 40% to 45% means low risk.

For decades we chased ectopy with drug therapy. Then the Cardiac Arrhythmia Suppression Trial (CAST) tested whether suppressing premature ventricular contractions (PVCs) lowers the risk of SCD in post-MI patients with low LVEF. The surprising result was an increase in SCD with antiarrhythmic drug therapy, even though Holter monitoring showed suppression of PVCs. The proarrhythmia effect of the drugs apparently outweighs the arrhythmia suppression effect.[20] (CAST was among the earliest multicenter trials in the era of evidence-based medicine.)

CAST also suggested a disconnect between the generation of PVCs, and the degeneration of ventricular ectopy to VF and SCD. This is further supported by studies showing that beta blockade after MI prevents SCD, but does not suppress PVCs.[21] Membrane active antiarrhythmic therapy is no longer prescribed for suppression of ventricular arrhythmias after MI; beta blockade is.

The MADIT II trial has changed the approach to SCD after MI: it is now device-based.[22] This randomized study compared conventional medical therapy with prophylactic automatic implantable cardioverter-defibrillator (AICD) treatment. It enrolled 1232 patients greater than 1 month after MI who had LVEF 30% or less. There was no upper age limit, although 95% were under 75 years old. Most patients received beta-blockers. There was no electrophysiology (EP) testing. The 3-year mortality rate was 28% lower with AICD therapy. The benefit of AICD treatment was not influenced by other conditions (advanced age, hypertension, diabetes, left bundle branch block, etc.).

The survival curves of the two treatment groups did not diverge during the initial 9 months, and at 1 year, the survival benefit with the AICD was minimal. Thus, it would not make sense to recommend an AICD for a patient whose expected survival is less than 1 year (i.e., because of advanced heart failure or another illness). Furthermore, those getting the AICD experienced more deaths from heart failure. With an AICD, a patient struggling with advanced CHF may lose the option of dying quickly and peacefully.

Symptomatic VT may respond to beta blockade. When it does not, consider adding amiodarone.[23] This may be an issue in patients with an AICD, because suppression of VT prevents frequent shocks. Although amiodarone is not as effective as the AICD for preventing SCD, it may be considered for the patient with VT who is not a candidate for device therapy (or who declines it).

Do not forget that the serum potassium is inversely proportional to the risk of VT during and after acute MI.[23]

New Systolic Murmur after Myocardial Infarction

Ventricular septal defect (VSD)—The incidence of septal rupture with MI was 2% in the pre-reperfusion era.[24] It is much lower with reperfusion therapy. It is more common with advanced age, hypertension, and multivessel CAD. Like free-wall rupture, thrombolytic therapy longer than 12 hours from the onset of MI predisposes to rupture of the septum.

The anterior descending and posterior descending arteries encircle the septum in the interventricular groove, and supply perforating branches into the septum. Thus, either anterior or inferior MI may cause VSD. The prognosis is worse with inferior MI, possibly because the basal location of the defect makes surgical repair difficult. A VSD caused by anterior MI usually is positioned nearer the LV apex. Proximal septal rupture following anterior MI is rare, probably because ischemic injury that extensive causes cardiogenic shock and death before rupture occurs.

Most VSDs develop during the first week after MI, with about 20% in the first day. A loud, harsh, holosystolic murmur is the rule, and many have a palpable thrill. Biventricular failure follows. With medical therapy, half die within a week, and 85% by 2 weeks.

A new murmur after MI is an indication for an urgent echocardiogram. The Doppler study demonstrates flow across the ventricular septum and excludes MR. The next step is prompt transfer for angiography and surgery.

While transfer is in progress, supportive care includes catecholamine and diuretics if there is pulmonary congestion. The IABP is usually inserted in the catheterization laboratory. Right heart catheterization confirms the diagnosis; the oxygen saturation in the pulmonary artery is higher than that in the vena cava or right atrium (there is a step-up in saturation at the site of left-to-right shunting).

Immediate surgical repair is indicated for the usual patient who is dependent on catecholamine and/or IABP support. Success is predicted by good LV function and brief duration of shock. A rare patient stabilizes without developing shock. In such cases, surgery may be delayed 3 to 4 weeks, hoping that partially healed tissue will be easier to repair. During this time, careful monitoring is needed, because rapid deterioration is possible.

Mitral regurgitation (MR)—The incidence of papillary muscle rupture with MI is about 1%. Most cases occur with inferior MI (the papillary muscles are supplied by the right and circumflex arteries). Unlike VSD, a tiny MI may cause MR, because infarction of just the tip of the papillary muscle can lead to rupture. The patient may have single-vessel CAD.

The onset of heart failure and pulmonary congestion is abrupt. Many have a loud, holosystolic murmur, but no thrill (which suggests VSD). When cardiac output and blood pressure are low, the murmur may be soft. Unlike chronic MR, there is no S_3 gallop. In fact, there may be an S_4, because the LV tends to be stiff and is not dilated.

When heart failure unexpectedly develops in a patient with a small MI, get an echocardiogram to rule out MR, regardless of the presence or absence of a murmur.

The echo demonstrates MR and often a flail mitral leaflet. LV function may be near normal. The pulmonary wedge tracing typically shows a tall V wave, analogous to the V wave in the venous pulse in patients with tricuspid regurgitation.

When pulmonary congestion is severe and there is low cardiac output, nitroprusside and the IABP provide a bridge to surgery. Immediate surgery is indicated.

Rupture of the Free Wall of the Left Ventricle

This is the second most common cause of death in patients hospitalized with MI (following heart failure), and is responsible for 10% of deaths. It occurs 3 to 7 days after MI, at about the same time acute VSD or MR develop. At this time after MI, the necrotic infarct zone is softest.

Rupture commonly happens after a first MI, and it may occur with small or large infarction (usually anterior or lateral in location). Single-vessel CAD and poorly developed collateral vessels are common. Risk factors for rupture are late thrombolytic therapy (>12 hours from onset of MI), hypertension, and advanced age. But it is not uncommon in young patients. Steroids and nonsteroidal anti-inflammatory drugs (NSAIDs) may increase the risk of rupture. Because anti-inflammatory therapy may alter healing and scar formation, NSAIDs probably should be avoided for 1 month after MI.

The clinical picture is one of acute tamponade and death. I have observed a number of cases with the patient still in hospital, and the bedside diagnosis is obvious. A patient with a small, or at least an uncomplicated MI, collapses unexpectedly. There may be mild agitation or other vague symptoms just before cardiac arrest, but no chest pain. Telemetry shows no arrhythmia. After the patient arrests, there is pulseless electrical activity—sinus rhythm may persist for a couple minutes. Resuscitation is unsuccessful and there is no time for emergency surgery. This is a cause of SCD for which there is no effective treatment. There are a couple case reports describing emergency surgical repair and survival, but I have never seen it, even when the clinical diagnosis was made immediately.

Rupture may occur soon after discharge from the hospital, and often in a patient with a small MI. For this reason, I tell patients with small infarction that the prognosis is good—especially when LV function is normal—but also indicate that there are rare complications of MI during the first month that prevent a guarantee of a benign course.

Pseudoaneurysm

An occasional patient with rupture has it contained by adherent pericardium, probably because of inflammation of the infarcted muscle and overlying pericardium. There is usually clot within the bulging aneurysmal sack that provides support but that also may embolize. A pseudoaneurysm tends to have a narrow neck where it communicates with the LV, distinguishing it from a true aneurysm. It may enlarge and rupture. There are no clinical findings indicating its presence, and it is usually an unexpected finding on an echocardiogram. Because of possible rupture, surgery is indicated.

The rare person who survives LV rupture probably has it contained by inflamed pericardium. Extravasated blood is thus localized, preventing tamponade, circulatory collapse, and immediate death.

Long-Term Treatment After Myocardial Infarction

Risk Stratification and Treatment of Late Complications

A patient preparing to leave the hospital after MI faces the possibility of sudden death, recurrent infarction, heart failure, or peripheral embolization during the next year. The standard of care includes laboratory evaluation to identify those at high risk for these late complications, and treatment to prevent them.

Sudden cardiac death—A normal LVEF excludes a risk for VF and sudden arrhythmic death. The management of late ventricular arrhythmias has been reviewed. MADIT II recommends AICD therapy for those with LVEF 30% or less at least 1 month after MI. This has not yet been incorporated into practice guidelines, and it will be interesting to see how the expert panel deals with this expensive therapy.

While a normal *predischarge* LVEF indicates low risk, low LVEF measured early can be misleading. Remember that MADIT II enrolled patients at least 1 month after MI. Some with low LVEF immediately after infarction have improvement during the first month, especially those who had reperfusion therapy.[25]

Other techniques to detect high risk for SCD include Holter monitoring, the signal averaged ECG, heart rate variability monitoring, T-wave alternans, and EP testing (they are reviewed in Chapter 6). These test results tend to be abnormal when LVEF is low. They are less important for screening purposes than the measurement of LVEF.

The most important medical therapy to prevent SCD is beta blockade. Long-term therapy is indicated for all patients after MI, regardless of LV function.[26]

Residual or recurrent ischemia—Patients who have not had reperfusion therapy need screening for the possibility of a future ischemic event, regardless of how small or uncomplicated the MI. Most patients, especially those who are young, have coronary angiography at some point.

If that is not done, noninvasive testing is indicated. A meta-analysis showed that ST-segment depression on a stress ECG was 44% sensitive in predicting cardiac death or reinfarction within the year after MI. Sensitivity improved to 80% with the exercise perfusion scan, to 71% with a pharmacologic perfusion scan, to 62% with a stress echocardiogram, and to 55% with a pharmacologic stress echo.[27] Most studies of exercise testing excluded patients with large MI and low LVEF. In such cases, angiography is safer.

The timing of noninvasive study is a fielder's choice. Testing while the patient is in hospital, within 4 to 6 days of MI, rules out ischemia that may occur early after discharge. There is also the logistic advantage of getting it done while the patient is still in the hospital. But the early exercise test should not push the patient hard— the target heart rate in most studies of early testing was 120 beats per minute. Exercise tolerance is not tested with heart rate limited testing.

The advantage of later testing, more than 10 days after MI, is that exercise tolerance may be measured with a symptom-limited study. That is important, because poor exercise tolerance indicates poor prognosis, and is as sensitive for this purpose as ST-segment depression on the stress ECG. For the low-risk patient with a small MI, you may want the more complete study done 10 to 14 days after MI. If there is uncertainty about the patient's stability, a predischarge study would be preferred.

A positive exercise or imaging study result or clinical suspicion that the patient has not completed the MI are indications for angiography. Remember that thrombolytic therapy interrupts MI; the infarction is incomplete and further evaluation is mandatory. There are clinical trials that used stress imaging to test for residual ischemia after lytic therapy. In the United States, most patients have angiography, and it is best to accomplish it soon after thrombolytic therapy.[28]

Reocclusion of the infarct artery and extension of the MI has a bad effect on prognosis. Mortality and heart failure are both increased. This is true with clinically silent infarct artery reocclusion.

Remember that silent reocclusion of the infarct artery is common. In fact, it is probably more common than symptomatic reocclusion, because nociceptive dysfunction is the rule after prolonged ischemia.[17] While the patient is in hospital, consider recurrent ischemia if a patient has an unexplained increase in ventricular ectopy, has more elevation of ST segments on telemetry leads, or has unexpected or vague symptoms such as anxiety, restlessness, or dyspnea. Reocclusion of the infarct artery is promptly identified by re-elevation of ST segments on a 12-lead ECG. In the months after discharge, a decline in exercise tolerance or LVEF may be a consequence of reocclusion.

The medical therapy to prevent ischemia or reinfarction includes *beta blockade*.[26] We tend to overlook the value of beta blockade in the era of reperfusion therapy, yet it is still important and should be continued in all patients, even those who have had revascularization.

Antithrombotic therapy is equally important, and both aspirin and warfarin are effective. The WARIS II trial compared three therapies: 1) a combination of low-dose warfarin with an International Normalized Ratio (INR) of 2.0 to 2.5 plus aspirin 75 mg/day; 2) 160-mg aspirin/day, alone; and 3) higher dose warfarin (INR 3.0). The aspirin plus warfarin combination was better than aspirin alone or warfarin alone in achieving event-free survival—a live patient with no recurrent MI or stroke at 4 years—but with a threefold increase in bleeding when compared with aspirin alone.[29] While aspirin remains the standard therapy after MI, warfarin should be considered for those at high risk for thromboembolism, or for others with aspirin resistance.[30]

Left ventricular thrombus and peripheral embolization—Without anticoagulation, mural thrombus develops in as many as 20% with transmural MI; the incidence is higher with anterior MI and large infarction. Approximately 10% of patients with mural thrombus have peripheral embolization. Thus, the risk of embolization ranges from 1% to 4% after acute MI, depending on the size and location of infarction.

The pathogenesis of ventricular clot is complex. A loss of wall motion may lead to stagnation of blood in contact with the surface. Normal contraction keeps blood moving along. It has also been suggested that inflammation of the injured endocardium may be thrombogenic. LV thrombus is easily visualized on the transthoracic echocardiogram; transesophageal study is seldom needed. Embolization is more likely when the clot is mobile, protrudes more into the LV chamber, and is large enough to be seen in multiple echo views.

Heparin therapy during acute MI lowers the chance of LV thrombus by 50%. Early reperfusion therapy also lowers the risk. There has been a report of late thrombolytic therapy dislodging an LV thrombus.

Warfarin therapy is indicated for the prevention of embolization when the LV apex is akinetic, especially when thrombus is visible. It may be discontinued after 3 months if a follow-up echo shows no clot. With persistent thrombus, warfarin should be continued indefinitely. Practice guidelines also allow long-term anticoagulation for those with LV dilatation and low LVEF. As noted, full-dose warfarin, or lower dose warfarin plus aspirin are effective for prevention of ischemia.[29]

Preventing the progression of coronary artery disease—Therapies that promote survival with CAD have been reviewed in Chapter 4. Aspirin and beta-blockers both lower the risk of recurrent angina and infarction, and favorably influence survival. All patients should be on appropriate lipid-lowering therapy. All patients with vascular disease benefit from ACE inhibitor therapy (see Chapter 4). But prophylactic, long-acting nitrate therapy is of no benefit.[31]

Exercise Therapy and Activity after Myocardial Infarction

The training effect—The best measure of cardiovascular fitness is VO_2 max, or the maximum amount of oxygen the body is able to use during exercise. It can be measured with a metabolic stress test using a device that collects expired air and measures oxygen uptake, minute ventilation, and carbon dioxide production. VO_2 max is influenced by the oxygen-carrying capacity of blood, pulmonary function and the ability to raise cardiac output. When VO_2 max is reached, continued exercise becomes anerobic with an increase in CO_2 production and minute ventilation, but no further rise in VO_2.

Trained distance athletes have higher VO_2 max, partly the result of greater cardiac reserve. At any level of physical work VO_2 is accomplished with lower heart rate, blood pressure, and minute ventilation. That is a rough description of the training effect. With training, the body processes oxygen more efficiently. There is little measurable effect on myocardial contractility, at least at the levels of exercise commonly used in cardiac rehabilitation programs.

Cardiac rehabilitation—People with advanced heart disease can achieve the training effect. With regular aerobic exercise, VO_2 max increases, and for a given work load or VO_2, heart rate is lower. For a patient with severe exercise limitations, a small improvement in VO_2 max may be the difference between total disability and a return to simple activities outside the home.

Multiple studies have attempted to show a survival benefit of cardiac rehabilitation. These are tough studies to do. There is a lot of crossover of control patients into exercise programs, and the studies have been small with short-term follow-up. The magnitude of survival benefit in these studies has been similar to that found in beta-blocker trials, but with too few patients to achieve statistical significance.

Other benefits of supervised aerobic exercise include weight loss, better control of diabetes, increased high-density lipoprotein cholesterol, and lower triglycerides. The psychological effects are especially important. Patients in cardiac rehabilitation after MI or heart surgery recover more quickly.

Advanced heart disease is not a contraindication to supervised exercise. Those with low VO_2 max tend to have the greatest benefit in terms of percentage increase in exercise tolerance. We commonly send patients with low LVEF and mild heart failure to cardiac rehabilitation. The sicker patient requires closer surveillance, and this starts with a baseline stress test. Exercise-induced ischemia, arrhythmias, or severe dyspnea are contraindications to unsupervised training.

Supervised exercise training has a good safety record.[32] The risk of death is 1.3 per million patient hours of exercise, and of resuscitated cardiac arrest, 8.9 per million patient hours. High-risk patients should have ECG monitoring during exercise. This includes patients with severe LV dysfunction or heart failure, exercise-induced ischemia, ventricular arrhythmias, hypotension with exercise, poor exercise tolerance, or an inability to self-monitor heart rate. Those with a combination of ischemia and heart failure have the highest risk of complications. At the low level of exercise they can tolerate—below the ischemic threshold—they may not achieve a conditioning effect.

Counseling the Patient about Common Physical Activity

One advantage of stress testing is that it provides reassurance about the safety of exercise. Angiography provides an equally good assessment about the near-term risk of ischemia. When the risk of ischemia or ventricular arrhythmia is low, the patient may resume low-level activity and begin an aerobic exercise program 2 to 4 weeks after MI. For the first 6 weeks after MI, intense weight training should be avoided. Weight lifting raises LV afterload and blood pressure, and may adversely affect LV remodeling.

Many patients exercise at home, outside a supervised setting. This is safe for those who do not have exercise-induced ischemia or arrhythmias. They should exercise to a prescribed target heart rate. It helps to suggest limits on perceived exertion as well. I tell patients that as long as they can talk, whistle, or sing, they probably are not pushing too hard (at this level, heart rate is usually less than 130 beats per minute).

Heart rate 120 beats per minute—It is a number worth remembering. Ambulatory monitoring studies after uncomplicated MI have shown that activities such as walking up stairs and light housework push the heart rate to about 120 beats per minute, but rarely higher. That is one reason that predischarge exercise testing is performed with a target heart rate of 120 beats per minute. Tell the patient that it is a safety test. Reaching that level with no ECG abnormality or symptoms shows that walking up stairs, carrying a bag of groceries, sweeping the floor, or making a bed will be safe.

Sexual activity—The same monitoring studies found that sex with one's usual partner in a familiar setting pushes the heart rate to 120 beats per minute. On the other hand, sex in a novel setting or with an unfamiliar partner produces a much higher heart rate response. If the patient can walk up stairs without symptoms, routine sex is safe. Checking the pulse rate after sex provides useful objective information.

Patients who are being treated medically for angina with a history of MI may find that sublingual nitroglycerin just before sex prevents symptoms. There is no reason to recommend this when there is no angina.

Sildenafil (Viagra) is not contraindicated for the stable patient who is 4 to 6 weeks post-MI. Note the discussion in Chapter 4. It should not be prescribed for a patient receiving long-acting nitrates, or who is carrying nitroglycerin.

Return to work and disability evaluation—Those in sedentary occupations are able to return to work 6 weeks after an uncomplicated MI. The average patient returns to work in 2 to 3 months. Those doing heavy physical work require longer rehabilitation, and they should have exercise testing before they resume full activity. Occupation often figures into decisions about angiography.

Your attitude will have a major influence on return to work. When the doctor outlines a timetable and exercise strategy aimed at full recovery, the time off work is shortened. Earlier return has no adverse clinical effects, and there are financial and psychological advantages for the patient.

A number of patients seek *medical disability* after MI. The Social Security Administration has objective criteria for awarding benefits. The patient must have cardiac symptoms that limit activity (angina or symptoms of heart failure such as easy fatigue). In addition there must be objective evidence of disability: LVEF less than 30% in the case of heart failure, or evidence for ischemia with noninvasive testing or coronary angiography.

Driving—A patient with small, uncomplicated MI may safely drive within 3 weeks of MI. I advise against long trips that early, suggesting short and nonstressful outings until later in recovery. The patient with large or complicated infarction is best advised to wait 6 weeks before starting to drive. It is wise to exclude arrhythmias and ischemia before agreeing to resumption of vehicle operation, using the risk stratification approach described previously.

References

1. Phibbs BP. Perpetuation of the myth of the Q-wave versus the non-Q-wave myocardial infarction. J Am Coll Cardiol 2002;39:556–558.

2. Yousef ZR, Redwood SR, Bucknall CA et al. Later intervention after anterior myocardial infarction: effects on left ventricular size, function, quality of life and exercise tolerance: results of the Open Artery Trial (TOAT Study). J Am Coll Cardiol 2002;40:869–876.

3. Muller JE, Mittleman A, Maclure M, et al. Triggering myocardial infarction by sexual activity. Low absolute risk and prevention by regular physical exertion. Determinants of Myocardial Infarction Onset Study Investigators. JAMA 1996;275:1405–1409.

4. Zimetbaum PJ, Josephson ME. Use of the electrocardiogram in acute myocardial infarction. N Engl J Med 2003;348:933–940.

5. Newby LK, Alpert JS, Ohman EM, et al. Changing the diagnosis of acute myocardial infarction: implications for practice and clinical investigations. Am Heart J 2002;144:957–980.

6. Horwich TB, Patel J, MacLellan WR, Fonarow GC. Cardiac troponin I is associated with impaired hemodynamics, progressive left ventricular dysfunction, and increased mortality rates in advanced heart failure. Circulation 2003;108:833–838. (*Troponin T is elevated more commonly than Troponin I with renal insufficiency:* Freda BJ, Tang WH, Van Lente F, et al. Cardiac troponins in renal insufficiency: review and clinical implications. J Am Coll Cardiol 2002;40:2065–2071).

7. Torbicki A, Kurzyna M, Kuca P, et al. Detectable serum cardiac troponin T as a marker of poor prognosis among patients with chronic precapillary pulmonary hypertension. Circulation 2003;108:844–848.

8. Keeley EC, Boura JA, Grines CL. Primary angioplasty versus intravenous thrombolytic therapy for acute myocardial infarction: a quantitative review of 23 randomised trials. Lancet 2003;361:13–20.

9. Jacobs AK. Primary angioplasty for acute myocardial infarction—is it worth the wait? N Engl J Med 2003;349:798–800.

10. McKay RG. Evolving strategies in the treatment of acute myocardial infarction in the community hospital setting. J Am Coll Cardiol 2003;42:642–645. (*For further insight into delayed therapy and mechanisms of reperfusion see* Schomig A, Ndrepepa G, Mehilli J, et al. Therapy-dependent influence of time-to-treatment interval on myocardial salvage in patients with acute myocardial infarction treated with coronary artery stenting or thrombolysis. Circulation 2003;108:1084–1088.)

11. Berger PB, Ellis SG, Holmes DR, et al. Relationship between delay in performing direct coronary angioplasty and early clinical outcome in patients with acute myocardial infarction: results from the global use of strategies to open occluded arteries in Acute Coronary Syndromes (GUSTO-IIb) trial. Circulation 1999;100:14–20.

12. Kleiman NS. Combination therapy for acute myocardial infarction; Will it survive? J Am Coll Cardiol 2003;41:1261–1263. (*If thrombolysis is to be followed by stenting, best results come from stenting the same day rather than waiting a couple weeks:* Scheller B, Hennen B, Hammer B, et al. Beneficial effects of immediate stenting after thrombolysis in acute myocardial infarction. J Am Coll Cardiol 2003;42:634–641.)

13. Rezkalla SH, Kloner RA. No-reflow phenomenon. Circulation 2002;105;656–662.

14. Gibson CM. Has my patient achieved adequate myocardial reperfusion? Circulation 2003;108:504–507.

15. Gibson CM. Time is myocardium and time is outcomes. Circulation 2001;104;2632–2634. Also note, Kloner RA, Dai W. Glycoprotein IIb/IIIa inhibitors and no-reflow. J Am Coll Cardiol 2004;43:284–286.

16. Verstraete M. Third-generation thrombolytic drugs. Am J Med 2000;109:52–58.

17. Taylor GJ, Katholi RE, Womack K, et al. Increased incidence of silent ischemia after acute myocardial infarction. JAMA 1992;268:1448–1450. (*This includes a review of other studies that also describe silent infarct artery reocclusion after thrombolytic therapy. About 70% of patients who develop ischemia after reperfusion have no associated pain.*)

18. Webb JG, Lowe AM, Sanborn TA, et al. Percutaneous coronary intervention for cardiogenic shock in the SHOCK trial. J Am Coll Cardiol 2003;42:1380–1386.

19. Scheidt S, Wilner G, Mueller H, et al. Intra-aortic balloon counterpulsation in cardiogenic shock. Report of a co-operative clinical trial. N Engl J Med 1973;288:979–984.

20. Preliminary report: effect of encainide and flecainide on mortality in a randomized trial of arrhythmia suppression after myocardial infarction. The Cardiac Arrhythmia Suppression Trial (CAST) Investigators. N Engl J Med 1989;321:406–412.

21. Pratt CM, Waldo AL, Camm AJ. Can antiarrhythmic drugs survive survival trials? Am J Cardiol 1998;81:24D–34D. (*A review of all clinical trials of antiarrhythmic therapy after MI, including the beta blocker trials.*)

22. Moss AJ, Zareba W, Hall WJ, et al. Prophylactic implantation of a defibrillator in patients with myocardial infarction and reduced ejection fraction. N Engl J Med 2002;346:877–883.

23. Estes NA, Weinstock J, Wang PJ, et al. Use of antiarrhythmics and implantable cardioverter-defibrillators in congestive heart failure. Am J Cardiol 2003;91:45D–52D. *Also note,* Curtis AB. Filling the need for new antiarrhythmic drugs to prevent shocks from implantable cardioverter defibrillators. J Am Coll Cardiol 2004;43:44–46. And, Macdonald JE, Struthers AD. What is the optimal serum potassium level in cardiovascular patients? J Am Coll Cardiol 2004;43:155–161. (*During acute MI they recommend 4.5–5.5 mmol/L.*)

24. Birnbaum Y, Fishbein MC, Blanche C, Siegel RJ. Ventricular septal rupture after acute myocardial infarction. N Engl J Med 2002;347:1426–1432.

25. Hohnloser SH, Gersh BJ. Changing late prognosis of acute myocardial infarction: impact on management of ventricular arrhythmias in the era of reperfusion and the implantable cardioverter-defibrillator. Circulation 2003;107:941–946.

26. Gheorghiade M, Goldstein S. Beta-blockers in the post-myocardial infarction patient. Circulation 2002;106:394–398.

27. Weber KT. What can we learn from exercise testing beyond the detection of myocardial ischemia. Clin Cardiol 1997;20:684–696.

28. Guetta V, Topol EJ. Pacifying the infarct vessel. Circulation 1997;96:713–715.

29. Hurlen M, Abdelnoor M, Smith P, et al. Warfarin, aspirin or both after myocardial infarction. N Engl J Med 2002;347;969–974.

30. Becker RC. Antithrombotic therapy after myocardial infarction. N Engl J Med 2002;347:1019–1022.

31. Kanamasa K, Hayashi T, Takenaka T, et al. Continuous long-term dosing with oral slow-release isosorbide dinitrate does not reduce incidence of cardiac events in patients with healed myocardial infarction. Clin Cardiol 2001;24:608–614.

32. O'Connor GT, Buring JE, Yusuf S, et al. An overview of randomized trial of rehabilitation with exercise after myocardial infarction. Circulation 1989;80:234–244. (*An old report, but not dated. There have been no controlled trials of the effect of cardiac rehab on survival since the mid-1980s.*)

CHAPTER 6

CARDIAC ARRHYTHMIAS AND SYNCOPE

Abbreviations			
AF	atrial fibrillation	LVH	LV hypertrophy
AIVR	accelerated idioventricular rhythm	MI	myocardial infarction
		PAC	premature atrial contraction
AV	atrio-ventricular	PAF	paroxysmal atrial fibrillation
CAD	coronary artery disease	PSVT	paroxysmal supraventricular tachycardia
DC	direct current		
ED	emergency department	PVC	premature ventricular contraction
EP	electrophysiology		
ICD	implantable cardioverter-defibrillator	RA	right atrium
		RV	right ventricle
IHSS	idiopathic hypertrophic subaortic stenosis	SA	sinoatrial
		SCD	sudden cardiac death
INR	international normalized ratio	VA	ventricular arrhythmia
LA	left atrium	VF	ventricular fibrillation
LV	left ventricle (ventricular)	VT	ventricular tachycardia
LVEF	left ventricular ejection fraction	WPW	Wolff-Parkinson-White

Supraventricular Arrhythmias

Sinus Rhythms and Sinus Arrhythmia

*S*inus bradycardia—a rate less than 60 beats per minute—is usually an indicator of normal cardiac function, and rarely causes symptoms. It is common in trained athletes and active young people. Illnesses that may cause sinus bradycardia are hypothyroidism and the sick sinus syndrome. Sleep apnea is a common cause; during hypoxia the rate may slow. This is a common cause of long pauses in patients who are in sinus rhythm. On the other hand, it is common for the heart rate to slow during sleep, and when a 24-hour monitor flags a spell of bradycardia, check the time it occurred. Drugs are a common cause of sinus bradycardia, usually beta-blockers, diltiazem, and verapamil. This may limit the dose that can be tolerated, although a rate in the low 50s (beats per minute) without symptoms is no reason to back away from the medicine.

The key question for the patient with sinus bradycardia with an otherwise normal ECG is "Do you have dizzy spells, or have you blacked out?" In the absence of these symptoms, and especially if exercise tolerance has not changed, further cardiac evaluation is rarely necessary.

Sinus tachycardia may or may not be a benign rhythm, depending on the clinical setting. It is the normal response of a healthy person to exercise, stress, or excitement. On the other hand it may point to noncardiac conditions such as anemia, thyrotoxicosis or fever. Arteriovenous malformation is a rare cause, the fast rate suggesting high-output heart failure.

Sinus tachycardia in a patient with heart disease often indicates decompensation. After myocardial infarction (MI) it is a marker of low left ventricular ejection fraction (LVEF), and it also indicates a poor prognosis with congestive heart failure. Interestingly, ventricular fibrillation (VF) in the early hours of MI may occur with a small infarction, where LVEF is little affected and long-term prognosis is good. Thus persistent sinus tachycardia in a patient with a history of MI indicates a worse prognosis than VF at the onset of MI. Students and house officers commonly miss the significance of this arrhythmia.

Sinus arrhythmia and an irregular pulse occasionally prompt a cardiology referral. It is a benign rhythm that reflects normal cardiac function. The ECG shows normal P waves and PR interval, with variation in the R-R interval. It is a parasympathetic (vagal) rather than a sympathetic phenomenon. With inspiration and increased venous return to the heart, stroke volume rises. The vagus is activated and the rate slows for a couple beats, although without a change in cardiac output (recall that cardiac output = heart rate × stroke volume). During expiration there is a decrease in venous return to the chest and heart, and withdrawal of vagal tone leads to a temporary increase in heart rate. Again, cardiac output remains stable.

Changes in sympathetic tone also affect heart rate, but this system responds more slowly, over a period of seconds. Increased rate with exercise, stress, or pain— the fight or flight response—reflects a rise in serum catecholamines, which have a brief half-life. But it is not that brief. The catecholamine effect is too long to produce a beat-to-beat variation in rate. That is a parasympathetic function.

The normal response to poor LV function and reduced cardiac output is to shut down the parasympathetic system and to increase sympathetic tone. In addition to increased rate, there is a loss of respiratory variation in vagal output, and the rhythm becomes more regular. Thus, an absence of sinus arrhythmia is a marker of LV dysfunction. This has been found to be clinically useful after MI. Heart rate variability can be measured, and its loss indicates low LVEF and poor prognosis (vide infra).

Premature Atrial Contractions

Premature atrial contractions (PACs) are usually easy to recognize, as the QRS complex is narrow (that is to say, the right and left ventricles are activated simultaneously). An abnormal P wave may be seen before the QRS, possibly distorting the T wave of the preceding beat.

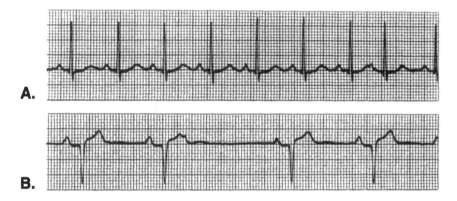

Figure 6.1 Two patients with premature atrial contractions (PACs). **A:** An ectopic P wave is seen before the premature QRS. **B:** Blocked PAC, causing a pause. The ectopic P wave is seen as a distortion of the preceding T wave. This is a common cause of pauses. In most cases, the ectopic P wave is harder to see; look for subtle changes in the preceding T wave. (Reproduced by permission from Taylor, GJ. *150 Practice ECGs*, 2nd ed. Malden, MA: Blackwell Science, 2002:21.)

A blocked PAC is a common cause of a pause on the ECG, and may be felt as a skipped beat by the patient. It happens when the PAC is early enough that the AV node is refractory and will not conduct it. The ectopic P may be buried in the preceding T wave, making it easy to miss. There usually is some distortion of the T wave, but it may be subtle (Figure 6.1). It is something to look for when telemetry shows pauses (especially on a board examination).

PACs are common in healthy people and do not indicate heart disease. If the ECG, cardiac history, and examination are normal, no further testing or treatment is necessary.

Paroxysmal Supraventricular Tachycardia

Paroxysmal supraventricular tachycardia (PSVT) is a rapid, regular rhythm with a rate of 120 to 200 beats per minute (Figure 6.2). Most cases are caused by reentry within the AV node. Reentry is a common mechanism of both atrial and ventricular tachyarrhythmias. Although often misunderstood, the concept is fairly simple (Figure 6.3). The reentrant focus is a region that is protected, or insulated, from surrounding tissue. Current enters one end of the focus and exits the other—conduction is unidirectional. Within the reentrant focus, conduction is slower than conduction in the surrounding tissue. By the time current exits the focus, the surrounding tissue has depolarized and has had time to recover. Thus, the current exiting the focus finds the surrounding tissue vulnerable and ready to be stimulated. This is just what happens, and a premature beat is generated. A reentrant focus in the atrium or AV node causes a PAC, and one in the body of the ventricle causes a premature ventricular contraction (PVC).

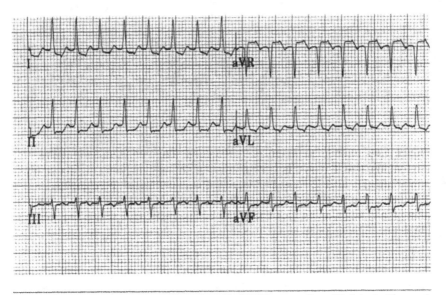

Figure 6.2 Paroxysmal supraventricular tachycardia (PSVT), a recording of limb leads. The rate is 200 beats per minute. The T waves appear distorted, and these distortions may be ectopic P waves. This episode lasted 45 minutes, plenty of time to get an ECG. (Reproduced by permission from Taylor, GJ. *150 Practice ECGs*, 2nd ed. Malden, MA: Blackwell Science, 2002:23.)

If the timing is perfect, the premature beat may slip back into the entrance of the reentrant focus, leading to another or even to a series of ectopic beats, usually at a rapid rate. A reentrant circuit is created.

AV nodal reentry is the usual mechanism of PSVT. Current exiting the focus passes normally through the common His bundle, and the resulting QRS complex is narrow. Again, the sequence of ventricular stimulation is normal with simultaneous LV and RV activation. PSVT is therefore a narrow QRS complex tachycardia (Figure 6.2). The P wave is often buried in the QRS; if it comes at the beginning or end of the QRS there may be subtle slurring of the complex or a pseudo R or S wave. Proof that this is from atrial depolarization requires comparison with a baseline ECG.

It is possible to have a wide QRS with PSVT. A patient may have coexisting bundle branch block with a wide QRS. Or a diseased infranodal conduction system may be stressed by the fast heart rate, causing aberrant conduction, usually right bundle branch block. The right bundle tends to be the weakest link in the conduction system, the first to fail at high heart rates. Right bundle branch block is a clue that a wide complex tachycardia is SVT with aberrancy rather than ventricular tachycardia (VT).

PSVT is a common arrhythmia in otherwise healthy young people. It is not dangerous, but it can be bothersome, causing palpitations, dizziness, and near syncope. Loss of consciousness is rare. Teach the Valsalva maneuver to terminate spells, although

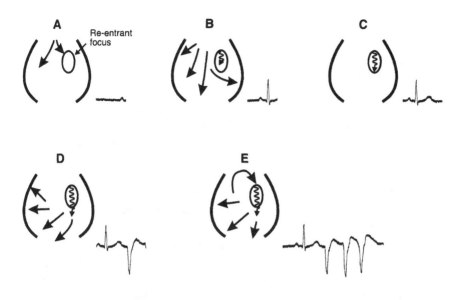

Figure 6.3 Reentry. Follow the sequence of events. **A:** The wave of depolarization comes from above (the atrium in the case of atrial arrhythmias, the ventricle in this case of ventricular reentry). **B:** As current moves through the myocardium, it also enters the reentrant focus, a region that is insulated from the surrounding tissue. **C:** Depolarization of the surrounding myocardium happens quickly, but conduction through the reentrant focus is slow. **D:** By the time current exits the reentrant focus, the surrounding tissue has been repolarized and is *vulnerable*. That is to say, it can be stimulated. This produces the *ectopic beat*. **E:** If the timing is perfect, current from the ectopic beat reenters the protected focus, travels through it, and again finds the surrounding tissue vulnerable when it exits. A circuit is established and the result is repetitive ectopic beats. Characteristics of the reentrant focus that makes this possible: (1) Insulation from the surrounding tissue, (2) unidirectional conduction, and (3) slow conduction. (Reproduced by permission from Taylor, GJ. *150 Practice ECGs*, 2nd ed. Malden, MA: Blackwell Science, 2002:22.)

many patients with palpitations will have learned it on their own. When PSVT occurs infrequently and spells are brief and easily terminated, other therapy may be unnecessary. Drugs that slow AV conduction may control symptoms, including beta-blockers, verapamil, diltiazem, or digoxin.[2] Intravenous adenosine, a strong AV node blocker, is used to interrupt the tachycardia in the emergency department (ED).

When symptoms are frequent and not easily controlled, catheter ablation of the reentrant focus is possible. Many patients find an electrophysiology (EP) cure preferable to life-long drug therapy. EP testing is needed to map the site of reentry. An ablation catheter is placed next to the reentrant focus, and radiofrequency energy is applied to create a mild burn that permanently interrupts conduction through it. (The intensity is about like sunburn; I reassure patients that we do not smell burning flesh or smoke in the catheterization laboratory.)

Preexcitation

Preexcitation is the archetypal reentrant rhythm, and the most common form is the Wolff-Parkinson-White (WPW) syndrome. The mechanism is described in Figure 6.4. Normally, there is a layer of connective tissue separating the atria and ventricles that serves as insulation, preventing free passage of neural impulses between upper and lower chambers. The AV node is the normal passage through this insulation. Slow conduction (the duration of the PR interval) through the AV node allows time for atrial systole to complete ventricular filling before ventricular systole.

The preexcitation syndromes occur because of an additional "defect" in the insulation between atria and ventricles. This defect is called a *bypass tract*. As the wave of depolarization passes through the atria, it leaks through the bypass tract as well as through the AV node.

Conduction through the bypass tract is usually faster than AV node conduction. As current exits the bypass tract it stimulates the ventricle—the ventricle is preexcited. An instant later, current exits the AV node and also stimulates the ventricle. The ventricular complex originating from two sites is a *fusion beat*. The QRS is wider than normal and starts earlier after the P wave, so the PR interval is short. The initial slurred portion of the QRS caused by preexcitation of the ventricle through the bypass tract is the delta wave (Figure 6.4).

A bypass tract can conduct both antegrade and retrograde. A PAC that finds the accessory pathway refractory may pass through the AV node, capture the ventricle, conduct retrograde through the accessory pathway, and establish a reentrant circuit. Because antegrade conduction is through the AV node, the reentrant rhythm looks like PSVT with a narrow QRS complex. A reentrant circuit moving in the opposite direction—retrograde through the AV node and antegrade through the accessory pathway—produces a wide QRS complex because the sequence of ventricular activation is abnormal. The resulting wide complex tachycardia looks like VT.

How can you tell whether the wide complex tachycardia is ventricular or supraventricular? At times you cannot, just from the ECG. The clinical setting helps. A young patient with a history of palpitations, no previous heart disease, and no alteration of consciousness is more likely to have PSVT with bypass tract reentry. An older patient with syncope or near-syncope plus a history of heart failure or MI should be treated assuming a diagnosis of VT. When in doubt, it is hard to go wrong treating an unstable patient with wide complex tachycardia as probable VT. DC cardioversion is appropriate.

A diagnosis of PSVT caused by preexcitation affects drug therapy. Digoxin should be avoided because it shortens the refractory period of the accessory pathway and blocks the AV node. If the patient has atrial flutter or fibrillation, these actions may favor antegrade conduction through the accessory pathway and lead to an unusually rapid ventricular rate. Verapamil, diltiazem, and beta-blockers may do the same thing. On the other hand, membrane active antiarrhythmic drugs

Preexcitation of the left ventricle through a bypass tract

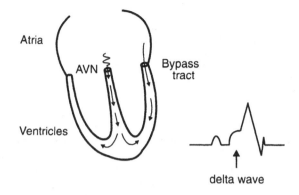

Two patterns of supraventricular tachycardia

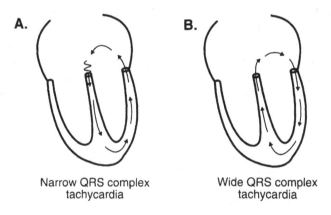

Narrow QRS complex   Wide QRS complex
tachycardia   tachycardia

Figure 6.4 Pre-excitation (or the Wolff-Parkinson-White syndrome). This cartoon illustrates the changes caused by a bypass tract between the atria and ventricles. The tract is located on the LV side and near the mitral valve in this particular patient, but bypass tracts may be located at any site where the atria and ventricles come into contact. Simultaneous activation of the ventricles via the bypass tract and the AV node produces a fusion beat. Conduction through the bypass tract is faster than through the AV node. Early activation of the ventricle produces the delta wave and makes the PR interval appear short. A reentrant circuit can develop between the bypass tract and the AV node, resulting in supraventricular tachycardia. There are two possibilities. **A:** The reentrant circuit moves antegrade through the AV node, retrograde through the bypass tract. The sequence of ventricular activation is therefore normal, and the QRS is narrow. **B:** The reentrant circuit is directed retrograde through the AV node and antegrade through the bypass tract. Because activation of the ventricles originates from the lateral wall of the LV, the QRS complex is wide. (Reproduced by permission from Taylor, GJ. *150 Practice ECGs*, 2nd ed. Malden, MA: Blackwell Science, 2002:27.)

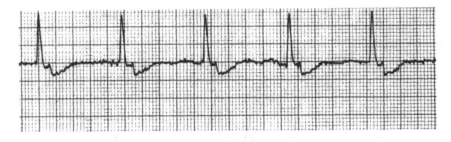

Figure 6.5 Nodal (or junctional) rhythm. The retrograde P wave distorting the T wave is prominent in this example. Usually it is more subtle and it may be absent. Even without retrograde P waves, the diagnosis of junctional rhythm may be made when the rate is regular, is less than 100 beats per minute, and there are no P waves. The QRS is usually narrow. (Reproduced by permission from Taylor, GJ. *150 Practice ECGs*, 2nd ed. Malden, MA: Blackwell Science, 2002:24.)

tend to slow accessory pathway conduction; intravenous procainamide is a good choice if drug therapy is needed.

Membrane active drugs have been used for long-term management as well. However, catheter ablation of the accessory pathway usually works and is preferable to life-long drug therapy. Radiofrequency energy is delivered to the region of the bypass tract, burns it and leads to a scar that plugs the defect in the insulation.

Nodal (Junctional) Rhythm

It is recognized by the absence of P waves preceding the QRS, and the rhythm is regular (Figure 6.5). A retrograde P wave following the QRS may be apparent, or it can be buried in the T wave. As the impulse originates above the bifurcation of the bundle branches, the QRS complex is narrow.

When the rate is less than 60 beats per minute, the mechanism usually involves depression of the sinus node, with the AV node assuming the role of dominant pacemaker—it is an *escape rhythm*.

An accelerated nodal rhythm above 100 beats per minute is less common. The mechanism is increased automaticity rather than reentry; the rate of spontaneous depolarization of the AV node increases and it become the dominant pacemaker. This is a common digitalis toxicity rhythm. It may also complicate MI. Inferior MI is the usual setting, and nodal rhythms have no influence on prognosis. On the other hand, nodal tachycardia with anterior MI is a marker of large infarction and therefore, poor prognosis.

Regardless of etiology, nodal rhythms are generally benign, transient, and seldom require treatment. As with all tachyarrhythmias, do not overlook hypokalemia or hypomagnesemia as a cause. Symptomatic tachycardia may be controlled with beta-blockers, diltiazem, or verapamil. Hemodynamic instability or tachycardia induced ischemia are indications for cardioversion.

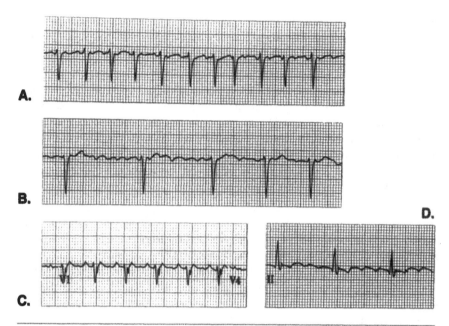

Figure 6.6 Four patients with supraventricular tachyarrhythmia. **A:** Atrial fibrillation (AF) with rapid ventricular response; at higher rates, the variation in the RR interval seen with AF may be subtle. **B:** AF with a controlled ventricular response; with drug therapy to slow AV node conduction, the ventricular rate is kept between 80 and 100 beats per minute. In this case, you can see the fibrillation waves as coarse undulation in the baseline. **C:** Atrial flutter with 2:1 block; note the sawtooth pattern in the baseline. **D:** Atrial flutter with 4:1 block; the flutter waves are more obvious. (Reproduced by permission from Taylor, GJ. *150 Practice ECGs*, 2nd ed. Malden, MA: Blackwell Science, 2002:25.)

Atrial Fibrillation

The incidence of atrial fibrillation (AF) has increased over the past couple decades, for reasons that are not certain, and it is the most common arrhythmia requiring treatment. After chest pain, AF is the most common indication for cardiology consultation in my hospital. It is more common in older people; by age 80 the chance of developing it is approximately 3% per year.[2]

Pathophysiology

AF may be paroxysmal (PAF) or chronic (Figure 6.6). Patients with structurally normal hearts may have AF with electrolyte abnormalities (commonly low potassium or magnesium), alcohol intoxication (the holiday heart syndrome), or thyrotoxicosis. PAF is usually idiopathic, although many with this condition have hypertension, raising the possibility of elevated left atrial pressure.

Lone AF refers to the patient with no structural abnormalities on an echocardiogram (and that means a completely normal study), *plus no history of hypertension.* I emphasize hypertension, because many do not realize that it is a marker of stroke risk for those with AF, just like left atrial enlargement or mitral valve disease. Lone AF is actually uncommon, accounting for less than 3% of those with new AF.[2] But they are worth identifying, as theirs is a benign illness if they are 60 years old or younger; those who are older have a higher risk of stroke.

One of my mentors (J. O'Neal Humphries) taught that AF is a disease of the left atrium (LA), while flutter comes from the right atrium (RA). In 1975, he based this on the clinical observation that AF tends to complicate left heart disease, and flutter, right heart disease. AF occurs with mitral valve disorders, hypertension, and LV dysfunction, and LA enlargement on the echocardiogram is common. Cor pulmonale is a frequent cause of atrial flutter. More recently, EP has confirmed this observation. Ablation of fibrillation is an LA procedure, and flutter, an RA procedure.

Idiopathic AF begins with an atrial myopathy, possibly localized atrial myocarditis. Elevation of C-reactive protein has been observed. A change in autonomic tone or an increase in atrial wall tension with elevated LV afterload (e.g., hypertension) may trigger the arrhythmia. Most AF is reentrant. There are multiple, small reentrant circuits acting simultaneously. It is a chaotic situation, with these circuits colliding and either enhancing or extinguishing each other. AF develops if there is enough enhancement, which also means that a critical mass of atrial tissue is supplying reentrant circuits.

LA contractility and function decline with prolonged AF, but there may be recovery after cardioversion.[2] This mechanical recovery is usually delayed, and may take weeks. That may be the mechanism for thromboembolism in the weeks after cardioversion.

We previously believed that recovery of atrial contraction eliminated the risk of thromboembolism. This turns out to be wrong. An important discovery of the AFFIRM trial is that the risk of stroke persists *long-term* after restoration of sinus rhythm.[3] About half of the strokes in this study occurred after patients stopped warfarin. This suggests a different pathogenesis of thromboembolism: No longer do we assume that clot is the direct result of the atrium quivering. Rather, the atrial myopathy—perhaps inflammatory—is responsible for clot formation, just as it is the cause of AF, and the myopathy persists after cardioversion (Figure 6.7).

Note the parallel with ventricular arrhythmias (VAs); ventricular myopathy is the usual cause of VF, just as atrial myopathy causes AF.

Evaluation of New Atrial Fibrillation—Hospitalization is not necessary for the hemodynamically stable patient with few symptoms. Those who are symptomatic with a rapid rate, or patients with congestive heart failure who have a higher risk of thromboembolism require inpatient stabilization and evaluation. An occasional patient who presents immediately after the onset of AF is admitted for early cardioversion.

The laboratory evaluation includes thyroid function studies. Recall that George Bush had AF complicating thyrotoxicosis while he was president. In fact, AF is the most common presenting symptom in older people with hyperthyroidism. Other signs of thyrotoxicosis may be absent, and a nursing home patient may even appear

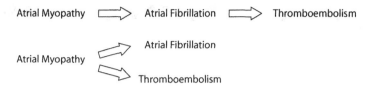

Figure 6.7 Our understanding of the pathogenesis of thromboembolism and stroke with atrial fibrillation (AF) has evolved. Top: We previously believed that the atrial abnormality (myopathy) caused AF, which, in turn, caused clot formation and embolism. This implies eradication of stroke risk with correction of the arrhythmia. Bottom: Based on the AFFIRM trial, it seems that the atrial myopathy can cause clot formation in the absence of AF. AF is a marker of atrial myopathy, and thus indicates increased risk of thromboembolism. The AFFIRM has shown that anticoagulation is needed after successful cardioversion of AF.[3]

sluggish or depressed. This apathetic hyperthyroidism is usually discovered during the evaluation of new AF.

In addition to an ECG, the other cardiac test that is needed is an echocardiogram. You are looking for structural abnormalities including valvular disease, LA enlargement, and LV disorders (hypertrophy, enlargement, or dysfunction). The house staff often wants to screen for coronary artery disease (CAD) (inexperienced doctors believe that CAD causes most heart problems). Although AF may complicate a large, acute MI, asymptomatic CAD rarely causes it. A history and ECG are adequate workup.

Routine pacemaker interrogation may unexpectedly detect paroxysmal AF. The device clinic may report episodes of mode switching—the dual chamber pacer stops pacing the atrium (the DDD mode), and instead paces just the ventricle (the VVI mode). The usual cause of this is AF and loss of the P wave. An asymptomatic patient with mode switching probably should be on warfarin (vide infra).

Treatment

There are three treatment issues that are addressed simultaneously at the time of initial evaluation: anticoagulation, rate control, and cardioversion.

Anticoagulation—*The first goal of therapy is to protect the brain.* Although the mortality rate with AF is above normal, I generally tell patients that AF itself is not dangerous. I know patients who have done well with AF for decades. Morbidity and mortality are usually the result of embolic stroke or the heart condition that caused AF.

Both paroxysmal and sustained AF may cause stroke, and the benefits of anticoagulation are similar with both clinical patterns. The risk of stroke is related to the company AF is keeping. Here is the approximate risk for subsets of patients with AF:

- Mitral stenosis—an 8% per year risk of stroke;
- AF without mitral stenosis—1% to 6% per year risk of stoke

Table 6.1 Anticoagulation for Atrial Fibrillation		
Age (yr)	Risk Factors for Stroke*	Therapy
≤65	None	Aspirin 325 mg or none (there is no proof that aspirin is better)
66–75	None	Warfarin or aspirin 325 mg (it depends on the risk of warfarin—if the bleeding risk is low, warfarin is preferable)
All ages	One or more	Warfarin unless there is a definite contraindication.

*Risk factors for stroke in patients with AF: mitral stenosis, hypertension (even if it is controlled with treatment), previous stroke or transient ischemic attack, heart failure or LV dysfunction, age >75 years. (To these some would add a "structurally abnormal" heart on the echocardiogram, including left atrial or ventricular enlargement, and left ventricular hypertrophy.)

Modified with permission from Falk RH. Atrial fibrillation. N Engl J Med 2001;344:1067–1078. Copyright © 2001, Massachusetts Medical Society. All rights reserved.

- Within this range, the incidence of stroke is higher for those with these risk factors: advanced age, hypertension, prior stroke or transient ischemic attack, diabetes and LV dysfunction (Table 6.1). These risk factors are additive.
- Lone AF: a patient younger than 60 years old with a normal echocardiogram and no hypertension—1% per year risk of stoke.

Based on data from multiple anticoagulation trials, we can identify patients at highest risk for stroke, and they require anticoagulation (Table 6.1). There are intermediate risk patients, age 65 to 74 with no other risk factors for stroke, who do not have to be on warfarin. It's a fielder's choice, and the patient should be in on the decision. The EP community (arrhythmia specialists) leans toward treatment. If the bleeding risk is low and the patient is highly motivated, consider warfarin. But if there is any reason to avoid warfarin therapy—including a history of medicine noncompliance, or an increased chance of falling or bleeding—aspirin is adequate.[3]

Another gray zone in decision-making is the patient with a first, brief episode of AF. Many of them will have no recurrence. The usual evaluation of new AF is warranted, including electrolytes, thyroid function studies and an echocardiogram. A correctible cause of AF would argue against warfarin therapy, as would a normal echocardiogram. Findings indicating an increased risk of recurrence, such as marked LA enlargement or mitral valve disease, would weigh in favor of anticoagulation.

Warfarin should be given to bring the international normalized ratio (INR) to 2.0 to 3.0, and this reduces the risk of stroke by approximately 85%. Aspirin is half as effective, and the optimum dose is uncertain. One placebo controlled trial showed a 42% reduction in stroke with 325 mg aspirin per day, while another using lower dose therapy showed no significant benefit over placebo.[2] Current practice guidelines make no definite recommendation about the dose of aspirin, but I currently prescribe 325 mg/day. As noted above, cardioversion does not eliminate the need for anticoagulation.

Direct thrombin inhibitors will probably replace warfarin. Ximelagatran has been found superior for prevention of stroke, with no increase in bleeding.[4] About 6% had elevation of liver enzymes within 6 months of starting therapy, and which resolved when it was stopped (liver function probably will need to be monitored). Dabigatran is a newer agent that may have less hepatotoxicity. Unlike the vitamin K inhibitor, warfarin, the dose of thrombin inhibitors is the same for all patients. Monitoring the prothrombin time is unnecessary. (This story may parallel that of low-molecular-weight heparin, which has been found superior to unfractionated heparin for most clinical indications. I expect that the direct thrombin inhibitors will consistently outperform warfarin.)

Control of hypertension lowers the risk of thromboembolism. The left atrial appendage is the usual location of thrombus. It is not visible on the transthoracic echocardiogram, but is easily seen using transesophageal echo. (Examination of the appendage is the major reason for doing transesophageal echo in a patient with AF.) There is a correlation between uncontrolled hypertension, stasis of blood in the atrial appendage and thrombus formation.[5] Flow velocity in the atrial appendage improves with control of blood pressure.

Clinical trials of anticoagulation have also found that the risk of bleeding on warfarin is higher with uncontrolled hypertension. Regulation of anticoagulation should be accompanied by vigorous efforts to control blood pressure.

A related issue is *cognitive dysfunction* in some patients with AF. While this occurs in a minority, elderly patients and those with uncontrolled hypertension or CAD are at higher risk. This is another reason for careful attention to blood pressure control and anticoagulation. Cerebral micro-infarction may be the mechanism.

Surgical isolation of the left atrial appendage may prevent thromboembolism. The indication would be AF plus another risk factor for stroke, and a contraindication to anticoagulation. Presently, a number of surgeons routinely amputate the appendage for stroke prophylaxis during heart surgery, especially mitral valve surgery. Thoracoscopic removal of the atrial appendage is being studied as a new approach to prophylaxis.[5] Early experience indicates that it is safe, but its effectiveness in preventing stroke has not been tested in controlled trials.

Rate control—An occasional elderly patient has abnormal AV node conduction, and has a ventricular rate less than 100 beats per minute, but most with AF require an AV nodal blocking agent to prevent tachycardia. Beta blockade, diltiazem, verapamil, and digoxin are effective, and your first choice may be influenced by other conditions. For example, if the LVEF is low, beta blockade would be good to begin with, followed by digoxin. Verapamil should be avoided because it depresses contractility enough to precipitate congestive heart failure.

Another patient with LV hypertrophy (LVH) and/or hyperdynamic contractility might avoid digoxin, and instead benefit from either beta blockade or verapamil. Difficult hypertension may respond to either a beta-blocker or diltiazem, or both.

Patients with healthy AV nodes commonly require two drugs to control the ventricular rate. The goal of therapy is prevention of excessive tachycardia during normal activity, not just at rest. Adding a second drug is preferable to pushing the first to toxicity. At an earlier time we were taught that there was no upper limit to the dose of digoxin that could be given: the proper dose was the one that controlled the rate. In current practice it is more common to treat the patient with digoxin 0.25 mg/day, and titrate the dose of another drug to reel in the heart rate (the safety of digoxin and use of the digoxin level is discussed in Chapter 1). With this approach, the non-cardiac toxic effects of digoxin (nausea, anorexia, malaise, or visual changes) are avoided, particularly in elderly patients. Note that adding verapamil to digoxin raises the serum digoxin level, and toxicity is possible. Be prepared to lower the digoxin dose.

I find that house officers often prescribe an inadequate dose of diltiazem. Unless the patient is small or elderly, start with 240 mg/day. Although diltiazem depresses LV contractility slightly, it is rare to see worsening heart failure. As noted, verapamil may precipitate congestion in a person with low LVEF and should be avoided.

An occasional patient has persistent tachycardia despite multiple drug therapy. Rate control may be achieved using *AV node ablation*, a relatively straightforward EP procedure. Destruction of the AV node creates complete heart block. This requires a permanent ventricular pacemaker for the patient with persistent AF, or a dual chamber pacer with paroxysmal AF. Atrial pacing may prevent recurrence of AF. In practice, the pacer is inserted first, and the ablation is done a week or more later. All rate lowering drugs may then be stopped. There is speculation that some patients feel better with a more regular rhythm, as well as a slower rate, and ventricular pacing provides that.

For a short time after AV node ablation there is an increased risk of sudden death. This is attributed to the slower heart rate leading to a lower threshold for torsades de pointes (see subsequent discussion). To avoid this complication, the pacemaker is initially set at 90 beats per minute, and the rate is cut back a few months later.

Cardioversion—The indication for cardioversion is symptomatic AF (intolerable fatigue, worsening CHF, etc.). Approximately two thirds of patients have spontaneous return of sinus rhythm within a day of developing AF. After that the rate of conversion is low, and beyond 1 week of persistent AF spontaneous conversion is rare. A patient with a first, brief episode of AF may not have a recurrence, and drug therapy to prevent AF is unnecessary.[2] If the first episode is complicated by stroke, or there are multiple risk factors for stroke, anticoagulation is needed, and some would argue for antiarrhythmic therapy hoping to suppress AF.

Practice guidelines allow cardioversion without anticoagulation if the duration of AF is less than 48 hours—using either drugs or DC countershock.[2] Watch for that to change, as a number of those involved in anticoagulation trials feel that the window of safety is shorter. When the duration of AF exceeds 2 days, the patient should be anticoagulated and have a therapeutic INR (>2.0) for 3 weeks before cardioversion. An alternative to this is to perform a transesophageal echocardiogram. If no left atrial thrombus is present, immediate cardioversion is safe, and it should be followed by anticoagulation.[6]

Table 6.2 Antiarrhythmic Drugs for Converting Atrial Fibrillation or Maintaining Sinus Rhythm

Drug	Dose* Cardioversion	Maintenance	Comment
Flecainide Propafenone	300 mg 600 mg	50–150 mg bid 150–300 mg every 8 hrs	Class IC drugs used for PAF with a normal echocardiogram and no CAD. Oral dosing only.†
Sotalol	‡	120–160 mg bid	Hospitalization needed when starting Rx.
Dofetilide	0.5 mg bid (lower the dose with renal insufficiency)		Hospitalization needed when starting Rx.
Amiodarone	1200 mg IV over 24 hours	600 mg/day for 2 wks, then 200–400 mg/day	Slow onset of cardioversion, even with IV therapy. It is a beta-blocker, and slows the ventricular rate. Hospitalization not required when starting.
Ibutilide	1 mg IV over 10 min to start. For cardioversion only (see package insert for weight adjustment).		Contraindicated with hypokalemia, long QT interval or history of torsades de pointes.

IV, intravenous; bid, twice daily; PAF, paroxysmal atrial fibrillation; CAD, coronary artery disease; Rx, treatment.
*Oral dose unless otherwise noted.
†Hospitalization is not required when starting class Ic drugs or raising the dose, as long as LV function is normal and there is no history of ventricular arrhythmia.
‡Sotalol has a low conversion rate and is not used for that purpose.
Modified with permission from Falk RH. Atrial fibrillation. N Engl J Med 2001;344:1067–1078. Copyright © 2001, Massachusetts Medical Society. All rights reserved.

The drugs that block the AV node and slow the ventricular rate are no more effective than placebo in converting AF to sinus rhythm. However membrane-active antiarrhythmic drug therapy increases the chance of cardioversion by 90%.[2] Drugs that are commonly used for AF are summarized in Table 6.2. Amiodarone, ibutilide, and dofetilide may be used for cardioversion. Sotalol has poor conversion efficacy, but is effective for maintenance of sinus rhythm. Hospitalization and monitoring for 48 to 72 hours after starting drug therapy has been recommended for all of the drugs except amiodarone.[2]

The class IC agents, flecainide and propafenone, are approved for those with lone AF. That excludes their use in patients with structural heart disease, including CAD. But do not write them off. There are few side effects with these medicines.

Amiodarone is as effective as the IC agents for cardioversion, but it is a bit slower and conversion may not take place until 24 hours after starting it.[7] Consider this strategy for a patient with AF who has been anticoagulated for the requisite 3 weeks: begin a loading dose of amiodarone as an outpatient. Have the patient come in 4 to 7 days later and if AF persists, go on with DC cardioversion.

For the patient who develops AF in hospital—particularly one with postoperative AF—intravenous ibutilide is fast acting and about 50% successful. If it does not work, it increases the chance of successful DC cardioversion. Do not forget to check electrolytes, including magnesium (the forgotten cation). Replacing potassium and/or magnesium may lead to cardioversion. If not, it will increase the effectiveness of drug or DC cardioversion.

After conversion, antiarrhythmic therapy increases the chance of staying in sinus rhythm (Table 6.2). This is not necessary with a brief, first episode that converts spontaneously. Although sotalol is not effective for cardioversion, it is for the purpose of maintaining sinus rhythm. The IC agents may be used when the echocardiogram is normal, and there is no CAD. Hypertension is not listed as a contraindication to propafenone or flecainide.[2] Quinidine is approved for AF suppression, but I rarely use it. When a patient has been on it for years, I do not stop it. Quinidine should be avoided when there is LVH. Procainamide is not approved for AF.

Amiodarone is the most effective drug for maintaining sinus rhythm. It causes less proarrhythmia than other drugs, and may be used by those with depressed LV function (as can dofetilide).

Paroxysmal AF also responds to antiarrhythmic drugs. It may not be abolished, but the intervals between spells lengthen and there is symptomatic improvement. An advantage of sotalol and amiodarone is rate control in addition to prevention, so that when AF occurs it causes fewer symptoms.

"Sinus rhythm begets sinus rhythm." With suppression of AF, there seems to be a conditioning effect, and the atrium learns to stay in sinus rhythm. This is the rationale for implantable atrial defibrillator therapy, currently in clinical trials. An occasional patient stops having PAF with drug therapy, and there is a question about whether to stop the medicine. The trend is to continue anticoagulation if it is easily tolerated. Most would agree with a trial off antiarrhythmic drugs after the patient has had a number of symptom-free months.

Ablation—The EP team offers three approaches. The first is a palliative, rate control approach. Creation of complete heart block with AV node ablation plus ventricular pacing is commonly performed for persistent AF and an inability to control the ventricular rate with the usual drug therapy. This may be important for the prevention or correction of tachycardia-related cardiomyopathy (see Chapter 1). A regular rhythm may contribute to symptom relief, beyond the effects of rate control.

The second, and newest EP approach is curative, ablation of the reentry circuit(s) needed for the initiation and propagation of AF.[8] Most AF originates in the posterior LA, near the ostia of the pulmonary veins. Isolating the pulmonary veins with radiofrequency catheter-induced burn lines works in patients with PAF. Chronic AF does not respond as well. For this reason, the patient must have shown an ability to be in sinus rhythm. The Italian group with the largest experience has reported improved quality of life as well as reduced rates of stroke and cardiovascular death in a nonrandomized study comparing ablation with medical therapy.[9] In this study, ablation was offered to those with PAF with more than two previous ineffective trials of antiarrhythmic therapy, or more than two

AF-related hospitalizations in the previous 2 years, *or* at least 2 years of antiar-rhythmic drug treatment.

The third approach is the atrial cardioverter-defibrillator. The device monitors the atrial rate, and delivers DC countershock in the event of AF. Unlike the implantable ventricular defibrillator, it does not cardiovert at the onset of the arrhythmia. The patient is warned and has an opportunity to take medicine for pain before initiating the shock. The goal of defibrillation plus drug therapy is to train the atrium to stay in sinus rhythm. This seems to work, as the frequency of countershock therapy decreases with time.

Postoperative Atrial Fibrillation

This disorder develops in about 20% of patients after heart surgery, but it may occur after any large operation.[10] It may increase the length of hospitalization, and some have suggested an increased risk of perioperative stroke. Beta blockade and amiodarone have been shown to reduce the incidence of AF after heart surgery, but it is not clear that prophylactic therapy reduces length of stay or prevents other complications of surgery.[10]

Many with AF in the early postoperative period have hypomagnesemia, and this can develop after any major operation. The mechanism is uncertain, with some suggesting that "cut surfaces either soak up or weep magnesium." Correcting elec-trolyte abnormalities—usually magnesium and potassium depletion—is at least a physiologic approach to rhythm management. Aggressive prophylactic magnesium replacement has been shown to prevent AF in one small study, and there has been no study testing this plus drug therapy.

There are no clinical guidelines for the treatment of postoperative AF.[10] The gen-eral principles of management outlined previously apply. It often responds to amio-darone therapy. There is no reason to continue this long term, as a late recurrence of AF is uncommon. I have the patient stop the amiodarone at the 1-month visit.

Likewise, transient postoperative AF is not an indication for long-term antico-agulation. Warfarin should be considered for those at high risk for recurrence or thromboembolism (e.g., a history of recurrent AF, mitral valve disease, marked LV enlargement or dysfunction, prior thromboembolism). As noted previously, ampu-tation of the LA appendage at the time of surgery lowers the risk of thromboem-bolism.

Atrial Flutter

Although AF may develop in patients with atrial flutter, and vice versa, they are quite different in mechanism. AF involves multiple, small reentrant circuits, usually in the LA. Atrial flutter, on the other hand, is usually an RA macroreentrant rhythm.[11] That is to say, there is one, large circuit that involves most of the RA.

The recognition of atrial flutter is relatively easy (Figure 6.6). The rhythm is regular, and the atrial rate is close to 300 beats per minute. In the absence of AV node blocking agents, 2:1 AV block is common, and the patient has a rate of

150 beats per minute. When evaluating a patient at the bedside with abrupt onset of tachycardia that is regular and about 150 beats per minute, atrial flutter is a good guess. The ECG shows flutter waves.

Chronic atrial flutter is less common than AF. Acute onset of atrial flutter raises the possibility of a rise in RA pressure. For example, new flutter in an elderly, bedridden patient may be an early sign of pulmonary embolus. Atrial flutter often accompanies an exacerbation of obstructive lung disease, with hypoxia leading to a rise in pulmonary artery pressure. It may be resistant to drug therapy until the patient's pulmonary illness improves.

The drug therapy of atrial flutter and AF are similar, but not identical. Control of ventricular rate with AV node blockade is the same, requiring digoxin, beta blockade, diltiazem, or verapamil. Drugs for cardioversion of atrial flutter include ibutilide (best in the acute situation), amiodarone, and sotalol. Note that sotalol works for flutter, but is less effective for conversion of AF (Table 6.2).

Preventing a recurrence of atrial flutter requires preventing the premature atrial beat that precipitates it. Beta-blockers may work, although they are not useful for preventing AF. Also effective are the class IC drugs (flecainide and propafenone), sotalol and amiodarone. Associated obstructive lung disease may limit the use of beta-blockers.

A major issue is anticoagulation. Unlike AF, there are no clinical trials data to guide us. Observational trials suggest a risk of thromboembolism, though not as great as that with AF.[12] As with AF, there is a delay in a return of atrial contractility after cardioversion of atrial flutter, increasing the risk of thrombosis.[11] Most cardiologists apply the AF anticoagulation guidelines for those with chronic atrial flutter, or intermittent flutter with frequent recurrences.

Catheter ablation of atrial flutter is less complicated than AF ablation. The success rate is high, and the cure tends to be permanent. Radiofrequency burns are generated on the right atrial wall to interrupt the reentrant circuit. Because it is a right atrial procedure it is relatively safe; in general, left heart catheterization is riskier because of the chance of systemic thromboembolism, including stroke. Many think that catheter ablation should be first-line therapy for chronic atrial flutter, preferable to long-term drug treatment. Warfarin can be stopped 4 to 6 weeks after successful catheter ablation.[11]

Ventricular Arrhythmias and Sudden Cardiac Death

The clinical setting determines the prognosis in patients with VAs. Premature ventricular contractions, also called ventricular premature beats (VPBs), may be a normal variant in the healthy person with normal LV function.

During the acute phase of MI, a complex VA, including VT or VF, may occur with minimal LV injury. The reentrant arrhythmia is purely an electrical event. Long-term prognosis—assuming successful treatment of the arrhythmia—is not influenced by the electrical storm during the acute phase of infarction.

But later after MI, complex VAs occur in those with severe LV dysfunction and thus indicate poor prognosis. On telemetry or a 24-hour monitor, *complex VA* is defined as a high frequency of paired PVCs or runs of VT (at least three PVCs in a row). The evaluation and treatment of VAs after MI—which applies to all with chronic CAD—are reviewed in Chapter 4.

Pathophysiology

Isolated PVCs may come from either an automatic focus or a reentrant focus. Repetitive ectopic beats, with three or more defined as VT, are usually reentrant. That is the case with VF.

An exception to this is accelerated idioventricular rhythm (AIVR). The rate may be less than 100 beats per minute, and the ectopic focus works like a fixed rate pacemaker. When the sinus rate falls below the ectopic rate, it takes over and paces the ventricle until the sinus rate increases. AIVR commonly occurs at the moment of reperfusion during MI, and is a reliable indicator of successful reperfusion therapy. It is considered benign as it rarely degenerates to VF. It tends to be transient, and is resistant to antiarrhythmic drug therapy (which is not needed, in any event).

VAs are aggravated by low potassium or magnesium. Community-based studies of sudden cardiac death (SCD) have found that it is more common in patients taking diuretics, and that hypokalemia is often present in those who are resuscitated. These patients also have other heart disease, usually LV dysfunction, but the electrolyte abnormality is the last straw. The first step with all rhythm consults is to check electrolytes, an easy problem to fix. Plus, if you do not fix electrolyte abnormalities, the arrhythmia will be tough to control. Do not overlook magnesium; like potassium it falls with diuretic therapy and also is low after surgery (the earlier discussion of postoperative AF applies to VAs after surgery).

The most common cause of VF and SCD is ischemic cardiomyopathy. Nonischemic dilated cardiomyopathy is responsible for about 10% of cases. Although reentry is the mechanism of VF with both diseases, there are some differences. For example, with ischemic heart disease electrophysiologic testing using paced PVCs provoke VT in those at high risk for SCD. Inability to provoke VT indicates low risk. Electrophysiologic testing is not as reliable for those with dilated, nonischemic cardiomyopathy.

Laboratory Evaluation

Evaluating LV function is the first step.[13] Normal LVEF usually excludes VAs as a cause of palpitations, dizziness, or syncope. We used to do a lot of 24-hour ECG (Holter) monitoring. As a screening test, complex VAs on a Holter monitor indicate a risk of SCD. With normal LVEF, the yield is low and there is little need for 24 hour monitoring. A monitor may be used to confirm complex VAs in the patient with a depressed LV, but the findings usually do not change management.

There are other noninvasive tests that identify high risk of complex VAs. All of them also are markers of low LVEF in patients with prior MI, and they add little to the assessment of risk once LV dysfunction is identified.[13] The *heart rate variability* (HRV) test measures sinus arrhythmia (discussed previously). Beat-to-beat variation with respiration is governed by vagal activation. With LV dysfunction, the parasympathetic system shuts down, and the heart rate becomes more regular. Most ECG machines are now equipped with a program that allows measurement of R-R intervals. It collects a 5- to 10-minute rhythm strip and computes the mean R-R interval; the standard deviation of that mean is a measure of HRV. HRV is low in patients with MI and low LVEF, and indicates a higher risk of SCD.

The *signal-averaged ECG* (SAECG) is a computer summation of a large number of QRS complexes that allows measurement of late potentials, low voltage deflections at the end of the QRS. This small current may come from the reentrant focus itself (Figure 6.3). When present, late potentials correlate with complex VAs after MI, a higher risk of SCD, and—of course—low LVEF.

Microvolt *T-wave alternans* is the latest of the noninvasive studies, and is of special interest as it may identify those with nonischemic cardiomyopathy who are at risk for SCD.[13] Other predictors of SCD work well for those with prior ischemic injury, but have not been as effective in nonischemic cardiomyopathy. The beat-to-beat alteration in T-wave morphology reflects an alteration in action potential voltage in the failing heart. When present, this heterogeneous pattern of repolarization is the substrate for reentry. Heterogeneity is ubiquitous in those with previous infarction, as normal muscle is interspersed with scar. When present in those with nonischemic cardiomyopathy, an uneven pattern of repolarization is probably the result of scar or fatty tissue infiltration, and it identifies a subset of patients at risk for reentry.[14] T-wave variation is measured both at rest and during low-level exercise, as it is more prominent with a rise in serum catecholamines. Beta blockade may abolish it.

Electrophysiology testing has been the best test for a risk of SCD, but it may be less important in the future. As noted, stimulation of the ventricle—introducing PVCs to provoke VT—is sensitive and specific for the risk of SCD for those with ischemic cardiomyopathy. However, the MADIT-2 trial found that patients with previous MI and LVEF of 30% or less had improved survival with an implantable cardioverter-defibrillator (ICD), and this study did not use EP testing.[15] Because of this, many think that an expensive EP study is unnecessary. The counter-argument is that a negative EP study may identify a subset of patients with low LVEF who have a low risk of SCD, and who do not need an ICD. Thus, the role of EP testing is unresolved at this time. Remember that provocative testing is less sensitive for those with nonischemic cardiomyopathy.

Wide QRS tachycardia—A patient with a rapid rhythm that looks like VT, and who has low blood pressure and altered sensorium probably is having VT. Immediate cardioversion is needed. It makes no difference whether the rhythm is ventricular or supraventricular with aberrant conduction—hemodynamic instability mandates cardioversion.

There are some patients with wide QRS complex tachycardia who are clinically stable. They may not feel well, and may be aware of palpitations, but the blood

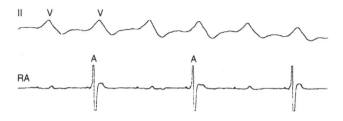

Figure 6.8 Wide QRS tachycardia; simultaneous recording of ECG lead II and a right atrial (RA) electrogram. There is not an atrial (A) beat with each ventricular complex (V). AV dissociation indicates VT. (Reproduced by permission from Taylor, GJ. The Cardiology Rotation. Malden, MA: Blackwell Science, 2001:232.)

pressure is stable. How do you determine the origin of the rhythm? Tachycardia stresses the infranodal conduction system, and may cause *aberrant conduction*—a bundle branch block pattern with a wide QRS. It is important to distinguish between atrial and ventricular rhythms, as the prognosis and treatment are different. If it is supraventricular, it is relatively benign and AV nodal blockers and/or membrane active antiarrhythmic agents may work. But if it is ventricular, there is a risk of SCD and defibrillation may be needed. As noted, the right bundle is the weakest link in the conduction system, and right bundle branch block suggests aberrant conduction. Monophasic QRS complexes are more likely ventricular in origin.

To make a certain diagnosis requires identification of the relationship of P waves and QRS complexes. A rare patient has identifiable P waves on the surface ECG, and if they are not related to the ventricular (QRS) rhythm, VT is the diagnosis. More commonly, an intracardiac electrogram is needed to magnify the P waves (Figure 6.8). If it shows AV dissociation, the rhythm is VT. If there is a P wave before or after each QRS complex, it is supraventricular tachycardia.

Another way of guessing the origin of the arrhythmia is the clinical setting. An older person with a history of MI or heart failure or known LV dysfunction is more likely to have VT. SVT is the likely arrhythmia in a young patient with no history of ventricular disease (i.e., MI). In such cases, a history of palpitations is common.

Treatment of Ventricular Arrhythmias and the Prevention of Sudden Cardiac Death

We no longer try to suppress PVCs or even nonsustained VT with drug therapy. The routine use of beta-blockers after MI lowers the risk of SCD and thus is considered prophylactic. Because beta blockade improves survival with nonischemic cardiomyopathy, it is possible that it prevents VF in this population (see Chapter 1).

Before the MADIT-2 trial, symptomatic or sustained (>30 seconds) VT was the indication for EP testing for those with CAD. Inducible, sustained VT was the indication for ICD therapy. Following MADIT-2 the indication for ICD insertion is previous MI, LVEF of 30% or less and an expected survival greater than 1 year.[15]

I argue against ICD therapy for some with end-stage ischemic cardiomyopathy. MADIT excluded patients who were functional class 4. Furthermore, there was no survival benefit for the first 10 months after ICD insertion, suggesting little point to this treatment for a patient who is not expected to live 1 year. A desire to die peacefully should be an important consideration for the end-stage patient. More than half who die with ischemic cardiomyopathy die suddenly (it is often what happens when an old person "dies in his sleep"). The ICD prevents that. Rather than dying quickly, the patient is subjected to painful shocks, and is more likely to die with pump failure symptoms. Practice Guidelines list "terminal illness" as a contraindication to ICD therapy.[16]

ICD therapy effectively prevents SCD, with 95% survival at 5 years. It works by first identifying a rapid rate. The device usually incorporates a pacing function to overdrive-pace the ventricle and interrupt the VT circuit. If this does not work, the ICD fires, delivering 15 to 20 J to the endocardial surface. It records the rhythm before firing. Later interrogation of the device allows documentation of the arrhythmia. The longevity of the battery is related to the number of discharges, and with average use they tend to last 4 to 8 years before a battery change is needed.

The engineering has become quite sophisticated.[16] An ICD may include a dual chamber pacemaker. This may be considered for the patient who could not tolerate an adequate dose of beta-blocker because of slow rate. Pacemakers are not inserted just for this indication, but if an ICD is required, there is no additional risk with one that also paces. A number of our patients with heart failure are getting units that provide biventricular pacing and an ICD (see Chapter 1).

Many patients with an ICD also are on VT-suppressing drug therapy. Although drug therapy does not improve survival when used alone, preventing VT at least prolongs battery life and prevents ICD discharge, which is painful.[16]

Management after ICD discharge—Between 50% and 70% of patients with an ICD have it fire within 2 years of insertion.[17] Most of these are appropriate, a single shock converting VT. A smaller number have ICD storm, with multiple discharges. This can be a response to recurrent VT, but an occasional patient is shocked because of AF (misdiagnosed by the ICD as VT), or lead fracture, or electromagnetic noise leading to malfunction.

There are a few things to check after ICD discharge (Table 6.3). The first is to interrogate the unit to determine that discharge was an appropriate response to VT. If the patient has a history of intermittent firing, is clinically stable, and there are no other red flags (Table 6.3), hospital admission is not needed. Hospital admission is warranted when there is a change in the clinical pattern. This would include an increase in the frequency of discharge, ICD storm, or abnormalities that need correction (e.g., electrolyte abnormalities or a mechanical malfunction). Drug therapy may be adjusted to prevent VT, usually amiodarone and beta-blockers.[16]

Table 6.3 Management After ICD Discharg	
Steps	Comment
1. Interrogate the ICD	• Determine that firing was an appropriate response to VT • Exclude AF or PSVT as the inciting tachyarrhythmia • Detect unit malfunction
2. Exclude treatable cause of VT	• Low potassium or magnesium • Acute MI or unstable angina* • Proarrhythmia from antiarrhythmic drug therapy • Torsades de pointes with a long QT interval
3. Indications for hospital admission	• A broken ICD (lead fracture, etc.) • Frequent discharges (ICD storm) • Another medical condition that requires admission (MI or unstable angina, electrolyte abnormality, change in the arrhythmia, proarrhythmia, etc.)

ICD, implantable cardioverter device; MI, myocardial infarction; VT, ventricular tachycardia; AF, atrial fibrillation; PSVT, paroxysmal supraventricular tachycardia

*Acute ischemia causing increased VT frequency is an indication for aggressive evaluation, including angiography.

Do not forget the importance of correcting hypokalemia and hypomagnesemia; keeping the potassium 4.5 to 5.5 mEq/L has been suggested for patients with heart failure.[17]

It is important to emphasize that intermittent cardioversion of VT does not indicate a worse prognosis—it is just the machine doing its job. ICD storm with multiple discharges is painful, and may induce something akin to post-traumatic stress disorder. Careful debriefing of the patient and family may help to prevent this. Psychological assessment should be considered early to prevent anxiety disorders and avoidance behaviors.[17]

Driving after ICD placement—The American Heart Association currently recommends a 6-month wait before a patient resumes driving.[16] This restriction may not be consistent with the data, which show a low motor vehicle accident (MVA) rate among these patients.[18] In this relatively large trial, most patients who had a symptomatic arrhythmia did not have a MVA, but were able to control their vehicles. The annual risk of an MVA that could be attributed to an arrhythmia was 0.4%. Compare that with the 7.1% annual probability of MVA for all drivers in the United States. Nevertheless, the Heart Association guideline is still the 6-month wait, and your state may have requirements that you should be aware of.

Other Sudden Cardiac Death Syndromes

Long QT interval and torsades de pointes—This is a peculiar form of VT with wide polymorphic QRS complexes that become larger and then smaller as the axis shifts (Figure 6.9). It is like the QRS axis is turning about a point; hence, the ballet term "torsades de pointes." It is a triggered arrhythmia, not reentrant, that

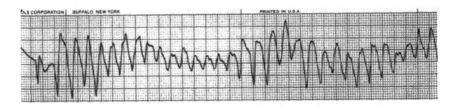

Figure 6.9 Torsades de pointes, an undulating, polymorphic VT in which the axis of each successive beat is different from that of the preceding one. (Reproduced by permission from Taylor, GJ. *150 Practice ECGs*, 2nd ed. Malden, MA: Blackwell Science, 2002:34.)

occurs in patients with QT interval prolongation (Table 6.4).[19] The first case I saw in the early 1970s was a patient with quinidine syncope who had been started on the drug for AF. At about that time I encountered another patient with intractable VT who had been on chronic tricyclic antidepressant therapy and had her first episode a couple days after starting antihistamines.

Table 6.4 Prolonged QT Interval*	
Familial	Jervell and Lange-Nielsen syndrome (congenital deafness, autosomal recessive) Romano-Ward syndrome (normal hearing, autosomal dominant)
Acquired (drugs)	Quinidine Procainamide and its metabolites Sotalol Amiodarone (uncommon) Disopyramide Phenothiazines and derivatives (including some antihistamines) Tricyclic antidepressants Erythromycin (especially when combined with antihistamines) Pentamidine Some antimalarials Cisapride (Propulsid)
Electrolyte abnormalities	Hypokalemia and hypomagnesemia (complicating diuretic therapy or extreme diets) Hypocalcemia (a less common cause of VT; the T wave is delayed but the T wave duration is not prolonged as it is with other causes of long QT)
Others	Acute myocardial ischemia Central nervous system lesions Hypothermia Bradycardia

*The conditions and drugs that cause QT prolongation and VT are synergistic. Thus, a patient who is on sotalol who develops low magnesium and potassium because of diuretic therapy may experience QT prolongation and torsades de pointes.

Torsades is thus a common form of proarrhythmia—or drug-induced VT—and it tends to develop early after starting a new drug. It is idiosyncratic rather than dose-dependent.[19]

Lability of the QT interval is a predictor of SCD in those with long QT. The QT interval may lengthen after a pause. Treatment may include increasing the heart rate with temporary pacing or with isoproterenol. This prevents pauses, and at higher rates the QT shortens. First line therapy for torsades is intravenous magnesium, which also shortens the QT interval. Other antiarrhythmic drugs are avoided. VT that is hemodynamically unstable requires DC cardioversion.

Proarrhythmia without QT prolongation—The class IC antiarrhythmic drugs, flecainide and propafenone, slow intraventricular depolarization and widen the QRS, but have little effect on repolarization (the QT interval). The mechanism of arrhythmia is reentry, and it is dose-dependent. This complication of therapy may be avoided by getting an ECG a couple weeks after starting therapy to check the QRS duration. QRS prolongation may be present only with exercise, and treadmill testing may be considered for the patient who is having spells.

Unlike torsades, which occurs soon after starting the medicine, this drug-induced monomorphic VT may occur late. VT is more common when LV function is depressed, so class IC drug therapy is limited to those with normal LVEF.

Arrhythmogenic right ventricular dysplasia—This rare familial disorder causes fatty infiltration of the right ventricle (RV), with some loss of muscle.[19,20] The ECG usually is abnormal with T wave inversion in precordial leads. The VT has a left bundle branch block pattern. The RV may appear abnormal on the transthoracic echocardiogram, and the MRI demonstrates increased thickness of the RV wall. The diagnosis is confirmed with endomyocardial biopsy.

VT may be prevented by beta blockade, class IC antiarrhythmic agents, calcium blockers, or amiodarone. Ablation of an arrhythmogenic focus has been described, but ICD therapy often is needed. Markers of poor prognosis include exercise induced VAs or syncope, a dilated RV and sustained VT.

Brugada syndrome—This is an autosomal dominant disorder that is characterized by ST-segment elevation right precordial leads (Figure 6.10). The heart is structurally normal, the workup for ischemia is negative, and electrolytes are normal.[21] The diagnosis of Brugada syndrome requires the ECG changes plus clinical evidence of VAs, or a family history of the syndrome.

It is a cause of SCD. The usual arrhythmia is polymorphic VT, which may degenerate to VF. SCD occurs most commonly in early morning hours, during sleep. The illness is endemic in southeast Asia, and more common in men at about age 40 (although cases have been reported at all ages, including infancy). SCD may be the initial symptom. VT may cause syncope, and most who develop VF have a history of syncope.

The molecular disorder is a defect in the membrane's sodium channel. Sodium channel blockers—including flecainide, procainamide, and ajmaline—cause a worsening of the right precordial ST segment changes. These drugs may also trigger VT.

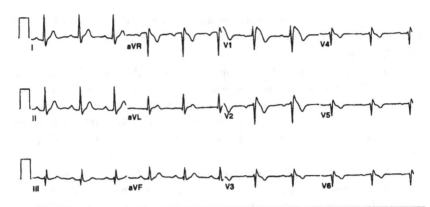

Figure 6.10 Brugada syndrome; unusual ST elevation in right precordial leads (usually V_{1-3}) that looks a bit like right bundle branch block. Normal QRS duration in limb leads excludes bundle branch block.

There are other possible causes of right-precordial ST elevation, and a drug challenge may be needed to make the diagnosis.[21]

Hypertrophic cardiomyopathy—Predictors of sudden death with hypertrophic cardiomyopathy include a family history of SCD and a history of syncope. SCD may be the presenting symptom. The severity of outflow tract obstruction is not related to arrhythmia or sudden death risk. Reducing outflow tract obstruction with alcohol infusion or surgical ablation has not been shown to lower the risk of death. There have been observational trials suggesting amiodarone may help those with documented VT, but the current approach is ICD therapy for high-risk patients.

SCD in young athletes—*Hypertrophic cardiomyopathy* is the most common cause.[22] Collapse and death often occurs during exertion. Outflow tract obstruction is worse when the LV is small, so a reduction in vascular volume—dehydration—may trigger SCD (see Chapter 2). Limiting water intake as an aid to conditioning—a common practice during spring training a couple decades ago—is clearly a bad idea.

A systolic murmur that is heard during the Valsalva maneuver suggests LV outflow tract obstruction (idiopathic hypertrophic subaortic stenosis, or IHSS). It would seem that checking for this on routine physical examinations would allow identification of the SCD candidate. However, this is usually a subtle physical finding that may or may not be present depending on the level of hydration during the examination. Sudden death in young athletes is rare enough that no one has suggested routine echocardiography screening in the United States.

An *anomalous coronary artery* is the second most common structural abnormality that causes SCD in young athletes. Usually the left main artery originates from the right sinus of Valsalva, then courses between the pulmonary artery and aorta. With exercise, the great vessels pinch the left main artery, creating ischemia. Consider it when there is a history of chest pain or syncope with exertion. Stress testing results may not be positive, because ischemia may be episodic. Transesophageal echo and

MRI are good noninvasive tests for this anomaly, and angiography is the next step. If there are symptoms, particularly VT, bypass surgery is indicated.

The variety of other cardiac conditions that may cause sudden death in young people include myocarditis, the Marfan's syndrome with rupture of an aortic aneurysm, long QT interval syndromes, occult mitral or aortic valve disease, infiltrative cardiomyopathies (i.e., cardiac sarcoidosis), dilated cardiomyopathy, a tunneled (bridged) coronary artery, and premature atherosclerotic CAD. There are non-cardiac causes that show up in most series, but account for small numbers of the deaths: drug abuse, asthma, heat stroke, and ruptured cerebral artery.

Commotio cordis is a recently described cause of death in young teenagers, just behind hypertrophic cardiomyopathy as a cause of SCD.[22] VT is caused by an apparently minor blow over the sternum, not severe enough to cause bruising or injure the ribs. For example, the shortstop is hit by a ground ball. Energy from the blow is transmitted to the heart, provoking VT and VF. Animal studies indicate that contact must just before the peak of the T wave, at the so-called vulnerable phase of repolarization. Mechanical energy creates an "R on T" PVC, which precipitates VT. This is truly a freak accident, as the vulnerable phase occupies just 1% of the cardiac cycle. Strategies to prevent it include softer baseballs, and chest protective devices for some youth sports (hockey, lacrosse, baseball).

The task of screening young athletes for SCD is a large one, because there are 8 million participants in organized sports in the United States.[22] Here is my recommendation: Listen to the heart squatting, then after standing for a minute—a new systolic murmur suggests IHSS. Ask specifically about syncope or near syncope, and check the family history for sudden death. If uncertain, get a 12-lead ECG (most with IHSS have some abnormality). If there is a systolic murmur, or if the ECG is not normal, order an echocardiogram.

Hypertrophic cardiomyopathy is the usual criterion for disqualification from high-intensity sport (that would not include golf or bowling). Exercise-induced VAs with any other condition would also contraindicate intense exercise. Myocarditis is an indication for temporary withdrawal from sports, with resumption based upon recovery. While there are no guidelines defining recovery, it would require the passage of time, normal LV function and sedimentation rate, and no symptoms with resumption of normal activity.

Bradyarrhythmias

Heart Block

The term *block* often confuses patients, not to mention medical students. We glibly refer to blocked arteries, valves and nerves, and these can be unrelated illnesses. The term, heart block, is usually reserved for nerve conduction disorders. It may occur at any level of the cardiac nervous system. Block is possible though uncommon within sinoatrial (SA) node, or in the body of the atrium. It is most common in the

AV node and the nerves below it. These infranodal nerves include the His–Purkinje system.

Blocked conduction may alter intervals on the ECG, and may cause bradycardia and syncope. When block is complete there is no transmission to distal structures, but the heart rarely stops. Instead, an auxiliary pacemaker below the level of block takes over. The intrinsic rate of the takeover pacemaker is progressively slower the farther it is from the SA node. Control of heart rate reminds me of the children's game, King of the Mountain. Pacers highest on the mountain, nearest the SA node, get the first chance to rule because they have the fastest rate of spontaneous depolarization. When the conduction beyond the pacer is blocked, those just below take over. As you go lower on the mountain, the pacers have a slower intrinsic rate. In addition, these lower level pacers are less influenced by the autonomic nervous system.

As an example, when complete block develops in the AV node, a pacemaker in the bundle of His, just below the node, paces with an intrinsic rate of 35 to 45 beats per minute (Figure 6.11). It would be hard to exercise with a rate that slow, but at that rate syncope is uncommon. If complete block occurs farther down, within the interventricular septum and beyond the division of the two bundle branches, the takeover pacer is in the body of the ventricles. The beat it generates looks like a

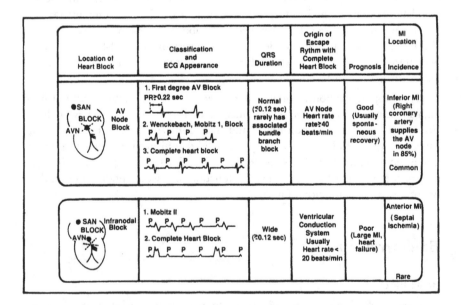

Figure 6.11 Heart block after MI. It is important to distinguish between block at the level of the AV node and block below AV node. The takeover pacemaker with AV nodal block has an adequate intrinsic rate and responds to atropine. Deep ventricular pacemakers that take over after infranodal block are less responsive and are too slow. (Reproduced by permission from Taylor, GJ. *150 Practice ECGs*, 2nd ed. Malden, MA: Blackwell Science, 2002:20.)

PVC, with a wide QRS. These deeper, ventricular pacers have a much slower intrinsic rate, occasionally as slow as 10 to 20 beats per minute. In this case, syncope and even sudden death are possible.

Furthermore, a takeover pacer in the body of the ventricle is unresponsive to the autonomic nervous system. A higher pacer, near the AV node, may respond to catecholamine stimulation with an increased rate of firing.

From this outline of general principles, you begin to see that the level of block determines prognosis, and identification of this level is critical.

First-degree AV block—The site of conduction delay is the AV node, and the PR interval is prolonged, measuring at least 0.22 seconds. Increased vagal tone, hyperkalemia, digitalis, diltiazem, verapamil, and beta-blockers all may slow AV conduction. It is common in elderly patients who may have a sick AV node with no associated CAD. Right coronary artery occlusion—acute inferior MI—may also cause first degree heart block, as the right coronary supplies the AV node (Figure 6.11).

Second-degree AV block—Second degree block is the failure of some beats to reach the ventricles—the ventricles are not activated. On the ECG there is a P wave that is not followed by a QRS complex.[23]

Second-degree block is classified as two types, *Mobitz I* or *II* (also called type I or II block). *Mobitz I block* occurs within the AV node, and is associated with the Wenckebach phenomenon. The dysfunctional node tires with each succeeding beat until it is so tired that a P wave is completely blocked. On the rhythm strip there is progressive lengthening of the PR interval until a P is not followed by a QRS (Figures 6.11 and 6.12). The PR interval of the cycle following the blocked

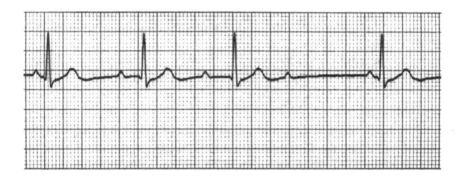

Figure 6.12 Second-degree AV block, Mobitz type I (or Wenckebach). The level of block is the AV node. There is progressive lengthening of the PR interval until the P wave is not conducted. After the dropped beat, the PR interval is short (the AV node has had time to recuperate). An additional feature, not mentioned in the text, is progressive shortening of the RR interval before the dropped beat. Note that the QRS complex is narrow, more evidence that the level of block is the AV node. (Reproduced by permission from Taylor, GJ. *150 Practice ECGs*, 2nd ed. Malden, MA: Blackwell Science, 2002:16.)

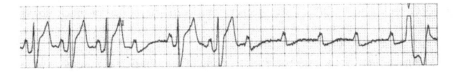

Figure 6.13 Second-degree AV block, Mobitz type II. The patient initially drops a single beat, and this dropped beat is an example of Mobitz II block. He then goes into complete heart block. The last beat is a ventricular escape beat. The PR interval of conducted beats is fixed; there is no evidence of the Wenckebach phenomenon. In addition, the QRS complex is wide; the 12-lead ECG showed bifascicular block. A wide QRS, indicating abnormal intraventricular conduction, is a consistent feature of infranodal heart block. (Reproduced by permission from Taylor, GJ. *150 Practice ECGs*, 2nd ed. Malden, MA: Blackwell Science, 2002:17.)

beat is shorter, reflecting recuperation of the AV node. In some cases, progressive lengthening of the PR is subtle. However, if the PR following the blocked beat is obviously shorter, the diagnosis is Wenckebach (Mobitz I).

The conduction system below the AV node is usually normal in patients with Mobitz I, so the QRS complex is narrow (Figure 6.11). In fact, a narrow QRS excludes block below the AV node.[23] On the other hand, a wide QRS does not guarantee that block is infranodal, as it is possible for a patient to have conduction abnormalities in the node and below it (e.g., a person with bundle branch block may develop delayed conduction in the AV node). Most cases of drug induced heart block are nodal, not infranodal.

Mobitz II block is caused by block below the AV node. It does not cause progressive prolongation of the PR in the beats before the blocked P wave (Figure 6.13). Because the infranodal conduction system is diseased, the QRS is wide. Mobitz II block often precedes symptomatic complete heart block and is an indicator for pacemaker therapy. Most who have it are symptomatic, but pacing is justified even in the absence of symptoms.

2:1 block: is it Mobitz I or II?—Block in the AV node (Mobitz I) can be severe enough that every other beat is blocked. This eliminates progressive lengthening of the PR interval as a diagnostic marker of AV nodal rather than infranodal block. It is a common digitalis toxic rhythm.

There are a couple ways to determine the level of block. The easiest is QRS duration. If narrow, the block is nodal. If wide, it may be infranodal. Check an old ECG; a narrow QRS previously but a wide one now suggests new infranodal conduction disease.

A long rhythm strip may help. At times the block is less severe, and the 2:1 block is replaced by 3:2 or 4:3 conduction. During these times the typical variation of the PR interval indicates Mobitz I. With Mobitz II there is no PR variability.

When in doubt, a His bundle electrogram in the EP laboratory is diagnostic (Figure 6.14). A long H-V interval identifies infranodal conduction disease and is

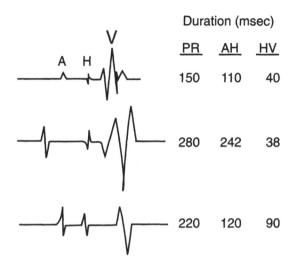

| Duration (msec) | | |
PR	AH	HV
150	110	40
280	242	38
220	120	90

Figure 6.14 His bundle recordings from three patients. The goal of EP study when evaluating heart block is to determine the anatomic level of conduction delay (see Figure 6.13). The His (H) spike is generated by depolarization of the His bundle, just below and adjacent to the AV node, and is recorded with a bipolar catheter positioned next to the tricuspid valve. The H spike essentially divides the PR interval into its AV nodal (the AH interval) and infranodal (HV) portions. **Top:** the PR interval is normal as is the HV interval (<55 msec). **Middle:** A patient with first-degree AV block (long PR). Marked prolongation of the AH interval indicates that the level of block is the AV node. Infranodal conduction (the HV interval) is normal, so there is no delay in the conduction in the AV node. **Bottom:** The prolonged HV interval indicates infranodal conduction delay. With infranodal disease, there is a higher risk of developing symptomatic heart block. (Reproduced by permission from Taylor, GJ. Primary Care Management of Heart Disease. St. Louis: Mosby, 2000:325.)

an indication for pacemaker therapy. This is a simple, low-risk study. A electrode catheter is advanced from the femoral vein to the RA—it takes about 10 minutes to complete.

Third-degree, complete heart block—Nothing gets through. There are P waves and QRS complexes, but they are unrelated (Figure 6.15). This is an example of AV dissociation (another is VT with a unrelated atrial rhythm; Figure 6.8). How can you tell whether complete block is at the level of the AV node or below it?

The principles are the same as those discussed previously with 2:1 heart block. When block is nodal, the QRS is narrow and the takeover pacing rate is above 40 beats per minute (Figure 6.15). The rate increases with catecholamine stimulation. Congenital heart block is usually AV nodal, and young people with this condition are often asymptomatic.

Infranodal complete heart block is more common with elderly patients. It may causes syncope (Stokes–Adams attacks), but also can present as fatigue or heart failure. Even if it is asymptomatic it is an indication for pacemaker therapy, as sudden death is possible. The etiology is often misunderstood. Senile heart block is not

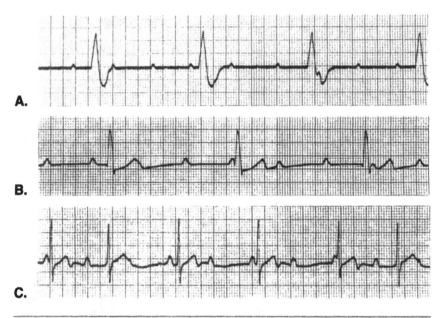

Figure 6.15 Three patients with complete heart block. The atria are being discharged at a regular rate (P waves), and the ventricles at a regular rate (QRS complexes). The two rhythms appear unrelated; there is *AV dissociation.* You may be tempted to say that P waves coming before QRS complexes could be conducted, but these do not alter the regularity of the ventricular escape rhythm. **Patients A and B** have wide QRS complexes and slow ventricular rates; they probably have block below the AV node, and the takeover pacemakers are ventricular in origin. **Patient C** has a more rapid escape rate (55 beats/min), and the QRS complex is narrow; the level of block is probably the AV node. (Reproduced by permission from Taylor, GJ. *150 Practice ECGs*, 2nd ed. Malden, MA: Blackwell Science, 2002:19.)

caused by ischemia. Instead, a degenerative, fibrotic process involving the cardiac nerves below the AV node is the usual cause—think of them as frayed wires. Most of these patients have bundle branch block on prior ECGs, before developing third-degree block. Unless there are other symptoms indicating ischemia, evaluation for CAD is unnecessary.

Sick Sinus Syndrome

Sick sinus syndrome, also called the brady-tachy syndrome, usually occurs in elderly patients and is the most common indication for pacemaker therapy in the United States. The patient usually has atrial tachyarrhythmias, which may include paroxysmal AF or PSVT, alternating with spells of marked sinus bradycardia. The bouts of tachycardia may be followed by disturbingly long SA pauses with syncope. An EP study is rarely needed to make the diagnosis. When performed it involves rapid atrial pacing, then determining how long it takes the SA note to fire when pacing is terminated (the "sinus node recovery time").

The rapid atrial rhythms are controlled using the therapies described earlier. Most patients need beta blockade, diltiazem, verapamil, or digoxin. However, these medicines aggravate the bradyarrhythmia—hence the need for both drug treatment and cardiac pacing.

Pacemaker Therapy

The most common indication for cardiac pacing is a symptomatic bradyarrhythmia. It is important to document the slow rhythm while the patient is having symptoms. Prophylactic pacing is justified for complete heart block, Mobitz II block (the patient usually has symptoms), asystolic pauses at least 4 seconds in duration, and after anterior MI when there is new left bundle branch or bifascicular block.[24]

As noted in Chapter 4, permanent pacing is rarely needed for third-degree block caused by inferior MI, because the level of block is the AV node, and spontaneous recovery is the rule (Figure 6.11).

Pacemaker nomenclature—A three-letter code is used. The first letter refers to the chamber paced, the second to the chamber sensed, and the third to the mode of response (inhibited or triggered). Single chamber, VVI pacing is the simplest pacing system: a lead in the RV paces the heart, and the same lead is the sensor. If the heart rate is adequate, the pacer senses this and is inhibited for a preset period. If it senses no ventricular beat (there is a pause), it paces the ventricle.

For some time, dual-chamber pacers had a pacing electrode in the ventricle and only a sensing electrode in the RA. This sensed a P wave and triggered a ventricular beat (VAT pacing).

The modern dual chamber pacer is DDD: it paces both the atrium and ventricle and senses with both electrodes. When the atrial lead senses a P wave, it inhibits atrial pacing. If the ventricular lead does not sense a QRS on time, it paces the ventricle.

Physiologic pacing—Single chamber ventricular pacing protects against a slow heart rate. However, it bypasses atrial contraction, and the atrial contribution to diastolic filling is lost (see Chapter 2). This may be intolerable for the patient with LV diastolic dysfunction. In such cases, stroke volume may fall 25% or more. This is a common problem for elderly patients who tend to have stiff left ventricles (and who are the major consumers of cardiac pacing).

The "pacemaker syndrome" is one consequence of VVI pacing and loss of atrial contraction. The patient describes spells of fatigue or weakness caused by an abrupt fall in cardiac output whenever the ventricular pacemaker turns on. The solution is dual chamber pacing, which preserves atrial contraction.

DDD pacing is thus useful when there is abnormal LV function. Note that DDD pacing is not possible when the underlying rhythm is AF. Intermittent AF leads to *mode switching*; the DDD pacer switches to the VVI mode. When this is noted by the device clinic, you will be notified that your patient probably is having paroxysmal AF (and should be treated—anticoagulation, rate control, etc.).

While physiologic, dual chamber pacing may have symptomatic benefits, it does not improve survival or prevent stroke.[25] Those with dual chamber pacing are less likely to develop AF, possibly by avoiding the atrial stretch associated with the LA contracting against a closed mitral valve.[25]

Pacemaker follow-up and troubleshooting—All patients should be enrolled in a telephone follow-up clinic. Regular telephone monitoring using a fingertip electrode and a transmitter allows remote troubleshooting. Pacemaker leads and batteries may fail unexpectedly, and failure is easily detected with telephone telemetry. A drop in the baseline pacing rate indicates that the battery is reaching end-of-life.

If the pacer is not firing at all, the patient places a magnet over the battery pack. This temporarily turns the sensing function off and the pacer fires at its fixed rate, ensuring that it is able to pace the heart. It is quite safe to use a magnet in the ED or office to establish fixed rate pacing (DOO or VOO pacing).

There is still some concern about electrical interference, although shielding is effective. Household appliances, microwave ovens, and cellular telephones are not a problem, although I recommend avoiding direct contact with the pacemaker battery. More powerful electromagnetic devices such as ham radio or arc welding equipment may be a threat, and the pacemaker company should be consulted when there is a doubt about safety.

DC cardioversion, electroconvulsive therapy, lithotripsy, and electrocautery during surgery are safe as long as they do not direct energy to the region of the pacemaker battery. On the other hand, magnetic resonance imaging subjects the pacemaker to intense magnetic fields and is generally contraindicated. Radiation therapy may alter pacer function if the battery is directly in the radiation beam. In both cases, if absolutely needed, contact the pacemaker company first.

Syncope

Sudden loss of consciousness occurs when systolic blood pressure falls below 70 mm Hg (and usually much lower). A drop in cardiac output or arterial dilatation are the usual causes, and common etiologies are reviewed in Table 6.5.[26] As a rule, syncope caused by heart disease conveys a worse prognosis, while vasovagal syncope is benign.[27]

The patient's other cardiac or medical history may point to an etiology. Thus, a history of MI or heart failure would be consistent with VT as the cause. An elderly person with no history of heart disease, but with left bundle branch block may have intermittent complete heart block.

The evaluation and treatment of cardiac arrhythmias has been reviewed. Arrhythmias are uncommon in otherwise healthy young people. Think instead of neurocardiogenic or carotid sinus syncope, and screen for other cardiac lesions that may not be apparent on physical examination.

I find that the house staff is quick to order carotid Doppler studies when evaluating new syncope. It is a waste of time, because carotid disease is an exceedingly

Table 6.5 Syncope

Cardiac Causes

Slow heart rate	Heart block (Stokes-Adams attacks), asystole, atrial fibrillation with a slow ventricular rate (common in elderly patients, and a feature of the brady-tachy syndrome). Most bradyarrhythmias may be aggravated by digoxin, beta-blockers, verapamil, and diltiazem.
Rapid ventricular rhythms	A normal LVEF excludes VT and VF as the cause of syncope (exceptions include hypertrophic cardiomyopathy, RV dysplasia, and the Brugada and long QT interval syndromes).
Mechanical causes of low cardiac output	Left heart: aortic stenosis, hypertrophic cardiomyopathy with LV outflow tract obstruction, atrial myxoma, prosthetic valve malfunction. Rarely syncope complicates mitral stenosis or aortic regurgitation. Right heart: pulmonary embolism, primary pulmonary hypertension, pulmonic valve stenosis, Eisenmenger's syndrome, tetralogy of Fallot (pulmonary outflow obstruction), pericardial tamponade.
Pacemaker failure	Loss of pacing and severe bradycardia
Neurocardiogenic syncope	See text. This is one time that beta blockade may not aggravate bradycardia.

Noncardiac Causes

Vasovagal syncope	The common faint. There are prodromal symptoms: sweating, pallor, nausea, blurred vision. This differentiates it from the drop attack that occurs with cardiac arrhythmias and (usually) neurocardiogenic syncope.
Orthostatic hypotension	Often associated with antihypertensive drug therapy, or with phenothiazines, antidepressants, and tranquilizers. Blood pressure tends to drop immediately upon standing (unlike the delayed fall in pressure with neurocardiogenic syncope).
Cerebrovascular disease	See text. Vertebrobasilar insufficiency is a rare cause of syncope, and other brainstem symptoms are usually present (vertigo, diplopia, dysarthria, paresthesia, ataxia).
Subclavian steal syndrome	Syncope follows upper extremity exertion. Look for a pulse deficit and bruit. Mechanism: stenosis or occlusion of the subclavian artery, with flow to the limb via collateral vessels from the vertebral artery. With exercise and vasodilatation, flow is stolen from the vertebral artery, and there is brainstem ischemia.
Carotid sinus syncope	Usually elderly patients. About 25% report symptoms with stimulation of the carotid sinus (sudden turns, shaving, a tight collar). Others have hypertension or CAD. A few have pathologic conditions of the neck (tumor, previous radiation, large lymph nodes, previous trauma or surgery).
Situational syncope	Micturition, cough or sneeze, defecation and straining, swallowing and Valsalva syncope. Vagal activation is the usual mechanism.
Migraine syndromes Metabolic	Syncope is possible, but other features of migraine are usually present Hypoglycemia, hypoxia, hyperventilation (with associated finger and circumoral tingling, etc).
Hysterical syncope	A diagnosis of exclusion

ICD, implantable cardioverter device; MI, myocardial infarction; VT, ventricular tachycardia; AF, atrial fibrillation; PSVT, paroxysmal supraventricular tachycardia

*Acute ischemia causing increased VT frequency is an indication for aggressive evaluation, including angiography.

rare cause of syncope. Ischemia of both cerebral hemispheres would be required for loss of consciousness. Instead, carotid disease causes transient ischemic attack, a syndrome characterized by lateralizing neurological symptoms or a transient speech disorder. Basilar artery ischemia can cause dizziness or syncope, and it is accompanied by other brainstem symptoms (Table 6.5). Furthermore, the basilar arteries cannot be evaluated with noninvasive studies in the vascular laboratory (this is not a part of the carotid Doppler study).

Neurocardiogenic Syncope

Before the discovery of this illness, about half of the cases of syncope were labeled idiopathic. Neurocardiogenic syncope is responsible for most of these, and it is the single most common cause of syncope.[26]

The initiating event is venous pooling with a shift to upright posture. Reduced venous return leads to lower cardiac output. Baroreceptors are stimulated, increasing adrenergic tone. Both heart rate and LV contractility increase. This is the normal response to the change in position.

For uncertain reasons, patients with neurally mediated syncope have an overshoot of the of LV mechanoreceptors to the increase in contractility. These receptors are connected to the central vasomotor center, and there are two responses to its activation: *vagal discharge*, leading to decreased heart rate (and rarely, asystole), and *withdrawal of sympathetic tone*, leading to vasodilatation and hypotension. In most cases, hypotension is the predominant mechanism leading to syncope (Figure 6.16).

This complex series of reflexes takes some time, leading to a characteristic delay in syncope after the change in posture. Most patients are upright for 2 to 5 minutes before dizziness begins. A typical history is, "I got up, walked to the kitchen, and fell while standing at the sink." Syncope can occur while sitting as well as with standing.

On the other hand, when a patient describes dizziness immediately upon standing, think of drug-induced hypotension or hypovolemia.

You may try to elicit neurocardiogenic syncope at the bedside, having the patient stand while monitoring blood pressure for 5 to 10 minutes. More sensitive is the *tilt-table test*, which monitors arterial pressure even longer. One study reported a mean time to syncope of 12 minutes after upright tilt. Strapping the patient to the tilt table avoids muscular activity that may prevent the initial vagal response. Repeating it with isoproterenol infusion may increase the sensitivity of this test, although this reduces specificity (more false positive results).

Increasing vascular volume may prevent vasodepressor syncope. Diuretics should be stopped if possible, and salt tablets may be added. Beta-blockers may work, blocking the increase in LV contractility that initiates the reaction (results of studies are mixed, but a therapeutic trial is reasonable). An occasional patient has prodromal symptoms. In such cases isometric exercise may abort the attack.[28,29]

An occasional young person with neurocardiogenic syncope has a long period of asystole. It is quite alarming to witness 4- to 7-second pauses on telemetry, and

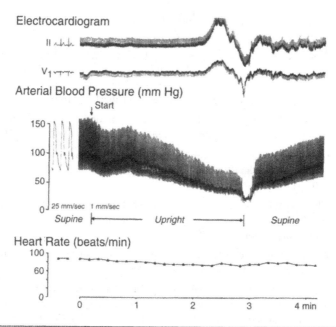

Figure 6.16 Tilt-table test in a 72-year-old woman with breast cancer metastatic to the glossopharyngeal region. This episode of syncope occurred despite a dual-chamber pacemaker and stable heart rate. Note that pressure fell slowly but steadily with head-up tilt, and syncope occurred 3 minutes later. She was successfully treated with disopyramide. (Reproduced by permission from Osswald S, Troutan TG. Images in clinical medicine. Neurocardiogenic (vasodepressor) syncope. N Engl J Med 1993;329:30. Copyright © 1993, Massachusetts Medical Society. All rights reserved.)

such pauses usually causes a loss of consciousness. These spells usually respond to beta blockade, and pacemaker therapy is rarely needed.

References

1. Ferguson JD, DiMarco JP. Contemporary management of paroxysmal supraventricular tachycardia. Circulation 2003;107:1096–1099.

2. Falk RH. Atrial fibrillation. N Engl J Med 2001;344:1067–1078. Also note, Wattigney WA, Mensah GA, Croft JB. Increasing trends in hospitalization for atrial fibrillation in the United States, 1985 through 1999: implications for primary prevention. Circulation 2003;108:711–716. (*During that time the rate of AF in hospitalized patients more than doubled.*) Also note, Aviles RJ, Martin DO, Apperson-Hansen C, et al. Inflammation as a risk factor for atrial fibrillation. Circulation 2003;108:3006–3010.

3. Wyse DG, Waldo AL, DiMarco JP, et al. A comparison of rate control and rhythm control in patients with atrial fibrillation. The AFFIRM trial. N Engl J Med 2002;347:1825–1833. Also note, Olshansky B, Rosenfeld LE, Warner AL, et al. The Atrial Fibrillation Follow-up Investigation of Rhythm Management (AFFIRM) study: approaches to control rate in atrial fibrillation. J Am Coll

Cardiol 2004;43:1201–1208. (*Beta-blockers use most effective for rate control, but combination drug therapy was often needed.*)

4. Executive Steering Committee on behalf of the SPORTIF III Investigators. Stroke prevention with the oral direct thrombin inhibitor ximelagatran compared with warfarin in patients with non-valvular atrial fibrillation (SPORTIF III): randomised controlled trial. Lancet 2003;362:1691–1698.

5. Halperin JL, Gomberg-Maitland M. Obliteration of the left atrial appendage for prevention of thromboembolism. J Am Coll Cardiol 2003;42:1259–1261.

6. Klein AL, Grimm RA, Murray RD, et al. Use of transesophageal echocardiography to guide cardioversion in patients with atrial fibrillation. N Engl J Med 2001;344:1141–1420.

7. Chevalier P, Durand-Dubief A, Burri H, et al. Amiodarone versus placebo and class Ic drugs for cardioversion of recent-onset atrial fibrillation: a meta-analysis. J Am Coll Cardiol 2003;41:255–262.

8. Ellenbogen KA, Wood MA. Ablation of atrial fibrillation: awaiting the new paradigm. J Am Coll Cardiol 2003;42:198–200.

9. Pappone C, Rosanio S, Augello G, et al. Mortality, morbidity, and quality of life after circumferential pulmonary vein ablation for atrial fibrillation: outcomes from a controlled nonrandomized long-term study. J Am Coll Cardiol 2003;42:185–197.

10. Kim MH, Eagle KA. Importance of limiting atrial fibrillation after heart surgery. Cardiology Review 2002;19:19–21.

11. Wellens HJ. Contemporary management of atrial flutter. Circulation 2002:106:649–652.

12. Seidl K, Hauer B, Schwick NG, et al. Risk of thromboembolic events in patients with atrial flutter. Am J Cardiol 1998;82:580–583.

13. Kunavarapu C, Bllomfield DM. Role of noninvasive studies in risk stratification for sudden cardiac death. Clin Cardiol 2004;27:192–197. Also note, Hohnloser SH, Klingenheben T, Bloomfield D, et al. Usefulness of microvolt T-wave alternans for prediction of ventricular tachyarrhythmic events in patients with dilated cardiomyopathy: results from a prospective observational study. J Am Coll Cardiol 2003;41:2220–2224. (*The discussion provides an excellent summary of risk stratification for SCD in this illness.*)

14. Verrier RL, Tolat AV, Josephson ME. T-wave alternans for arrhythmia risk stratification in patients with idiopathic dilated cardiomyopathy. J Am Coll Cardiol 2003;41:2225–2227.

15. Moss AJ, Zareba W, Hall WJ, et al. Prophylactic implantation of a defibrillator in patients with myocardial infarction and reduced ejection fraction. N Engl J Med 2002;346:877–883.

16. DiMarco JP. Implantable cardioverter-defibrillators. N Engl J Med 2003;349:1836–1847. Also note, Curtis AB. Filling the need for new antiarrhythmic drugs to prevent shocks from implantable cardioverter-defibrillators. J Am Coll Cardiol 2004;43:44–46.

17. Sears SE, Conti JB. Understanding implantable cardioverter defibrillator shocks and storms: medical and psychosocial considerations for research and clinical care. Clin Cardiol 2003;26:107–111. Also note, Saksena S, Madan N. Management of the patient with an implantable cardioverter-defibrillator in the third millennium. Circulation 2002;106:2642–2646. And, Macdonald JE, Struthers AD. What is the optimal serum potassium level in cardiovascular patients? J Am Coll Cardiol 2004;43:155–161.

18. Akiyama T, Powell JL, Mitchell LB, et al. Resumption of driving after life-threatening ventricular tachyarrhythmia. N Engl J Med, 2001;345:391–397.

19. Roden DM. Drug-induced prolongation of the QT interval. N Engl J Med 2004;350:1013–1022.

20. Kinsara AJ, Zaman L, Gorgels A. Arrhythmogenic right ventricular dysplasia. Am J Emerg Med 2001;19:67–70.

21. Wilde AA, Antzelevitch C, Borggrefe M, et al. Proposed diagnostic criteria for the Brugada syndrome: consensus report. Circulation 2002;106:2514–2519.

22. Maron BJ. Sudden death in young athletes. N Engl J Med 2003;349:1064–1075.

23. Barold SS, Hayes DL. Second-degree atrioventricular block: a reappraisal. Mayo Clin Proc 2001;76:44–57.

24. Gregoratos G, Abrams J, Epstein AE, et al. ACC/AHA/NASPE 2002 guideline update for implantation of cardiac pacemakers and antiarrhythmia devices. Circulation 2002;106:2145–2161.

25. Kerr CR, Connolly SJ, Abdollah H, et al. Canadian trial of physiological pacing; effects of physiological pacing during long-term follow-up. Circulation 2004;109:357–362.

26. Kapoor WN. Syncope. N Engl J Med 2000;343;1856–1862.

27. Soteriades ES, Evans JC, Larson MG, et al. Incidence and prognosis of syncope. N Engl J Med 2002;347:878–885.

28. Krediet CT, van Dijk N, Linzer M, et al. Management of vasovagal syncope: controlling or aborting faints by leg crossing and muscle tensing. Circulation 2002 106:1684–1689.

29. Brignole M, Croci F, Menozzi C, et al. Isometric arm counter-pressure maneuvers to abort impending vasovagal syncope. J Am Coll Cardiol 2002;40:2053–2059.

CHAPTER 7

VALVULAR HEART DISEASE

Abbreviations

A_2	aortic second heart sound	MS	mitral stenosis
ACE	angiotensin-converting enzyme	MVP	mitral valve prolapse
AF	atrial fibrillation	PA	pulmonary artery
AR	aortic regurgitation	P_2	pulmonic second heart sound
AS	aortic stenosis	RHD	rheumatic heart disease
CHF	congestive heart failure	RV	right ventricle (ventricular)
ECG	electrocardiogram	S_1	first heart sound
IE	infective endocarditis	S_2	second heart sound
LA	left atrium	S_3	third heart sound
LV	left ventricle (ventricular)	S_4	fourth heart sound
LVEF	LV ejection fraction	SCD	sudden cardiac death
LVH	LV hypertrophy	TR	tricuspid regurgitation
MR	mitral regurgitation		

Young clinicians tend to believe that managing valvular heart disease is more complicated than it is. Taking a logical, physiologic approach simplifies it. Evaluate the patient's heart murmur with the following questions in mind:

1. What cardiac chamber is most affected by the valve lesion (Table 7.1)?

2. What is the effect on the chamber? Does the lesion change left ventricular (LV) preload, afterload, or contractility, leading to dilatation or hypertrophy?

3. What diagnostic study will identify the altered chamber size and function, and thus define the hemodynamic significance of the lesion?

4. What changes in LV size and function necessitate valve surgery, and how will surgery affect function? If LV function is not jeopardized, then the indication for surgery must be intolerable symptoms.

Mitral Stenosis

Mitral stenosis (MS), for practical purposes, can be equated with rheumatic heart disease (RHD). All patients with RHD have scarring of the mitral valve apparatus. This has a typical appearance on the echocardiogram, and you may therefore use the echocardiogram to diagnose or exclude RHD. Isolated aortic valve disease, with a normal mitral valve, is not caused by rheumatic fever.

Table 7.1 Overview of Valvular Heart Disease

Lesion	Chamber/Effect	Indications for Surgery
Mitral stenosis	LA pressure overload and dilatation. The LV is spared (normal afterload, and normal or low preload). There is pulmonary congestion, but no gallop.	As there is no unusual loading of the LV, and no risk of LV injury, surgery may be delayed until there are symptoms (congestion, fatigue).
Chronic mitral regurgitation (MR)	LA and LV volume overload (high preload). The LA gives, absorbing the LV pressure wave, so there is no V wave on the pulmonary wedge tracing. Eventually there is LV contractile dysfunction, and an S_3 gallop reflects volume overload and dysfunction.	Net afterload is low (see text), falsely elevating LVEF. The LV is not as good as it looks. Surgery is considered when LVEF ≤ 60%, or LV end-systolic dimension ≥ 4.5 cm, even without symptoms. Repair is better than replacement for papillary muscle preservation.
Acute MR	LA and LV volume overload, with high preload. LV pressure is transmitted to the lungs, and there is a V wave on the wedge pressure tracing. Because of acute onset, there is no time for LV or LA dilatation.	Severe congestion necessitates urgent surgery in most cases.
Aortic stenosis	LV pressure overload (a pure afterload condition). LVH and associated findings. With calcification, A_2 eventually softens and disappears.	Valve replacement reduces afterload, so LV function improves after surgery. The usual indication for surgery is symptoms.
Aortic regurgitation	LV volume overload. Afterload is increased as well, so there is both LV dilatation and hypertrophy. Wide pulse pressure due to peripheral vasodilatation.	As with MR, do not delay surgery until CHF develops. Indications for surgery: LVEF ≤ 55% or LV end-systolic dimension ≤ 5.5 cm. Because afterload is up, there may be improvement in LV function after surgery.
Tricuspid regurgitation	RV and RA volume overload. The RV pressure wave is transmitted to the jugular veins (V wave). Think of TR when there is right side congestion.	TR usually complicates left heart failure or mitral valve disease. The tricuspid valve may be repaired if TR remains severe after mitral valve repair.

LA, left atrium; LV, left ventricle; LVH, LV hypertrophy; LVEF, LV ejection fraction; RA, right atrium; RV, right ventricle.

MS has become an unusual illness in western medicine because of the widespread treatment of strep throat with antibiotics and because of antistreptococcal prophylaxis after rheumatic fever. It remains a common illness in lesser-developed countries. In rural Latin America or India, RHD often has a more aggressive course, with symptomatic MS (and other valvular lesions) appearing at an earlier age. In the United States, young people seldom have hemodynamically significant MS. The usual history is rheumatic fever in the early teens and then onset of symptomatic MS when the patient reaches middle age.

An occasional elderly patient—usually a woman—with new-onset congestive heart failure (CHF) is found to have MS on the echocardiogram. It usually is a surprise diagnosis, as low cardiac output and reduced flow across the stenosed valve results in a soft or absent murmur. She may present with fatigue or weight loss (the dwindles) and relatively little pulmonary congestion. An echocardiogram to screen for occult valvular or myocardial disease may thus prove useful for an old person with vague, unexplained symptoms.

Pathophysiology, History, and Physical Examination

The blocked mitral valve causes pressure overload of the left atrium (LA). Unlike the ventricles, pressure overload of the atria leads to dilatation rather than hypertrophy (Table 7.1). Increased LA pressure is transmitted to the pulmonary capillary bed. As one of my teachers said, "mitral stenosis is a disease of the lungs."

Dyspnea on exertion and winter bronchitis are early symptoms. A patient may ask for antibiotics for a "chest cold that is hard to shake." Fatigue is a common result of low cardiac output. The onset of symptoms tends to be insidious. Patients may be unaware of how sick they have been until symptoms are relieved by surgery.

A minority of patients with advanced disease develops pulmonary hypertension, and with it symptoms of right heart failure: edema, ascites, and fatigue.

Most of these symptoms are common to other forms of heart failure. Hemoptysis is more specific for MS, and is caused by the rupture of small bronchial veins. It may be substantial, with cough producing a few ounces of blood—more than just blood-streaked sputum. With bleeding, the veins decompress and the bleeding stops. Hemoptysis is rarely a fatal complication of MS.

With time, most patients with LA enlargement caused by mitral valve disease develop atrial fibrillation (AF).

The left ventricle is unaffected by MS. LV afterload is normal. The stenosed valve inhibits LV filling, and a poorly compensated patient with low cardiac output has a low preload. But the asymptomatic patient does not; adequate LV filling is accomplished by raising LA pressure, thus forcing blood across the stenosed valve. This pressure gradient across the valve is the definitive hemodynamic finding in MS (Figure 7.1).

The LV is usually small and contracts normally. The high LA pressure and limited cardiac output can lead to the CHF syndrome, mimicking the effects of cardiomyopathy. The neurohumoral response to low cardiac output is the same (see Chapter 1).

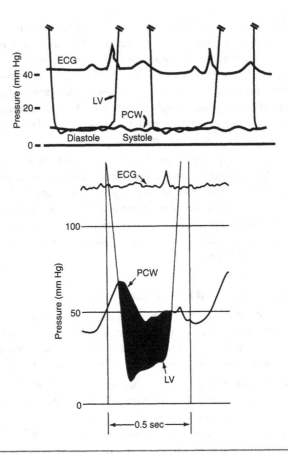

Figure 7.1 Pressure tracings from the cardiac catheterization laboratory. **(A)** Normal. The pulmonary capillary wedge (PCW) pressure is identical to left atrial pressure during diastole (there is no valve separating the pulmonary artery from the left atrium). There is no difference, or gradient, between left atrial and LV diastolic pressure when the mitral valve is open. **(B)** Mitral stenosis. Even when the mitral valve is open during diastole, there is a pressure gradient caused by stenosis (shaded area). (Reproduced by permission from Carabello BA, Grossman W, eds. Cardiac Catheterization and Angiography, 3rd ed. Philadelphia: Lea & Febiger, 1986.)

On physical examination, the apical impulse is normal. With pulmonary hypertension, there may be a right ventricular lift. Because LV loading is normal, there is no gallop. Recall that gallops occur during diastole and reflect LV filling abnormalities: rapid early diastolic filling of a big flabby LV causes the S_3, and atrial contraction at the end of diastole forcing a column of blood against a stiff ventricle causes the S_4. With MS, the LV is neither dilated and flabby nor hypertrophied and stiff.

The earliest physical finding is a loud, snapping S_1, and this physical finding is easier to detect than the soft murmur. With time the valve stiffens and becomes less mobile, and S_1 softens. The diastolic murmur is low-pitched, probably because flow velocity across the stenosed valve is relatively low given a pressure gradient of 10 to 15 mm Hg (compared with the higher flow rate and pressure gradient across a stenosed aortic valve).

The opening snap (OS) is an interesting physical finding, created by the movement of the calcified valve. It is high-pitched, and that distinguishes it from the much lower pitch of the S_3 gallop; both are heard best at the apex. Opening of the mitral valve occurs shortly after closure of the aortic valve, so the OS follows S_2. With more severe stenosis the OS occurs earlier, and an S_2-OS interval less than 0.11 seconds indicates severe stenosis. Measuring this interval using the phonocardiogram was the best noninvasive test for gauging MS severity in the days before echocardiography. That test is no longer used, but you can estimate the S_2-OS interval at the bedside using an old-fashioned diagnostic trick: When you say the words, the interval between the letters b and l in *blah* is 0.10 seconds, and between the b and t in *butter* is 0.14 seconds. Admittedly low-tech, but this works (and using physical diagnosis to determine the severity of a valvular lesion is still great sport for clinicians).

Diagnostic Studies

The ECG shows left atrial enlargement, usually with a P mitrale pattern (Figure 7.2B). Another common finding is AF. On the chest x-ray, LA enlargement straightens the left heart border and creates a double density at the right heart border.

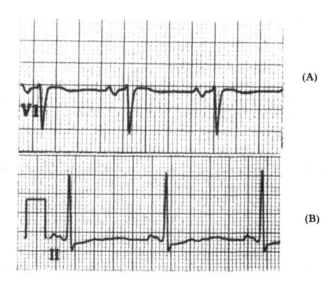

Figure 7.2 Left atrial abnormality. Two ECG findings may be used to make the diagnosis. **(A)** Biphasic P wave in lead V1; the negative deflection should be 1 mm deep and wide. **(B)** Broad notched P wave in one of the limb leads, most commonly II, III, or aVF (as the P wave vector is aimed inferiorly). (Reproduced by permission from Taylor GJ. The Cardiology Rotation. Malden, MA: Blackwell Science, 2001:47.)

The echocardiogram demonstrates the typical rheumatic deformity of the valve, reduced leaflet mobility, and calcification. All patients have LA enlargement. There are three methods for measuring the severity of MS with the echo-Doppler study. The first is visualization of the valve in cross-section and measuring the size of the opening. Two Doppler measures of severity come from flow velocity across the valve. First, flow velocity, in meters per second, is proportional to the valve gradient. This is analogous to increased flow velocity at the end of a garden hose as the nozzle is tightened. Second, the flow velocity remains high for a longer time with more severe stenosis, decaying at the very end of diastole. The pressure half-time is a measure of the time to decay of the flow velocity curve, and is proportional the pressure gradient.

Cardiac catheterization is seldom needed to make the diagnosis of MS, but may be performed to exclude coronary artery disease in older patients. The pressure gradient across the valve is measured using catheters in the pulmonary artery (PA) and the LV (Figure 7.1). Valve area is calculated using Gorlin's formula: area is proportional to flow across the valve (cardiac output) divided by pressure difference across the valve (gradient).

Timing of Surgery

As a consultant, I am rarely asked if the patient has MS (or another valve problem). That is usually obvious from the physical examination and noninvasive studies. Rather, the patient is sent to the cardiologist to determine whether surgical repair is needed. The timing of surgery is the issue you face in clinic, and will encounter on board exams.

A key issue in timing surgery for valvular disease is the state of the left ventricle (just as it tends to be a fundamental issue with most of the adult cardiac illnesses). With MS, the left ventricle is protected. Thus, surgery is not required prophylactically to save the LV. For this one reason, the usual indication for surgery is symptoms. Prognosis also tends to worsen when there is pulmonary hypertension, and this is a second indication for surgery. Pulmonary artery pressure can be estimated from echo-Doppler measurements.

Some have recommended surgery when AF develops. Correction of MS may allow the LA to shrink, restoring sinus rhythm. But this not a predictable effect, and at present, AF is not a standard indication for surgery.

When the valve is mobile and there is little calcification—often the case with young patients—repair is possible. Closed balloon valvulotomy in the catheterization laboratory works well, with an average doubling of the valve area that is maintained long-term. Associated mitral regurgitation (MR), thrombus in the LA, and valve calcification are contraindications to balloon repair, and indicate a need for surgery.

Medical Therapy

The asymptomatic patient in sinus rhythm requires only antibiotic prophylaxis for infective endocarditis (IE). When symptoms develop, surgery is indicated. But if surgery is not to be done, for whatever reason, diuretic therapy lowers LA pressure and relieves congestion. There is no role for measures to lower afterload or increase contractility. The only reason for digoxin therapy is the control of ventricular rate in the patient with AF.

AF is common. Reduced flow across the mitral valve and the enlarged LA make the risk of thromboembolism much higher than it is with other causes of AF. Warfarin is indicated (see Chapter 6). The control of ventricular rate with digoxin, beta-blockers, or calcium blockers is especially important for control of symptoms. Tachycardia reduces total diastolic time, a big problem for the patient with LV inflow obstruction who needs extra time for ventricular filling.

Mitral Regurgitation

The mitral valve prolapse (MVP) syndrome—not RHD—is the most common cause of chronic MR. RHD always cause MS; there may be a mild leak as well, but the echo usually shows that stenosis is the dominant lesion (e.g., LV size is normal). Isolated MR may also be caused by ischemic injury of papillary muscles, IE, or LV dilatation, which changes the orientation of the papillary muscles and slightly dilates the valve ring.

Chronic Mitral Regurgitation

Pathophysiology, History, and Physical Examination

There is volume overload of the LA and LV, and both chambers dilate slowly. The large, flabby LA gives, absorbing the shock of the regurgitant jet. Thus, LA pressure does not rise that much during systole—there is no substantial V wave on the pulmonary wedge tracing (in contrast to acute MR, vide infra).

LV afterload is low (Figure 7.3). Normally, systemic arterial resistance constitutes the impedance to LV ejection (afterload). With MR, the ventricle is able to unload into both the low-pressure LA and the higher-pressure aorta. Net impedance to ejection is thus low. Low afterload makes it easy for the LV muscle to shorten, so LV ejection fraction (LVEF) is artificially high. When the mitral valve is repaired and the LV can no longer dump its load into the low-pressure LA, there is a net increase in afterload.

Afterload *increasing* therapy? That doesn't sound good for the LV, and it is not. In fact, LVEF often declines following surgery for MR. For this reason, the risk of surgery for chronic MR has been high.

The eventual symptoms of MR are those of left heart (pulmonary) congestion and low cardiac output. On examination, the apical impulse is displaced and has a volume overload quality; it is rocking and occupies more than one rib interspace. There may be an S_3 gallop caused by the rapid filling wave early in diastole.

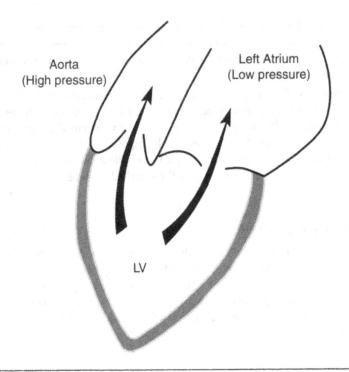

Figure 7.3 MR and left ventricular afterload. In the absence of MR, the ventricle empties into the aorta, a high-pressure system. But with MR the left ventricle (LV) can also empty into the low-pressure left atrium. The net afterload, or impedance to injection, is therefore low. Replacing the valve may be expected to increase net afterload, and left ventricular function suffers.

The murmur is holosystolic, extending to S_2, and is audible at the apex and axilla. The plane of the valve is perpendicular to a vector aimed from the apex impulse to the axilla, and a fish-mouth, fixed orifice would direct the murmur along that vector. On the other hand, a dysfunctional lateral leaflet may prolapse and serve as a baffle, directing the jet—and murmur—toward the base of the heart along the sternum. It may be audible at the right base rather than to the axilla. Thus, a loud systolic murmur at the base of the heart that *does not radiate to the neck* may be MR rather than aortic stenosis (AS). Furthermore, MR from papillary muscle dysfunction may generate a diamond-shaped murmur (crescendo-decrescendo), as peak dysfunction occurs at peak LV systolic pressure.

Diagnostic Studies and Timing of Surgery

The echocardiogram is the key study: it identifies the source of the systolic murmur (mitral vs. aortic valve), defines the valvular anatomy (prolapse, chordal rupture and flail leaflet, vegetation, calcification, etc.), and provides critical LV size and function data. Preoperative cardiac catheterization examines coronary anatomy and measures PA pressure, but it is seldom needed to determine a need for surgery.

Many patients with MR are asymptomatic and tolerate it for years. But waiting for symptoms to develop is a disaster, for symptoms may not occur until the LV is irreversibly damaged. The basic problem is overestimation of the quality of the LV preoperatively, because of low afterload.

Because LVEF is expected to decline with repair, a preoperative LVEF less than 50% is a poor prognostic sign. Dilatation of the LV during diastole is not a problem if the ventricle contracts down to a normal volume at end-systole. This, of course, also indicates a normal LVEF. With volume overload disease, both MR and aortic regurgitation (AR), an elevated end-systolic volume predicts higher operative mortality, more postoperative heart failure, and persistent LV enlargement after surgery.[1]

The LV end-systolic dimension is easily and accurately measured with the transthoracic echocardiogram, and it is a good substitute for end-systolic volume. This is the measurement that we follow when monitoring patients with volume overload valvular disease. An LV end-systolic dimension greater than 4.5 cm indicates a higher risk of surgery.

Best surgical results are obtained when the LV end-systolic dimension is 4.5 cm or less, or the LVEF is 60% or greater, even when there are no symptoms. Asymptomatic patients have serial echocardiograms to follow these LV measurements. Surgery is indicated when LV size and function approach these levels. Serial Doppler studies are unnecessary, because the diagnosis of MR is established. Order the less-expensive echo without Doppler. Insist on good measurements; a qualitative description of LV size like "moderate LV enlargement" is useless. Some patients are difficult to study, but the technician should be aware that the LV dimension is critical.

Repair of the mitral valve is better than replacement with a prosthesis. It is now clear that the mitral valve supporting structures contribute to LV function. Physiologists speak of the papillary muscles and chordae tethering the ventricle on its long axis, contributing to stroke volume by preserving normal LV shape during contraction. One study found a decline in LVEF from 55% to 35% with mitral valve replacement, but no significant decline with valve repair and salvage of chordal structures.[2] Most patients with mitral prolapse are candidates for repair.

Advanced LV dysfunction—Is it ever too late to attempt to correct MR? Mitral valve *replacement* with loss of the chordae tendineae and papillary muscles usually leads to catastrophe in patients with LVEF less than 30%.

On the other hand, mitral valve *repair* has been successfully performed in patients with LVEF as low as 15%.[3] With advanced disease, it must be certain that valve repair and chordal preservation is possible. Otherwise surgery should be avoided.[4]

Medical Therapy

Vasodilator therapy has been found to be helpful in patients with AR, and it seems intuitively correct that afterload reduction would promote forward flow in patients with MR. Angiotensin-converting enzyme (ACE) inhibition has been found to reduce LV size in patients with *symptomatic* MR.[4] However, the standard therapy for such patients is surgical correction, and vasodilator therapy is no substitute.

The more common question is whether to treat *asymptomatic* patients with afterload reduction therapy, hoping to delay a need for surgery. Recall that LV afterload is already low with MR. A further reduction to subnormal levels has not been supported by clinical trials. A small study found no reduction in LV size with vasodilator therapy in the absence of clinical heart failure.[5]

Symptomatic patients with MR who are not candidates for surgery benefit from standard therapy for heart failure including diuretics, vasodilators and digoxin (see Chapter 1). The role of beta blockade is uncertain.

Acute Mitral Regurgitation

MR after acute myocardial infarction has been reviewed in Chapter 5. Think of it when acute pulmonary edema develops after a relatively small MI because little injury is required to disrupt papillary muscle function.

Spontaneous rupture of chordae may occur in the absence of coronary artery disease, most commonly in middle-aged men with MVP. The history often includes a single, brief episode of non-anginal chest pain at the time of rupture. Over the next few days there is progressive dyspnea, and severe pulmonary congestion is apparent at the time of initial evaluation.

Pathophysiology, Physical Examination, and Laboratory Evaluation

Because of the abrupt onset of symptomatic MR, there is insufficient time for the LA and LV to dilate. Therefore, the apical impulse is not displaced. As the LV is not large and flabby, there is no S_3 gallop. In fact, the large volume of blood hitting the relatively small LV at end-diastole may cause an S_4 gallop. A small and stiff LA is unable to absorb the regurgitant wave, so there is a marked rise in LA pressure during ventricular systole. This V wave is transmitted to the pulmonary capillary bed, aggravating congestive symptoms (Figure 7.4). It is also an important finding in the catheterization laboratory, supporting the diagnosis of acute rather than chronic MR.

The systolic murmur is usually loud. As noted previously, it may radiate medially, rather than to the axilla (the prolapsing leaflet works as a baffle). A patient with severe pulmonary congestion may have a soft or inaudible murmur. The echocardiogram shows the MR jet, and may also identify a flail leaflet.

Treatment

Acute MR with associated pulmonary edema requires urgent surgery. Most patients have damage to valve support structures, yet valve repair is possible. As noted previously, this is preferable to replacement because anticoagulation is not required, and LV function is better preserved.

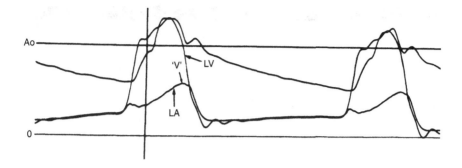

Figure 7.4 Simultaneous left atrial (LA), LV, and aortic (Ao) pressure tracings from a patient with *acute* MR. During LV systole, the LV pressure wave is transmitted back to the LA through the defective mitral valve and measured as a V wave. In the absence of MR there is a tiny V wave caused by the slight posterior bowing of the mitral valve. With chronic MR the large flaccid left atrium absorbs the pressure wave, and the V wave is not as prominent. (Reproduced by permission from Kern, MJ. The Cardiac Catheterization Handbook. St. Louis: Mosby, 1991.)

Mitral Valve Prolapse

MVP has been over-diagnosed. Thin young girls have stretchy connective tissue, and their chordae tendineae and mitral leaflets are as flexible as their joints. It is common to see a small amount of prolapse on their echocardiograms. But they do not have myxomatous degeneration of the valve, true MVP.

The diagnostic criteria have been refined in recent years. Pathologic MVP includes posterior motion of the valve beyond the plane of the mitral ring plus a thickened and redundant valve, the typical floppy or parachute valve. The presence of a mid-systolic click on examination is considered diagnostic, even when the echocardiographic findings are unimpressive.

Primary MVP can be inherited. It commonly accompanies other connective tissue disorders such as Marfan's syndrome. Most patients with Marfan's syndrome have prolapse on the echocardiogram. In such cases other features suggest abnormal connective tissue, including pectus excavatum, straight back, high arched palate, and an enlarged aortic root. Secondary MVP may complicate disorders of papillary muscle dysfunction (ischemic heart disease) or orientation (a dilated LV).

Although serious complications are possible (Table 7.2), they are rare. Recent studies suggest that a diagnosis of MVP does not convey an increased mortality risk.[6] Cardiovascular death is predicted by advanced age, more severe MR, and AF.

Pathophysiology and Physical Examination

The excursion of the prolapsing valve is increased when the LV is smaller. Thus, the findings of MVP are magnified by maneuvers that reduce venous return and LV size, such as standing. Amyl nitrate, a venodilator, is used for this purpose in the echocardiography laboratory.

Table 7.2 Complications of Mitral Valve Prolapse		
Complication	Risk	Risk Factors
Infective endocarditis	1% by age 75; No MR: 1/22,000 patients/yr MR: 1/2,000 patients/yr	MR, thickened valve
MR	Men: about 5% by age 75 Women: 1% by age 75	Male sex, obesity, hypertension, age >50
Sudden death	MR: 0.2%–1.0% No MR: 2/10,000	Severe MR, long QT interval, family history of MVP with complications
Embolic stroke	Rare; the best population studies indicate no risk with mild MVP	Atrial fibrillation, LA enlarge- ment, thickened valve

MR, mitral regurgitation; MVP, mitral valve prolapse; LA, left atrium,

The click is mid-systolic and the murmur follows it. When you hear a mid-to-late systolic murmur, the usual cause is MVP. Listen carefully for the click; it may be localized to a small area near the lower sternum or apex.

Diagnosis and Treatment

Avoid over-diagnosis. Healthy young people often have vague symptoms, including chest pain and palpitations. Do not assign a diagnosis of MVP and heart disease when the physical examination is normal, and the echocardiogram shows trivial prolapse but normal mitral valve thickness and shape. Population studies have shown that the prognosis is good for those with mild prolapse, with little risk of stroke, sudden death, or progression to severe MR.

On the other hand, serious illness is possible for those with real MVP (Table 7.2). Interestingly, it is not the thin young woman who is at risk for severe MR, but the middle-aged man with hypertension (a board question). Antibiotic prophylaxis to prevent endocarditis is recommended for those with a systolic murmur or a thickened valve on the echocardiogram. Mild MVP with no murmur does not require prophylaxis. Although untested, many prescribe aspirin for those with severe prolapse to prevent thromboembolic stroke. It is not indicated for mild MVP.

Although uncommon, it is possible for severe MVP to cause angina. The parachute valve increases papillary muscle tension, creating ischemia. This can lead to an abnormal stress ECG, with a perfusion abnormality in the region of the papillary muscle. In such cases, beta blockade may help.

A common treatment issue is the patient with mild MVP and vague, nonanginal chest pain or palpitations. Monitoring usually shows no arrhythmia during symptoms. Treating either symptom with beta-blockers rarely helps. In the absence of convincing angina, I try to avoid stress testing; false-positive results are common and add to the confusion. Most now believe that anxiety is the usual cause of these symptoms. One randomized study showed improvement with prescribed aerobic exercise. That seems a sensible approach, as exercise is good for stress management and is not bad for the heart. Reassure the patient that such symptoms tend to resolve with time.

Aortic Stenosis

Etiology, Pathophysiology and History

About 1% to 2% of the population has a bicuspid aortic valve and may develop AS. Most who do are men, and they become symptomatic in the fourth or fifth decades of life. Typically, a murmur is present from childhood reflecting increased turbulence, and with turbulence the valve degenerates prematurely. The degenerative process in vascular structures—including cardiac valves—involves the deposition of calcium. I tell patients that it is like a carpenter's hand developing callus after years of using a hammer.

Most of our adult patients with AS have tricuspid valves. I used to teach that a minor abnormality of valve shape leads to increased turbulence (and a murmur). This turbulence leads to premature stiffening of the valve and stenosis in the seventh or eighth decades of life. Those with a normally streamlined valve and no murmur could go a few decades longer before the aortic valve wears out. This degenerative model of senile AS is consistent with the usual history of heart murmur in middle age.

More recently, it appears that vascular inflammation contributes to the genesis of AS. Supporting this are studies showing that the early valvular lesion is similar to early atherosclerotic plaque, and that patients who develop AS also have risk factors of coronary artery disease including elevated C reactive protein (CRP).[7] Calcification of the aortic valve parallels calcification in coronary arteries. Perhaps most important, there have been reports that statin therapy retards the progression of AS.[7] This effect of statins cannot be attributed to the degree of cholesterol lowering. Rather, the vascular anti-inflammatory effect of statins is credited.[8] Although practice guidelines do not include statin therapy, many are recommending it for those with early AS.

While it may contribute, I do not buy inflammation as the sole cause of AS. There are many people who develop advanced coronary artery disease with associated inflammation, but never have valvular disease. Conversely, many with senile AS have no vascular disease. Finally, the common history of a murmur earlier in life suggests that longstanding turbulence—and a structural abnormality—caused premature degeneration of the valve. Perhaps turbulence around the valve provokes inflammation, which then contributes to progression of the disease. As with other medical conditions, the pathophysiology probably is multifactorial.

The term, aortic sclerosis, is commonly used to describe the asymptomatic patient with a murmur and reduced valve mobility on the echocardiogram.

The natural history of this condition is benign. Progression to AS occurred in 16% in one study, and only 2.5% developed severe AS.[7] In this small subset, the average time for progression to severe AS was 8 years.

AS primarily affects the LV. It is pure afterload, and the echocardiogram documents concentric LV hypertrophy (LVH). The earliest symptoms are those of left heart failure, including dyspnea on exertion or easy fatigue. A patient may describe a mild decline in exercise tolerance, and only after probing.

The second of the triad of symptoms is angina pectoris. This may occur without associated coronary artery disease; the hypertrophied LV has outrun its blood supply. However, about half of those with AS and angina are found to have a significant coronary stenosis at the time of catheterization.

Syncope is the last of the triad of symptoms. When syncope occurs at rest, it may be the result of a transient tachyarrhythmia, either ventricular tachycardia or AF (with severe diastolic dysfunction either can lead to a drop in blood pressure and cerebral perfusion, see Chapter 2). Syncope during exercise suggests another mechanism: Cardiac output is fixed because of AS, and thus fails to increase with exercise. Yet there is peripheral arterial dilatation with exercise, and the result is hypotension. An abnormal baroreceptor response of the hypertrophied LV, similar to that of neurocardiogenic syncope, may also contribute (see Chapter 6).

Physical Examination

AS is easy to diagnose; a loud systolic murmur that radiates to the neck cannot be much else. The critical issue is whether it is severe. The physical examination usually provides an answer, and the expected findings of severe stenosis are easily deduced from the pathophysiology of AS (Figure 7.5):

1. LVH. The apex impulse is forceful yet still in the midclavicular line as hypertrophy is concentric (e.g., from the outside in). Atrial contraction provides the last increment of ventricular filling at the end of diastole, and this atrial wave encounters a stiff LV producing a shudder, the S_4 gallop. It may be palpable as an apical A wave (roll the patient to the left side while feeling the apex, and feel for a glitch on the upstroke). LVH may be confirmed by the ECG, and will certainly be present on the echocardiogram.

2. The quality and length of the murmur. A mid-systolic, diamond-shaped murmur is typical with mild AS. With more severe disease, ejection is delayed and the murmur peaks later. Eventually the murmur is loud and occupies most of systole, without the crescendo-decrescendo pattern. A palpable murmur (thrill) indicates severe stenosis.

3. Evidence for a calcified valve. My favorite physical sign in elderly patients is the quality of the aortic second sound, A_2. When the valve is heavily calcified, as is usual with senile AS, A_2 softens, and then disappears. An audible A_2 is good evidence against clinically significant AS. How do you tell the difference between A_2 and the pulmonic second sound, P_2? In the absence of pulmonary hypertension P_2 is relatively soft, and can only be heard to the left of the sternum.

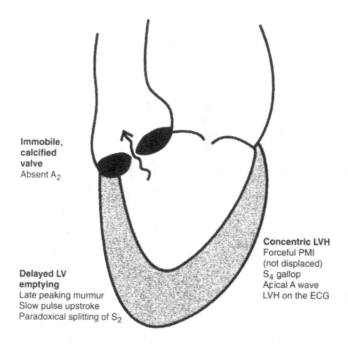

Immobile, calcified valve
Absent A_2

Concentric LVH
Forceful PMI
(not displaced)
S_4 gallop
Apical A wave
LVH on the ECG

Delayed LV emptying
Late peaking murmur
Slow pulse upstroke
Paradoxical splitting of S_2

Figure 7.5 Calcific (senile) aortic stenosis and the physical examination. The physical findings that indicate severe AS reflect LVH, delayed LV emptying, and a heavily calcified, immobile valve. PMI, point of maximum impulse. (Reprinted with permission from Taylor GJ. The Cardiology Rotation. Malden, MA: Blackwell Science, 2001:61.)

AS rarely causes severe pulmonary hypertension. If you hear an S_2 over the aortic area, you are hearing A_2. If the second sound is absent, then A_2 is missing.

4. Evidence for delayed LV emptying. In addition to a longer murmur, prolonged ejection causes a delay in the carotid upstroke. This is a reliable finding in younger patients. It is less so in the elderly who have stiffer arteries, which can mask the delay in the upstroke. I am cautious about mashing on the carotid arteries of elderly patients. There are stories of inexperienced and aggressive examiners provoking stroke.

When these physical findings are present you may count on a high gradient across the aortic valve (Figure 7.6), and on a small valve area (less than 0.8 cm²).

Diagnostic Studies and Timing of Surgery

Echo-Doppler study provides an accurate diagnosis for most patients. It also excludes idiopathic hypertrophic subaortic stenosis or MR, although neither causes a murmur that radiates to the neck. The flow velocity across the aortic valve is a key measurement; 70% of asymptomatic patients with a jet velocity above 4 m per second (corresponding to a peak gradient of 64 mm Hg) become symptomatic and require valve replacement within 2 years.[7]

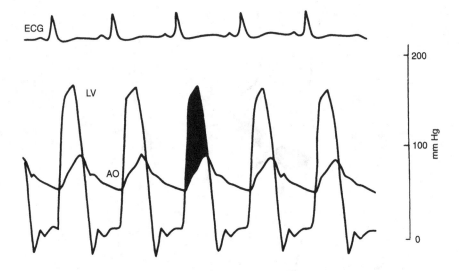

Figure 7.6 Aortic stenosis. Simultaneous LV and aortic (AO) recordings show a pressure gradient across the valve (blackened area). That is the excess pressure that the left ventricle must generate to maintain stroke volume. (Reproduced by permission from Grossman W, ed. Cardiac catheterization and angiography, 2nd ed. Philadelphia: Lea & Febiger, 1980.)

Exercise testing is contraindicated for those with *symptomatic* AS. It is being used more frequently to evaluate *asymptomatic* patients with borderline echocardiographic findings. Exercise-induced symptoms are considered an indication for surgery. In one study, one third of those tested had symptoms for the first time with treadmill testing. This makes sense, as older patients with valvular disease tend to attribute a gradual decline in exercise tolerance to aging, and have learned to avoid activities that provoke symptoms.

Cardiac catheterization allows accurate measurement of the valve gradient (Figure 7.6). Given a technically adequate echocardiogram, this usually is not needed. Coronary angiography is required before surgery.

Symptomatic AS—The onset of symptoms is a definite indication for surgery, because the mortality risk increases following the appearance of symptoms (Figure 7.7). As noted, symptoms may be subtle, and it is important to ask carefully about changes in exercise tolerance.

Sudden cardiac death (SCD) is possible with AS, but this is rarely the initial symptom. It is usually preceded by severe pulmonary congestion. A classic early British study found that 16 of 135 patients with tight AS died during the 6-month wait for surgery. All of those with SCD had a history of CHF, and elevated LV end-diastolic pressure at catheterization.[9] Because the risk of SCD increases substantially

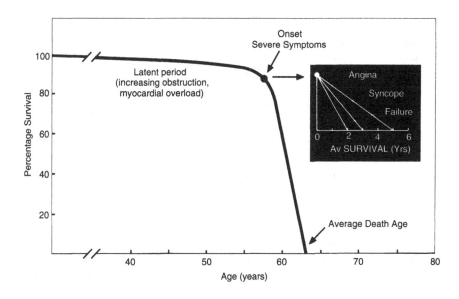

Figure 7.7 The natural history of aortic stenosis. In the absence of symptoms, survival is normal. However, once the symptoms of angina, syncope, or congestive heart failure develop, the survival curve plummets. As seen in the inset, average survival is 5 years after developing angina, 3 years with syncope, and just 2 years with heart failure. (Reproduced by permission from Ross J Jr, Braunwald E. Aortic stenosis. Circulation 1968;38[suppl]:61.)

after the onset of other symptoms, a recommendation that surgical repair should be accomplished within 1 month is sensible.[7]

Asymptomatic AS with a high gradient—The prognosis is excellent in the absence of symptoms, even when AS is severe. As noted, the risk of sudden death is low, perhaps under 1%. That compares favorably to the risk of surgery, which is at least 1% in older patients, plus the 1% per year risk of complications following valve surgery (i.e., thromboembolism, bleeding on warfarin, IE, failure of the valve prosthesis). Thus, the standard of care still favors observation in the absence of symptoms.

As noted, high flow velocity across the stenosed valve, greater than 4 m per second, identifies those at risk for rapid progression of disease, and exercise testing may help when the history is unclear.

Low gradient AS plus low LV ejection fraction—This is a difficult problem. A gradient below 40 mm Hg is considered nonsignificant AS. But the gradient can be low because of low cardiac output. That is a possibility with advanced AS; high afterload depresses the LV, so that EF is low, cardiac output is low, and the gradient and calculated valve area are low. In this case, fixing the valve lowers the afterload. LVEF and cardiac output rise, and there is clinical improvement.

On the other hand, it is possible that LVEF is low because of coexisting cardiomyopathy. In this case a low calculated valve area is the result of low cardiac output.

This has been called *aortic pseudostenosis*.[7] Because afterload is relatively normal, the LV fails to improve after surgery. As a group, those with a transvalvular gradient below 30 mm Hg plus low LVEF have a 20% operative mortality, and less than half are alive 4 years later.[7]

What we would like to do is identify the patient whose low LVEF and gradient are the result of high afterload (bad AS), but who has an intrinsically good LV. This can be sorted out in the catheterization laboratory by increasing cardiac output with dobutamine. With aortic pseudostenosis, the aortic valve gradient changes little as cardiac output increases. With severe AS, raising cardiac output raises the valve gradient. Nitroprusside has also been used: with arterial vasodilatation, downstream resistance falls but there is little change in cardiac output if AS is severe (e.g., all the afterload is in the valve). With cardiomyopathy, cardiac output increases with vasodilatation and afterload reduction.

Dobutamine stress echocardiography may also sort it out. Dopamine increases ejection fraction and cardiac output. The valve gradient will increase when there is true AS. If AS is mild and the patient has a cardiomyopathy, the ejection fraction increases but there is no change in the valve gradient.

Elderly patients—There appears to be no age limit for correction of AS in the absence of comorbid conditions. Surgical correction gives an 80-year-old person a normal life expectancy, on average about 6 years.[7] Coronary artery disease, other valvular heart disease, advanced renal and neurological diseases all increase the risk of surgery and must be considered.

An occasional old person declines surgery, most commonly one with poor general health. With the onset of symptoms, survival with AS can be as long as 2 to 5 years (Figure 7.6). It is probably less than that for a frail octogenarian.

Medical Therapy

Mechanical conditions require mechanical solutions, and medical therapy is no substitute for surgery. Asymptomatic, presurgical AS requires no specific therapy. As with other valve disease, antibiotic prophylaxis during dental and other invasive procedures is indicated.

HMG CoA reductase inhibitors have been reported to slow the progression of AS, but have not been tested in clinical trials. A possible mechanism is the potent vascular anti-inflammatory action of statins (see Chapter 3). At present, this use of statins does not fall within the standard of care.

Medical therapy does little to affect survival for those who are not to have surgery (for whatever reason). Symptomatic congestion should be managed with diuretics. Boosting cardiac output with digoxin may help. The use of afterload reducers has been reported, and is of clear benefit for those with aortic psuedostenosis (whose real illness is cardiomyopathy). However, with pure valvular AS, vasodilatation has little effect on cardiac output.

Aortic Regurgitation

Etiology, Pathophysiology, and History

AR is caused by diseases of the aortic root (Marfan's syndrome, ankylosing spondylitis, syphilis or the annuloaortic ectasia or aging), or by conditions affecting the valve leaflets (IE, rheumatic fever, congenital bicuspid valve, or collagen vascular disease).

Chronic AR—The LV responds to the volume overload with dilatation but also with eccentric hypertrophy. In contrast, MR—a pure volume overload disease—leads to dilatation with little hypertrophy. Whenever there is hypertrophy, afterload is high (the exception being infiltrative disease), and afterload is elevated with AR. The explanation for this is that the high stroke volume of AR is ejected into the aorta causing a rise in systolic pressure, and thus an increase in LV afterload. In a sense, there is not enough room in the central circulation for the high stroke volume. With MR the higher stroke volume (inevitable with any LV volume overload) is shared by the LA and aorta, so there is no increase in aortic systolic pressure.

Interestingly, the eccentric hypertrophy of AR is inadequate to normalize LV wall stress. Recall Laplace's law:

Wall stress or tension = (pressure × radius of the chamber)/wall thickness

Physiologists call the failure of the LV to thicken enough to normalize stress *afterload mismatch*, a term I find confusing. The phenomenon may cause mild short-term contractile dysfunction, and it contributes to decompensation over the long run.

The enlarged LV accommodates the regurgitant volume with little increase in diastolic pressure, so there is no pulmonary congestion. This chronic compensated phase of AR may persist for years. Eventually, the LV fails. There is a decline in contractility and a marked increase in LV end-systolic volume (e.g., LVEF declines). LV diastolic pressure increases, leading to pulmonary congestion. Surgery early in this phase of decompensation may restore normal LV function, but there is also a chance that LV dysfunction will persist.

An important peripheral circulatory response to AR is vasodilatation with low diastolic blood pressure. Pulse pressure is wide. With chronic AR and a valve that is still somewhat competent, there is a considerable difference between LV and aortic diastolic pressure. (If you think about it, LV diastolic pressure must be normal if there is no pulmonary congestion.) Wide pulse pressure is responsible for a number of physical signs: Corrigan's pulse (sharp upstroke and rapid descent of the carotid pulse), DeMusset's sign (head bobbing), Quincke's pulse (pulsating color in the nail bed with pressure on the nail), Hill's sign (augmentation of the systolic pressure in the leg by more than 40 mm Hg compared with the arm), and others. *If the pulse pressure is normal, AR probably is not hemodynamically significant.* That is a simple and useful fact; moderate-to-severe AR is common on echo-Doppler reports, but with normal blood pressure, a soft or absent murmur, and normal LV dimensions, the patient does not have significant AR.

The usual symptoms of AR are those of left heart failure with pulmonary congestion or declining exercise tolerance. Angina may occur with advanced disease.

Acute AR—The usual cause is endocarditis, most commonly with staphylococcal infection in a setting of drug abuse. Consider it when there is abrupt onset of heart failure in a young person. Look for peripheral signs of endocarditis (splinter or conjunctival hemorrhages, petechiae), and get blood cultures. A rash may indicate gonococcus sepsis.

The heart murmur may be soft or absent. Acute volume overload of the normal (not dilated) LV causes a marked rise in LV diastolic pressure and severe pulmonary congestion. The stiff pericardium helps to limit LV dilatation. LV diastolic pressure may be similar to aortic diastolic pressure, and arterial pulse pressure is not wide. With a small diastolic gradient across the valve, the volume of diastolic regurgitation is minimal, reducing murmur intensity.

Diagnostic Procedures and Timing of Surgery for Chronic Aortic Regurgitation

LV end-systolic size, accurately measured with the transthoracic echocardiogram, provides the best guide to timing of surgery, much as it does with MR. As long as the LV is able to contract down to a normal volume—or end-systolic diameter less than 4.0 cm—it is safe to continue observation. When the end-systolic dimension rises to 5.5 cm, it is time for surgery, even in the absence of symptoms. Between 4.0 and 5.5, any symptoms would indicate a need for surgery, and periodic echo surveillance is needed for the asymptomatic patient.

A summary statement: both of the LV volume overload conditions—MR and AR—require surgical correction before the onset of symptoms, and the timing of surgery is based on LV size and function. Get serial echocardiograms.

The LV size that requires surgery is higher with AR (LV end-systolic dimension 5.5 cm) than with MR (4.5 cm). The physiologic explanation is the higher afterload with AR; after surgery, the LV is more likely to improve. Correction of AR is possible when there is LV dysfunction, but the outcome is better with early surgery. A large Mayo Clinic series divided patients into groups with low (<35%), medium (35% to 50%), and normal (>50%) LVEF.[10] Surgical mortality was 14%, 6.7%, and 3.7% in the three groups, respectively, and 10-year survival was 41%, 56%, and 70%.

An additional indication for surgery is increasing aortic root diameter, a common complication of Marfan's syndrome. When the root diameter exceeds 5.5 to 6.0 cm, the risk of aortic dissection is high, and prophylactic valve plus ascending aorta replacement is needed.

Remember the "55 rule": fix AR when the LVEF falls below 55%, the end-systolic diameter exceeds 55 mm, or the aortic root is larger than 55 mm.[11]

Medical Therapy

Afterload reduction therapy favors forward flow. Vasodilatation with nifedipine has been shown to forestall the need for surgery in asymptomatic patients with good

LV function by as much as 2 to 3 years. ACE inhibition has been shown effective in children, and probably works for adults, although it has not been studied. Afterload reduction therapy is the mainstay for symptomatic patients who will not or cannot have surgery, and the dihydroperidine calcium channel blockers and ACE inhibitors may be used. Congestion is treated with diuretics, and many improve with digoxin.

It is important to treat systolic hypertension, as high central aortic pressure favors regurgitant rather than forward flow. But this is one situation where beta blockade may be harmful. Regurgitation takes place during diastole, and at a slower heart rate, the total diastolic time is increased. Thus, drugs that cause bradycardia may aggravate the symptoms of AR (beta-blockers, diltiazem, and verapamil).

On the other hand, beta blockade has been shown to prevent aortic dissection in patients with Marfan's syndrome, because reducing LV contractility blunts the shear stress of the ejection wave. Beta blockade is indicated for those with aneurysmal or dilated proximal aortas, but must be used carefully when there is significant AR.

Tricuspid Regurgitation

The most common cause of right heart failure is left heart failure. Left side failure is also the most common cause of tricuspid regurgitation (TR). Elevated left atrial and pulmonary venous pressure lead to high PA pressure. High right ventricular (RV) pressure and RV dilatation lead to TR. It is common for a patient having surgery for mitral valve disease to require tricuspid valve repair. Other causes of pulmonary hypertension, including cor pulmonale and primary pulmonary hypertension, may also cause TR.

Primary TR caused by structural damage to the valve is relatively uncommon. RV infarction, Ebstein's abnormality, endocarditis, and the carcinoid syndrome are illnesses you may encounter on board examinations. Levels of serotonin and its metabolites are higher in those with carcinoid plus TR than in others with a normal valve (drop that tidbit during morning rounds, and note the following discussion of appetite suppressant drugs). Clinically, the most common cause of isolated TR is endocarditis in drug users.

Presentation, Pathophysiology, and Examination

The typical symptoms are those of right heart failure, including edema, ascites, and fatigue. Hepatic congestion may lead to right upper quadrant pain, especially if the onset is rapid.

The apical impulse is not displaced unless there is LV disease. There is a parasternal lift (recall that the RV is the most anterior cardiac chamber, located just below the sternum and anterior to the LV). P_2 is loud when there is pulmonary hypertension, and this is one time you may hear both A_2 and P_2 at the right base (normally P_2 is soft and is heard only on the left side).

An RV gallop may be heard over the sternum, recognized as such by its increase with inspiration.

The murmur of TR is holosystolic and best heard along the right sternal border. It increases with inspiration. Negative intrathoracic pressure sucks blood into the chest, increasing RV filling and stroke volume, and increasing the TR volume. The murmur may not change with respiration if there is severe RV failure.

The jugular venous pressure is elevated, and it is important to examine the pulse wave. Normally, the dominant venous wave is the A wave, generated by atrial systole. But with TR there is no effective valve separating the RV from the jugular veins, so the pressure wave generated by RV contraction is dominant wave—the V wave. The key to examining the jugular pulse is to feel the brachial pulse. If the dominant venous pulsation is simultaneous with the arterial pulse, it is a V wave. If the venous pulse is just before the arterial pulse—presystolic—you are seeing an A wave. With TR, the V wave is greater than the A wave (frankly, this is about the only time I find the venous pulse wave helpful). The V wave may be reflected back through the great veins, leading to a pulsatile liver.

Treatment

The treatment of TR is centered on treating the primary illness (left heart failure, mitral valve disease, pulmonary hypertension caused by lung disease, etc.). When there is no left heart disease, therapy is aimed at relieving symptoms with diuretics. Isolated TR may be tolerated for years, and it is rare that surgical repair is needed.

TR often complicates mitral valve disease. The surgeon fixes the mitral valve, takes the patient off pump, and evaluates the tricuspid valve for persistent regurgitation. Traditionally this was done by sticking a finger through a hole in the right atrium and feeling the TR jet. Transesophageal echo is also used for this purpose during surgery. If TR remains severe, the patient goes back on bypass and tricuspid annuloplasty is performed.

Cardiac Valve Prosthese

No cardiac valve prosthesis is perfect. My surgical colleague with special insight—and a sense of humor—used a slide in lectures that assigned the different valves "units of disappointment." The major issues are durability and thromboembolic potential.

Tissue valves are the least thrombogenic, and there are a number of varieties (porcine aortic valves, bovine pericardial valves, etc). Aspirin therapy is adequate long term; warfarin is usually stopped 1 month after surgery. The problem is that the prosthetic devices begin to wear out after about 10 years, and much earlier in young patients with active calcium metabolism.

Tissue valves are currently used when there is a contraindication to warfarin therapy, or for the elderly patient where durability is less an issue. Deterioration of the valves tends to be gradual, and reoperation is rarely an emergency procedure. A patient who needs anticoagulation for chronic AF or previous embolism may as well have a mechanical valve.

The more durable mechanical valves have a thromboembolic rate of three to eight events per 100 valve-years, which is substantially reduced by warfarin therapy. Warfarin carries a risk of two hemorrhagic events per 100 valve-years, usually non-fatal gastrointestinal bleed. Most thromboembolic events are strokes. Thus, the evidence weighs in favor of warfarin therapy for all patients with mechanical valves. This is especially important for valves in the mitral position, where the embolic risk is higher than it is with an aortic valve prosthesis.

As noted earlier, mitral valve repair is preferable to replacement. Both procedures can now be performed endoscopically, and with good results.[12]

Anticoagulation

The target International Normalized Ratio (INR) with a mechanical valve is 3 to 3.5. The addition of low-dose aspirin further lowers the risk of stroke, and may be considered for higher risk patients: those with AF, history of stroke or transient ischemic attack (e.g., a previous embolus), or a valve in the mitral position. To these recognized risk factors, many would add a greatly enlarged LA or a cardiomyopathic LV, especially if the echocardiogram shows evidence for stagnant flow.

A common issue is what to do with anticoagulation when a patient with a mechanical valve needs a noncardiac surgical procedure. There are no clinical trials data to guide us. Before the late 1990s, most patients were admitted to the hospital for intravenous heparin before surgery, and it was used postoperatively as well. That aggressive approach does not appear necessary, and current recommendations suggest fitting anticoagulation needs to the patient's risk of thromboembolism (Table 7.3). Low-risk patients have warfarin stopped preoperatively, and restarted soon after surgery. Heparin coverage is not recommended either before or after surgery.[13]

When the risk of embolism is especially high, the time off anticoagulants is minimized by postoperative heparin therapy while warfarin is being restarted (Table 7.3). One review warns against starting heparin less than 12 hours after surgery, and another recommends starting heparin as soon as possible postoperatively.[13,14] In practice, the surgeon decides when hemostasis is adequate and it is safe to begin heparin. In most cases preoperative treatment with heparin is not required. Consider it for highest risk patients, particularly when there is a history of thromboembolism (Table 7.3).

Appetite Suppressant Drugs and Valvular Disease

Fenfluramine has been available since the early 1970s, but a report of the effectiveness of long-term therapy—in combination with phentermine—popularized its use in the early 1990s. Roughly two to four million people were treated with "fen-phen" for 4 to 12 months.[15] Reports of valvulopathy led to the withdrawal of fenfluramine and dexfenfluramine in 1997.

Early reports by the US Food and Drug Adminstration suggested that a new valve lesion developed in 30% of those exposed to fen-phen. Based upon larger experience, a more reasonable estimate is 15% to 20%, with the incidence of clinically significant disease much lower.[15]

Table 7.3 Anticoagulation in Patients with Prosthetic Valves Having Noncardiac Operations	
Low-risk patients (Bileaflet, St. Jude valve in the aortic position and no risk factors for thromboembolism*)	• Stop warfarin 4 days preoperatively • Surgery when the INR is <1.5 • Restart warfarin as soon as the patient can take pills • Consider heparin if the INR is <2.0 for 5 days or more
High-risk patients (Those with multiple risk factors for thromboembolism*)	• Stop warfarin 4–5 days preoperatively • Give full dose heparin when the INR is <2.0† • Stop heparin 10–12 hours before surgery • Surgery • Resume heparin soon after surgery (see text) • Resume warfarin as soon as the patient can take pills • Discontinue heparin when the INR is >2.0

*Risk factors for thromboembolism: double-position prosthetic valves, atrial fibrillation, severe LV dysfunction, previous embolus, hypercoagulable state, valve in the mitral position, an early generation prosthesis—a ball-in-cage (Starr-Edwards), or tilting disc (Bjork-Shiley) valve.
†Preoperative heparin is less important than postoperative coverage—consider it when there are at least 3 risk factors (the very highest risk patients).

Modified from Tiede DJ, Nishimura RA, Gastineau DA, et al. Modern management of prosthetic valve anticoagulation. Mayo Clin Proc 1998;73:665–680.

The usual lesion was AR. MR was reported early, but appears to be less common. Most of the patients affected were women. Higher dose and longer duration of therapy, plus combination drug use increased the risk of developing disease.

You will not encounter new cases because the drugs responsible for the syndrome are no longer in use. However, it is worth a brief summary because of the interesting pathophysiology. The fenfluramines are serotonin agonists; they suppress appetite by stimulating serotonin release and blocking its reuptake by nerve terminals in the hypothalamus. A few of the patients with AR had surgery, and the affected valves had pathology identical to that of AR caused by serotonin-secreting carcinoid tumor. Prolonged use of other serotonin analogues, methysergide and ergotamine, may also cause this cardiac manifestation of the serotonin syndrome. Another cardiac complication of serotonin is pulmonary vasoconstriction leading to pulmonary hypertension and right heart failure. Although reported, this is less common than the valvular complications of fenfluramine.

In vitro studies have shown that serotonin can stimulate the migration of fibroblasts to heart valve endocardium, and promotes the secretion of extracellular matrix. Although any heart valve can be affected, it is thought that AR is the usual problem because the aortic valve is exposed to the highest flow rates and shear stress.

The present guidelines for evaluating and diagnosing drug-induced valvulopathy begin with a physical examination. An echocardiogram is recommended only for patients with a murmur or with a history that suggests heart disease. The American Heart Association did not recommend echocardiogram for all patients who have taken diet drugs.[15]

You may reassure your patients who have taken fenfluramine in the past: valvulopathy is not a delayed reaction that can develop years after the use of the drug.

Those with valvulopathy tend to improve. The Mayo Clinic group that originally described the condition found that most patients had improvement in the appearance and function of the aortic valve 6 months after stopping the medicine.[16] Valve surgery is rarely needed.

Presently available appetite suppressants have no serotonergic properties, and do not cause valve disease. Thus, phentermine, sibutamine, orlistat, and diethylpropion have no direct cardiac toxicity.[17]

Infective Endocarditis

As with most infections, IE requires a susceptible host and exposure to an infecting organism. The major component of susceptibility is a roughened valve or endovascular surface, usually the result of increased turbulence. Fibrin and platelets attach to the roughened surface, and circulating bacteria stick to this thrombus, becoming an independent site of infection able to seed the rest of the body. Valve lesions with a high degree of turbulence are more likely to promote colonization than large defects with high flow, but low turbulence (e.g., atrial septal defect).

Almost all bacteria may reach the circulation, but only those able to adhere to thrombus cause IE. For example *Escherichia coli* and *Klebsiella pneumoniae* usually pass a roughened valve surface and do not stick, even though these are frequent causes of bacteremia in patients with cholangitis or pyelonephritis. On the other hand, *Staphylococcus aureus* is sticky, attaching to a roughened valve in the first circulatory pass and covering it within 24 hours.

Clinical Syndromes

Subacute IE—Fever and other constitutional symptoms such as weight loss, fatigue, and weakness are common with subacute IE. Virtually every organ in the body may be a target of emboli from the vegetation. Stroke occurs in about one fourth of cases.

On physical examination there is usually a heart murmur. Classic skin lesions include splinter hemorrhages, petechiae involving skin conjunctiva or mucous membranes, painful subcutaneous nodules on fingers or toes (Osler's nodes), and painless hemorrhagic macules on the palms and soles (Janeway lesions). Clubbing of the fingers is common with chronic endocarditis, but it is not specific (think of lung cancer as well). Roth spots are present in only 5% of cases, and can also be caused by leukemia, lupus, and profound anemia. Splenomegaly is found in as many as half the cases.

Acute IE—Rapid destruction of a valve is possible, most commonly with staphylococcal or gonococcal sepsis. Acute AR (or less commonly, MR) leads to severe pulmonary congestion or shock. As noted, the regurgitant murmur may be soft of absent.

Endocarditis is suggested by the abrupt onset of heart failure. Other clinical evidence of infection may include fever, a rash with gonococcal sepsis, and elevated white blood cell count. A history of intravenous drug use is common when the patient is young and has no history of heart disease. As with subacute IE, there may be evidence for peripheral embolus.

Associated Conditions

Right heart (usually tricuspid valve) endocarditis is most common with intravenous drug use. Think of it, as well, for those with indwelling catheters. In urban centers a common cause is methicillin-resistant *S. aureus*, although enterococcus, viridans streptococci, and *Pseudomonas aeruginosa* are possibilities. These patients are also at risk for candida endocarditis, with associated endophthalmitis and left-side valvular infection.

More than half the patients with *Streptococcus bovis* endocarditis have lesions in the colon, including malignancies. Other malignancies may predispose to bacteremia and valve infection with unusual organisms such as *Clostridium septicum*, *Listeria monocytogenes*, and group B beta-hemolytic streptococci.

Laboratory Studies

One of the first three blood culture results is positive in more than 95% of cases. When there has been antibiotic treatment in the previous 2 weeks, the yield falls to 65%. For the initial evaluation of the untreated patient, three sets of cultures are adequate. A patient who has had antibiotic therapy should have blood cultures 2 and 10 days after treatment ends.

Constitutional symptoms are usually accompanied by an elevated sedimentation rate or positive rheumatoid factor, but negative studies do not exclude IE. In Peterdorf's classic study, the mean Westergren sedimentation rate was 57 mm/hr. Normocytic anemia is present in most cases, and it worsens with time. The white blood cell count is elevated only occasionally.

The echocardiogram demonstrates valvular vegetations and is now included in diagnostic criteria for IE.[18] Small vegetations may be detected with transesophageal study. But the echocardiogram may have both false-positive and false-negative results. The test is more sensitive than specific. Vegetations may persist for 2 years or longer after successful treatment, so a vegetation does not prove active infection. Other imaging studies usually do not help (e.g., gallium scanning, although it is often ordered).

Treatment

A century ago viridans streptococcal endocarditis was the usual illness; now it accounts for less than one fourth of cases.[18] The causes of IE we encounter more frequently are less susceptible to antibiotics and are trickier to manage. Few cardiologists are up to it, and we rely on infectious disease colleagues for the treatment of the infection.

An acutely ill patient may require empiric therapy, pending the culture results. Start a combination of nafcillin or vancomycin plus an aminoglycoside.

Table 7.4 Risk of Infective Endocarditis (IE)	
Prophylaxis Recommended	
Highest risk	Prosthetic cardiac valves Previous endocarditis Cyanotic congenital heart disease
Moderate risk	Other congenital heart disease (note the following exceptions) Acquired valvular heart disease IHSS MVP with MR or thickened valve leaflets
Low risk (IE prophylaxis not recommended)	Isolated atrial septal defect* After surgical repair of atrial septal defect or patent ductus arteriosus (without residual after 6 months) After coronary artery bypass surgery or angioplasty Physiologic or functional heart murmur (no valve abnormality on echo) Previous rheumatic fever without valve abnormality Cardiac pacemaker or implanted defibrillator

*Primum ASD includes abnormal mitral and/or tricuspid valves, and the systolic murmur indicates valve regurgitation—prophylaxis is needed.

IHSS, idiopathic hypertrophic subaortic stenosis; MVP, mitral valve prolapse; MR, mitral regurgitation.

An issue for the cardiology consultant is the timing of surgery. The classic indications for valve replacement are heart failure, thromboembolism or persistent bacteremia. In recent years there has been a trend toward earlier replacement of infected valves. Difficult to treat organisms are relative indications for early surgery, including *P. aeruginosi* or fungi, especially when fever does not resolve with antibiotic therapy. Many believe that staphylococcal endocarditis requires early surgery, arguing that it is better to operate before perivalvular abscesses develop.

Prosthetic valve infection usually requires surgery. An exception is endocarditis more than 2 months after valve surgery with an especially susceptible organism such as viridans streptococci. Any dysfunction of the prosthetic valve, especially a perivalvular leak, indicates a need for surgery. A key part of the physical examination is listening carefully for the murmur of AR in a patient with an aortic valve prosthesis.

When there is an indication for surgery it should not be delayed. With time there is more opportunity for the organism to burrow into the myocardium, cause abscesses (heart block is a potential consequence of aortic valve endocarditis—watch the PR interval), and generate emboli. Infection of a replacement valve is infrequent, even when it is sewn to tissue that may not be sterile.

The new valve may not sit securely into the valve ring because of weakened tissue, and perivalvular leak complicates about 15%. Antibiotic therapy after surgery is a complex issue requiring infectious disease consultation (and management).

Prevention of Infective Endocarditis

Valvular disease with a murmur is the usual indication of antibiotic prophylaxis (Table 7.4).[19] Patients with MVP but no murmur rarely develop IE; however, Doppler evidence for moderate MR is an indication for prophylaxis. Another exception to the murmur rule is middle-aged men with MVP and a thickened valve. Their risk of IE is high and they should have antibiotic prophylaxis, even without a murmur.

Invasive dental, gastrointestinal, genitourinary, and upper respiratory tract procedures are indications for antibiotic prophylaxis. On the other hand, restorative dentistry (filling teeth), endotracheal intubation, esophageal endoscopy, and vaginal delivery are not, except for the highest risk patients. Antibiotic prophylaxis regimens are updated periodically by the American Heart Association and are found in most standard texts (the dentist usually has the information on his bulletin board).

References

1. Carabello BA. Mitral regurgitation: basic pathophysiologic principles. Mod Concepts Cardiovasc Dis 1988;57:53–58.

2. Rozich JD, Carabello BA, Usher BW, et al. Mitral valve replacement with and without chordal preservation in patients with chronic mitral regurgitation. Mechanism for differences in postoperative ejection performance. Circulation 1992;86:1718–1726.

3. Bach DS, Bolling SF. Improvement following correction of secondary mitral regurgitation in end-stage cardiomyopathy with mitral annuloplasty. Am J Cardiol 1996;78:966–969.

4. Otto CM. Clinical practice. Evaluation and management of chronic mitral regurgitation. N Engl J Med 2001;345:740–746.

5. Wisenbuagh T, Sinovich V, Dullabh A, Sareli P. Six month pilot study of captopril for mildly symptomatic, severe isolated mitral and isolated aortic regurgitation. J Heart Valve Dis 1994;3:197–204.

6. St John Sutton M, Weyman AE. Mitral valve prolapse prevalence and complications: an ongoing dialogue. Circulation 2002;106:1305–1307.

7. Carabello BA. Evaluation and management of patients with aortic stenosis. Circulation 2002;105:1746–1750. Also note, Carabello BA. Clinical practice. Aortic stenosis. N Engl J Med 2002;346:677–682. Also note, Otto CM. Why is aortic sclerosis associated with adverse clinical outcomes? J Am Coll Cardiol 2004;43:176–178.

8. Chandra HR, Goldstein JA, Choudhary N, et al. Adverse outcome in aortic sclerosis is associated with coronary artery disease and inflammation. J Am Coll Cardiol 2004;43:169–175. Also note, Otto CM. Why is aortic sclerosis associated with adverse clinical outcomes. J Am Coll Cardiol 2004;43:176–178. (*There is an association, but it is uncertain whether aortic sclerosis is the cause of inflammation or a marker of vascular inflammation.*)

9. Matthews AW, Barritt DW, Keen GE, Belsey RH. Preoperative mortality in aortic stenosis. Br Heart J 1974;36:101–103.

10. Chaliki HP, Mohty D, Avierinos JF, et al. Outcomes after aortic valve replacement in patients with severe aortic regurgitation and markedly reduced left ventricular function. Circulation 2002;106:2687–2693.

11. Carabello BA, Crawford FA. Valvular heart disease. N Engl J Med 1997;337:32–41.

12. Casselman FP, Van Slycke S, Wellens F, et al. Mitral valve surgery can now routinely be performed endoscopically. Circulation 2003;108(suppl 1):II48–II54.

13. Tiede DJ, Nishimura RA, Gastineau DA, et al. Modern management of prosthetic valve anticoagulation. Mayo Clin Proc 1998;73:665–680.

14. Kearon C, Hirsh J. Management of anticoagulation before and after elective surgery. N Engl J Med 1997;336:1506–1511.

15. Cannistra LB, Gaasch WH. Appetite-suppressing drugs and valvular heart disease. Cardiol Rev 1999;7:356–361.

16. Hensrud DD, Connolly HM, Grogan M, et al. Echocardiographic improvement over time after cessation use of fenfluramine and phentermine. Mayo Clin Proc 1999;74:1191–1197.

17. Glazer G. Long-term pharmacotherapy of obesity 2000; a review of efficacy and safety. Arch Intern Med 2001;161:1814–1824.

18. Mylonakis E, Calderwood SB. Infective endocarditis in adults. N Engl J Med 2001;345:1318–1330.

19. Osmon DR. Antimicrobial prophylaxis in adults. Mayo Clin Proc 2000;75:98–109.

CHAPTER 8

HYPERTENSION, AORTIC DISEASE, AND OTHER MEDICAL ILLNESSES WITH CARDIOVASCULAR EFFECTS

Abbreviations

AAA	abdominal aortic aneurysm	LVH	LV hypertrophy
ACE	angiotensin-converting enzyme	MI	myocardial infarction
ARB	angiotensin receptor blocker	MRFIT	Multiple Risk Factor Intervention Trial
BP	blood pressure		
CAD	coronary artery disease	P₂	pulmonic second heart sound
CHF	congestive heart failure	PA	pulmonary artery
CVD	cardiovascular disease	PPH	primary pulmonary hypertension
ECG	electrocardiogram		
HBP	high blood pressure (hypertension)	PVR	pulmonary vascular resistance
		RAA	renin-angiotensin-aldosterone (system)
HDL	high-density lipoprotein (cholesterol)		
		RA	right atrial
JNC	Joint National Committee	RBBB	right bundle branch block
LDL	low-density lipoprotein (cholesterol)	RV	right ventricle (ventricular)
		S₃	third heart sound
LV	left ventricle (ventricular)	S₄	fourth heart sound
LVEF	LV ejection fraction	TR	tricuspid valve regurgitation

Hypertension

About 50 million Americans are hypertensive, and it seems that most of us will be. According to the Framingham study, those who are normotensive at age 55 years have a 90% chance of developing high blood pressure (HBP) at some time.[1] You who are in primary care medicine spend a lot of time treating hypertension, and I suggest a review of the latest Joint National Committee report, JNC 7.[2] It is comprehensive yet avoids excessive detail, and it summarizes the clinical trials that have substantially changed our approach since the JNC 6 report in 1997. Box 8.1 summarizes the key points.

The reason to treat HBP is to prevent end-organ damage, primarily cardiovascular disease (CVD). Declining mortality rates from stroke and coronary artery disease (CAD) over the last 40 years have been attributed to more effective antihypertensive therapy. In the 1960s the most common cause of congestive heart failure (CHF) was hypertensive heart disease; now it is CAD, probably because of better therapy for HBP. In clinical trials antihypertensive lowers the rate of stroke by 40%, myocardial infarction (MI) by 25%, and CHF by more than 50%.

Yet we are not doing as well as we should. In the early 1990s, a rule of halves was described for the United States and Western Europe based on population surveys: half the hypertensive population was undetected, half of those diagnosed were untreated, and half of those treated had inadequate control. It is slightly better now, yet 30% with HBP are not aware they have it.[2]

Evaluating Hypertension

Blood pressure (BP) should be measured with the patient seated, at least 30 minutes after exposure to coffee or cigarettes. Smokers often stop for a last, furtive drag before coming into the office (attaching pejorative terms to this behavior seems unfair, but it is hard not to disapprove . . .). An elevated pressure should be reconfirmed in 5 to 10 minutes in the other arm. If still elevated, HBP should not be diagnosed until elevated pressure is confirmed with two subsequent visits. Have the office nurse check the pressure with the patient not scheduled to see the doctor; this may help avoid white coat hypertension. You and your staff should tell the patient what the BP measurement is.

JNC 7 provides a simplified classification for HBP, and introduces the prehypertension category (Table 8.1). The rationale for this is population data showing that increasing risk of CVD begins when BP is above 115/75 mm Hg, with the incidence of CVD doubling for each incremental increase of 20/10 mm Hg. Furthermore, those in the prehypertension category have a doubling of the risk of developing HBP. At lower levels, lifestyle modification is usually adequate. Both systolic and diastolic hypertension are indications for treatment, although elevated systolic pressure is a more potent risk factor for CVD.[2]

Examination and Laboratory Studies

The goal of the initial evaluation is to gauge the risk of CVD, detect end-organ disease, and screen for correctible causes of HBP. Risk factors for CVD, particularly the metabolic syndrome, have been reviewed in Chapter 3.

Abnormalities on physical examination that are noteworthy include retinal arterial narrowing, thyromegaly, arterial bruit (carotid, abdominal, or femoral),

Table 8.1 Classification and Management of Blood Pressure*			
Class	Systolic BP -or- Diastolic BP (mm Hg)		Treatment†
Prehypertension	120–139	80–89	Drug therapy only if another condition requires it (see Table 8.3)
Stage 1	140–159	90–99	Start with a thiazide, and add other drug(s) to reach BP goal†
Stage 2	≥160	≥100	Start two-drug therapy, including a thiazide

*Adults over age 18.
†All should have lifestyle modification (see text).

Modified with permission from Chobanian AV, Bakris GL, Cushman WC, et al. The seventh report of the Joint National Committee on Prevention, Detection, Evaluation and Treatment of High Blood Pressure (JNC 7). JAMA 2003;289:2560–2572.

depressed lower extremity pulses or BP (coarctation of the aorta), a forceful cardiac apical impulse or S_4 gallop, and an abnormal abdominal examination (bruit, enlarged aorta, masses).

As an exercise, try to justify each of the laboratory tests commonly recommended for newly diagnosed HBP. Do it before reading my explanation (and let me know if I miss something obvious).

Urinalysis. Urine glucose is a crude screen for diabetes. Albuminuria is a diagnostic criterion for kidney disease, even when serum creatinine is normal, and justifies a lower target BP (Box 8.1). Specifically, it is an indication for angiotensin converting enzyme (ACE) inhibitor therapy, which is antiproteinuric.[3] Proteinuria has also been identified as a risk factor for early CVD.

Chemistries. Serum *potassium* is especially important. When low off diuretics, it may indicate hyperaldosteronism, Conn's syndrome, as the cause of hypertension. Hypokalemia is a dangerous complication of diuretic therapy, and seems worse with thiazides than loop diuretics. Out-of-hospital cardiac arrest has been related to hypokalemia and to thiazide use. The MRFIT trial showed no mortality benefit with risk factor modification with early follow-up (there was a benefit later). There was an excess of sudden cardiac death (SCD) in the treated group that was later ascribed to thiazide therapy and hypokalemia.

Sodium measurement is less useful in patients with mild hypertension and who are otherwise healthy. In those with CHF, low sodium indicates poor prognosis and is a marker for high plasma renin activity (and increased sensitivity to ACE inhibition—start with low-dose therapy).

Creatinine and blood urea nitrogen are important as screens for underlying renal dysfunction, which changes the target BP (Box 8.1). *Glucose* is a better screen for diabetes when measured in a fasting state. Hyperglycemia may also be associated with secondary causes of HBP including Cushing's syndrome, pheochromocytoma, and primary aldosteronism.

Lipid analysis is a part of the CVD risk assessment. High triglycerides and low high-density lipoprotein (HDL) cholesterol are features of the metabolic syndrome (along with abdominal obesity, glucose intolerance and hypertension, Chapter 3). In this case the low-density lipoprotein (LDL) cholesterol level may be normal, but the LDL particles tend to be small and dense, and are more atherogenic.

Calcium and phosphate measurement is a screen for hyperparathyroidism, a potential cause of HBP. Uric acid may rise with diuretic therapy, and a baseline is useful.

The *hematocrit* has little direct relationship to HBP, but it is cheap and reasonable to screen for anemia if the patient is to have blood drawn.

The ECG is a crude tool. Its sensitivity for detecting LV hypertrophy (LVH) is less than 50%. The earliest sign of hypertensive heart disease is left atrial abnormality, usually a biphasic P wave in V_1 (see Figure 7.2). If you suspect LVH based on the ECG or physical examination (S_4 gallop or forceful apical impulse), get an echocardiogram to measure LV thickness. That is the gold standard, and increased thickness—LVH—indicates hypertensive heart disease. Making that diagnosis reinforces a need for aggressive BP control.

A *chest x-ray* is another sensible and relatively inexpensive screen for any middle aged person. It is relatively unreliable as a test for cardiac enlargement. Patients with LVH have concentric hypertrophy, with little chamber enlargement. Coarctation of the aorta may cause rib notching (collaterals vessels) and a "3" sign (dilated ascending aorta).

Secondary Hypertension

Hypertension is a complication of a number of illnesses, many of them apparent from the screening evaluation (Table 8.2).[4] There is an element of uncertainty when deciding how much farther to go when looking for a correctable cause of HBP. It is the conflict between too much testing and not wanting to miss disease. JNC 7 helps by stating that "more extensive testing for identifiable causes is not indicated generally unless BP control is not achieved."[2]

About 5% to 10% of HBP is secondary (Table 8.2). That does not seem like much, yet HBP is so common that we all see cases. In some series, renovascular hypertension accounts for 5%. Primary aldosteronism (0.5%), coarctation of the aorta (0.5%), pheochromocytoma (0.2%), and Cushing's syndrome (0.1%) are much less common. Sleep apnea and excessive alcohol use are often overlooked, and BP control may depend on their correction.

Treatment of Hypertension

The goals of therapy are aggressive and are based on clinical trials showing a reduction in CVD at these targets (Box 8.1). JNC 7 recommends focusing on the systolic BP; most patients reach the diastolic BP goal when the systolic pressure target is reached.[1]

Table 8.2 Secondary Causes of Hypertension

Disorder	Clinical Presentation	Laboratory Evaluation
Renal artery stenosis	HBP under age 20 New onset or worsening HBP in an older patient with increasing creatinine Abdominal/flank bruit	Magnetic resonance angiography Captopril augmented renal scan Angiography
Hyperaldosteronism	Hypokalemia, possibly hypernatremia	CT scan of adrenal glands
Sleep apnea	Snoring, daytime somnolence, obesity (thick neck)	Sleep study
Pheochromocytoma	Paroxysmal HBP, headache, flushing, tachycardia	Urinary catecholamine metabolites (metanephrines, VMA)
Hypothyroidism	Diastolic HBP, fatigue, weight gain, weakness	TSH level
Hyperthyroidism	Systolic HBP, heat intolerance, weight loss, tremor, new AF	TSH level
Hyperparathyroidism	Kidney stones, osteoporosis, weakness, lethargy	Serum calcium and parathyroid hormone levels
Chronic renal disease	Clinical setting	Creatinine clearance
Cushing's syndrome	Typical habitus	Dexamethasone suppression test
Coarctation of the aorta	Decreased or delayed femoral pulses, low leg BP	Chest x-ray findings, CT scan of the aorta
Excessive alcohol intake	Clinical history	Trial of abstinence
Drug side effects	Erythropoietin, cyclosporin, NSAIDs, COX-2 inhibitors, estrogen birth control pills, appetite suppressants, pseudoephedrine, monoamine oxidase inhibitors (Nardil), nicotine, amphetamines, testosterone	

HBP, high blood pressure; CT, computed tomography; VMA, vanillymandelic acid; NSAID, non-steroidal anti-inflammatory drug; COX, cyclooxygenase; CT, computed tomography; TSH, thyroid stimulating hormone.

It also emphasizes lifestyle modification, including weight loss, sodium restriction, physical activity, and reduced alcohol consumption. The Dietary Approach to Stop Hypertension (DASH) lowers the systolic BP about 10 mm Hg; it is rich in fruits and low-fat dairy products (and thus is high in potassium and calcium), and is low in saturated fats. The DASH diet plus a 1.6-g sodium intake is as effective as single drug therapy in reducing BP. We have little information about the long-term effects of popular low carbohydrate diets (e.g., the Atkins diet).

Drug therapy—Clinical trials evaluating CVD outcomes have continued to find no drug class superior to thiazide diuretics as initial treatment. Furthermore, diuretics enhance the actions of other drugs. One reason for failure of vasodilator therapy is inadequate diuresis. Sodium retention is a normal response to vasodilatation—it is perceived by the kidney as hypovolemia. Control of pressure requires correction of the consequent hypervolemia.

Most patients require multiple drugs to reach the BP goal, and JNC 7 suggests starting with two if the baseline BP is more than 20/10 mm Hg above goal. Angiotensin-converting enzyme (ACE) inhibitors, angiotensin receptor blocker (ARB), beta-blockers, and calcium channel blockers are effective antihypertensive agents, and all are reasonable as a second agent. The pharmacology of antihypertensives is the subject of standard texts and other reviews.[6]

Another illness often dictates the choice of therapy, which then has the dual purpose of lowering BP plus favorably influencing the progress of the disease (Table 8.3). Thus, a patient with known vascular disease should be on an ACE inhibitor for its vascular protective effects. Patients with a history of MI or heart failure with low LVEF have improved survival with beta blockade (as well as ACE inhibition and aldosterone blocking therapy). Diabetes is an indication for ACE inhibition. Prostatism is effectively treated with alpha blockers, although monotherapy in patients with CAD and a history of MI is associated with increased risk.[5]

Table 8.3 Choice of Antihypertensive Therapy for Patients with Other Illnesses

Condition	Drug Class Shown to Improve Outcome	Comments
Previous myocardial infarction	Beta-blocker, ACE inhibitor, aldosterone antagonist with low LVEF	The coronary event rate may be higher with alpha blockers and calcium channel blockers[5]
Congestive heart failure and low LVEF	Beta-blocker, ACE inhibitor, ARB, aldosterone antagonist (spironolactone)	Chapter 1; beta blockade has the most potent beneficial effect on survival
ASCVD	ACE inhibitor	See Chapters 4 and 5
Prior stroke	ACE inhibitor + thiazide	PROGRESS trial showed less recurrence of stroke[2]
Diabetes mellitus	ACE inhibitor or ARB, beta blocker, diuretics calcium blocker	All prevent CVD and stroke, and ACE inhibitors and ARBs reduce proteinuria and progression of nephropathy
Chronic renal disease	ACE inhibitor or ARB	Both lower the rate of progression, even for nondiabetic renal disease
Left ventricular hypertrophy	All classes reduce LVH, except direct vasodilators (hydralazine and minoxidil)	LVH is an independent risk factor for sudden cardiac death as well as CVD

ACE, angiotensin converting enzyme; ARB, angiotensin receptor blocker; CVD, cardiovascular disease including coronary artery disease, peripheral vascular disease and stroke; LVH, left ventricular hypertrophy; ASCVD, atherosclerotic CVD; LVEF, left ventricular ejection fraction.

A need for multiple drugs to treat these other illnesses may prevent the use of thiazides. If the pressure is still high after regulating the doses of other medicines, the diuretic can be added.

Chronic renal disease—Patients with kidney disease (creatinine >1.5 mg/dL for men, >1.4 mg/dL for women) tend to have a progressive decline in creatinine clearance. The rate of decline is slower when BP is lowered to 130/80 mm Hg or less. Multidrug therapy is usually needed, and should include blockade of the renin-angiotensin-aldosterone (RAA) system with an ACE inhibitor or ARB. The renal protective effect of RAA blockade applies to both nondiabetic and diabetic patients, and it is most pronounced for those with proteinuria. ACE inhibition reduces proteinuria. Those with mild renal dysfunction also have a higher incidence of CVD, and RAA blocking therapy lowers the rate of cardiac events.[3]

Renal dysfunction plus hyperkalemia is a contraindication to ACE inhibitors or ARBs. Monitoring serum potassium and creatinine is important for all patients, and I recheck a creatinine a couple days after starting RAA blocking therapy. A marked rise in serum creatinine during the first couple days of treatment suggests co-existing renal artery stenosis, which should be evaluated. If creatinine rises by less than 0.3 mg/dL, the ACE inhibitor or ARB can be continued with careful monitoring.

When the creatinine is above 1.5 mg/dL, thiazides are less effective and loop diuretics are needed. Diuretics and reduced sodium intake are especially important, as sodium retention is a common feature of renal dysfunction. Nonsteroidal anti-inflammatory drugs may provoke renal vasoconstriction and further lower glomerular filtration, leading to salt retention and possibly to hyperkalemia. They and potassium containing salt substitutes should be avoided.

Black patients—As a group, they have earlier onset HBP and are more likely to have severe (stage 2) disease. For years we thought that the RAA system played a minor role when compared with other racial groups. This was based upon the relative ineffectiveness of ACE inhibitors as monotherapy, when compared with diuretics and calcium channel blockers. The critical observation, however, is that monotherapy with any drug is ineffective for this group, and especially with ACE inhibitors or beta-blockers.

With appropriate combination therapy, both ACE inhibition and beta blockade are effective for black patients. The African-American Study of Kidney Disease (AASK) trial compared ramipril, metoprolol and amlodipine plus diuretic therapy in patients with moderate renal dysfunction (glomerular filtration rate 20 to 60 mL/min). The BP response was identical in the ramipril and amlodipine arms, but the rate of decline of renal function was substantially better with ramipril therapy.[3] Thus, for persons of color 1) ACE inhibition is as effective as calcium channel blockade in lowering BP when used as part of a multidrug regimen, and 2) it provides the best protection of renal function and thus should be the first choice of therapy. The study underscores an important management principle: drug therapy is about more than lowering BP. The other actions of drugs independent of BP effects—for example, renal or vascular protection—are as important.

Table 8.4 Causes of Inadequate Response to Antihypertensive Therapy	
Pseudoresistance	White coat hypertension Use of a regular cuff on an obese arm
Noncompliance to therapy	
Unrecognized secondary causes of hypertension	Table 8.2
Volume overload	Excess salt intake Fluid retention from vasodilator therapy and *inadequate diuresis*
Drug-related causes	Doses too low or incorrect dosing schedule Wrong type of diuretic (i.e., thiazide in a patient with advanced renal disease) Drug effects: Sympathomimetics, nasal decongestants, appetite suppressants, cocaine, oral contraceptives, adrenal steroids, cyclosporine, erythropoietin, antidepressants, nonsteroidal anti-inflammatory drugs
Associated conditions	Sleep apnea Smoking Increasing obesity Insulin resistance/hyperinsulinemia Alcohol intake >1 oz per day Arteritis with vasoconstriction Chronic pain

Elderly patients—As noted, most people older than 65 years have HBP. This is a group that is undertreated. Blood pressure goals, the workup, and choice of drugs are no different than those with younger patients. An abrupt and substantial rise in BP suggest atherosclerotic renal artery stenosis, especially when there is an increase in creatinine.

Postural hypotension is more common in older patients, and you may want to start with lower dose therapy to avoid this side effect. Volume depletion is a common cause. For this reason, targeting therapy to an upright BP makes sense for older patients. If the BP is borderline, measure it after a walk down the hall and while standing.

Women—Oral contraceptives raise BP, and this effect increases with the duration of therapy. Hormone replacement therapy, with its lower dose of estrogen, has no effect on BP (a broader discussion of hormone replacement is in Chapter 3).

During pregnancy, ACE inhibitors and ARBs should not be used because of fetal toxicity (avoid them if there is a chance of pregnancy). Methyldopa and nifedipine are safe. Beta-blockers may be used late in pregnancy, but can slow fetal growth.[3] Thiazides may be used, but furosemide may be embryotoxic.

Resistance to drug therapy—An inability to lower BP despite multiple drug therapy should prompt reconsideration of secondary hypertension (Table 8.2), or noncompliance with the medicine regimen. In the absence of these, consider other causes of drug resistance are outlined in Table 8.4. The most common of these in my experience are inadequate diuretic therapy, use of nonsteroidal anti-inflammatory drugs, excessive alcohol intake, and failure to recognize sleep apnea.

Diseases of the Aorta

Abdominal Aortic Aneurysm

About three fourths of aortic aneurysms are limited to the abdomen, originating below the renal arteries and usually sparing the visceral circulation. The size of the abdominal aortic aneurysm (AAA) determines the chance of rupture. There is a 50% chance of rupture in 1 year with a diameter greater than 6 cm, 15% to 20% when the AAA measures 5 to 6 cm, and less than 2% with a diameter less than 4 cm. Without surgery, the 5-year mortality rate with an aneurysm larger than 6 cm is at least 90%.

Most AAAs are detected during abdominal examination or with ultrasound screening studies. Because of the high mortality risk with undetected, large aneurysms, routine screening has been advocated for those older than 60 years of age.[7] There are few clinical trials data to support widespread screening, and it is not (yet) the standard of care, but patients are beginning to ask for it.

AAA is an atherosclerotic illness, and cigarette smoking, male gender, and family history are the major risk factors. Recall that wall tension = intraluminal pressure x radius (Laplace's law). Thus, hypertension—high intraluminal pressure—contributes to aneurysm growth. Because expansion occurs in 80% of patients, time is another risk factor for rupture. Gradual expansion is the rule, with only 20% enlarging rapidly (more than 0.5 cm per year).

Randomized trials have compared surveillance vs. early surgery for small AAA, and found no advantage with surgery for aneurysms less than 5.5 cm.[8,9] In addition to AAA size, the patient's general medical condition also influences the timing of surgery. When the general health is good, surgery is recommended for an AAA 5.5 cm or larger. On the other hand, a patient with multiple medical problems who is considered a poor surgical candidate may have repair delayed until the aneurysm approaches 6 cm. Mortality with elective surgery in the ADAM trial was just 1.8%, substantially better than that a decade ago.[8] Surgical mortality is higher with rapidly expanding aneurysms (5% to 15%), while surgery during acute rupture has a mortality risk closer to 40%.[7]

The newest approach is endovascular aneurysm repair using stents. The first devices were introduced in the early 1990s, and current models have been tested in more than 1000 patients. With proper patient selection stenting works well and appears a durable solution to AAA. Its role in treating rupture is uncertain.

The medical therapy of small AAA begins with risk factor modification and BP control. Beta blockade has not been found to have special benefits.[7] Reducing vascular inflammation may help, and trials of statins and antibiotics (doxycycline) therapy are in progress.

Thoracic Aortic Aneurysm

In young patients the usual cause is Marfan's syndrome, while older patients have atherosclerotic disease. Expanding aneurysms tend to cause pain or compression symptoms—hoarseness, cough, dysphagia, or the superior vena cava syndrome.

A diameter greater than 7 cm indicates a high risk of rupture. Surgery is recommended when thoracic aneurysms reach 6 cm. High surgical risk would favor delaying surgery in the absence of symptoms. Expansion tends to be slow with aneurysms smaller than 5 cm, and annual CT or MRI imaging is adequate. Above 5 cm, the expansion rate increases fourfold, and twice-yearly imaging is needed.

Medical therapy includes risk factor modification and control of hypertension. Beta blockade has a special role, because reducing the velocity of LV ejection protects the aorta. This has been proven for those with Marfan's syndrome, and beta blockade makes sense as initial antihypertensive treatment for all with thoracic aneurysm. (Small studies of AAA showed no benefit with beta blockade; the shearing force of LV ejection apparently dissipates by the time it reaches the distal aorta.)

Marfan's syndrome is the most common cause of thoracic aortic aneurysm in young people. Pregnancy increases the risk of dissection and should be avoided if the proximal aorta is larger than 4.0 cm.

Survival with elective surgery is above 90%. Inadvertent interruption of the vascular supply to the spine leads to paralysis in more than 5%. Decompression with spinal fluid drainage before surgery may lower the risk of paraplegia.[7]

Thoracic Aortic Dissection

Risk factors for dissection are poorly controlled hypertension, advanced age, and medial disease. A number of aortic diseases may cause it including Marfan's and Ehlers-Danlos syndromes, coarctation, bicuspid aortic valve, arteritis and Turner and Noonan syndromes.[10] Men are more commonly affected. Over age 50, hypertension is the usual etiology; under age 40, Marfan's syndrome is the most common cause.[10] While those with an aneurysm are at increased risk for dissection, not all dissections begin with a large aneurysm.

The standard classification of dissection is based on location: type A dissection begins in the proximal aorta, just above the aortic valve, and accounts for three fourths of cases. A type A dissection may extend all the way around to the distal aorta (DeBakey class 1), or may be limited to the proximal aorta (DeBakey class 2). Type B dissection (DeBakey class 3) begins distal to the left subclavian artery and involves the distal aorta (25% of cases).

Dissection causes chest pain. The diagnosis is often missed, as this is a less common cause of chest pain than CAD. The pain may be mid chest, and radiation to the back occurs in less than half of cases. The most useful diagnostic feature is that the pain is at maximum intensity at its onset (more than 80% of cases, and this figures into board questions routinely).[10] In contrast, the pain of MI starts slowly and crescendos.

The dissection may occlude major branches of the aorta. For example, chest pain plus stroke (carotid occlusion) suggests dissection. On physical examination, indications of limb ischemia, including diminished pulses or unequal BPs is evidence for dissection. Acute inferior MI with ST-segment elevation on the ECG may occur if the dissection occludes the right coronary ostium. Occlusion of the left coronary ostium is possible, but most with this complication die suddenly. Proximal dissection may cause aortic regurgitation. Neck vein distension suggests rupture into the pericardium and tamponade.

Diagnosis requires a transesophageal echocardiogram or imaging with CT or MRI. All are sensitive and specific, and the choice of technique is based on speed and availability. Abdominal ultrasound is a screening test for AAA, and it is not useful for the evaluation of possible dissection of the aorta (nor is transthoracic echocardiography). The mediastinum and/or aorta appear widened on chest x-ray in 80% to 90% of patients with thoracic dissection, making this a useful but not diagnostic test.

Management is aimed at stopping the progression of dissection. Medical therapy includes 1) decreasing the systolic BP to 100 to 120 mm Hg if there is adequate perfusion of vital organs (nitroprusside is the intravenous vasodilator of choice); 2) beta blockade to counter the shearing force of LV ejection, which may increase with vasodilator therapy; and 3) pain control.

Indications for emergency surgery are severe aortic regurgitation, threatened rupture, occlusion of a branch artery and persistent, uncontrollable pain.[10] In addition, surgery improves survival for those with proximal, type A dissection. It is no better than medical management for those with stable distal dissection. With type B dissection, a patient who has survived the acute phase and has no indication for emergency surgery has a 90% 1-year survival rate with both medical and surgical therapy.

Operative mortality ranges from 5% to as high as 70%, with highest risk predicted by cardiac tamponade, renal or visceral ischemia, the site of the tear, coexisting lung disease, and delayed time to surgery.[10] Tissue adhesives are now used to join the separated layers of aorta, eradicating the false lumen in more than half the cases.[10] Glue aortoplasty results in less bleeding, fewer postoperative complications, and probably improved survival (there have been no randomized studies, as there never are when a new surgical technique clearly makes things better).

Endovascular stenting has been tested in small numbers of patients who were poor surgical candidates, usually with descending aortic dissection (type B). Predictably, outcomes have been poor, and at this time stenting is considered a palliative procedure for those whose symptoms are from lower extremity ischemia.[10] Based on experience with most endovascular procedures, watch for the indications for stenting to expand with more experience and better equipment.

Residual aortic disease requires surgery within 10 years in 20% to 30% of patients who survive aortic dissection, with or without initial surgical therapy. Aggressive medical therapy is needed (risk factor and BP control, beta blockade, statins). They should have follow-up CT or MRI imaging at 3-month intervals for a year, then twice yearly, depending on the size of the aorta and rate of expansion.

Aortic Trauma

The most common cause is sudden high-speed deceleration during a motor vehicle accident. This creates shearing forces that are greatest where mobile and fixed portions of the aorta meet, most commonly, the aortic isthmus where the ligamentum arteriosum inserts (the former ductus arteriosus just beyond the left subclavian artery).

The diagnosis may be masked by other injuries. Localized hematoma can cause dyspnea or stridor, dysphagia or the superior vena cava syndrome. There may be an interscapular bruit on exam. The chest x-ray is abnormal in 90% (opacification between the aorta and pulmonary artery [PA] or mediastinal widening). Contrast CT or MRI confirms the diagnosis. Surgical correction is usually successful and may prevent sudden death.

Cardiac Complications of Other Medical Illnesses

Chronic Lung Disease (Cor Pulmonale)

Lung disease can cause pulmonary hypertension, leading to right heart failure. The three mechanisms are *hypoxic vasoconstriction* (especially with chronic bronchitis, cystic fibrosis, obesity hypoventilation—sleep apnea—and other hypoventilation syndromes), *obstruction of the vascular bed* (pulmonary embolism, primary pulmonary hypertension [PPH], sickle cell disease), and *obliteration of lung parenchyma* with loss of vascular surface area (emphysema, bronchiectasis, cystic fibrosis, interstitial lung disease).[11]

Hypoxia is a potent pulmonary vasoconstrictor. When prolonged, there is an increase in the thickness of the walls of small PA branches. These changes become permanent over time. A patient with chronic lung disease plus hypoxia, typically the blue bloater with bronchitis, is more prone to cor pulmonale than another with emphysema and equally severe airway obstruction, but with normal arterial oxygen saturation (the pink puffer). One of the indications for home oxygen therapy is right heart failure, because correction of hypoxemia relieves pulmonary hypertension.

Not everyone with bronchitis develops cor pulmonale. Some patients are susceptible but most are not. That also appears to be the case with some patients with left heart failure but predominantly right side CHF. A minority of those with mitral stenosis, atrial septal defect, or cardiomyopathy presents with edema (right heart failure) but no pulmonary congestion.

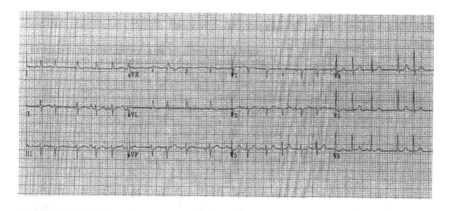

Figure 8.1 Multifocal atrial tachycardia. The rhythm is irregular, and there is variable P wave morphology. (Reproduced by permission from Taylor GJ. 150 Practice ECGs, 2nd ed. Malden, MA: Blackwell Science, 2002:196.)

It is a conundrum—how can the cause of right heart failure be left heart failure if there is no left heart failure? My impression is that there is a percentage of the population with hyperreactive pulmonary vasculature. When stressed with hypoxia (COPD) or hemodynamic overload (left side CHF), these patients develop pulmonary hypertension. Because the PA clamps down, the left heart is protected, and the clinical picture is isolated right heart CHF.

Clinical and laboratory findings—The syndrome is right heart failure—peripheral edema—in a patient with lung disease. The chest x-ray shows no pulmonary congestion, and the echocardiogram confirms normal LV function. Dyspnea is usual but is caused by the lung disease. Palpitations and atrial arrhythmias are common, especially atrial flutter and multifocal atrial tachycardia (Figure 8.1).

Other cardiac findings of right heart failure are subtle, and may be hard to detect when the chest exam is grossly abnormal. P_2 is accentuated with pulmonary hypertension. There may be a right ventricular (RV) lift and a right-side S_3 gallop (audible during inspiration). Jugular venous distension is a prominent finding. If there is also a V wave, consider tricuspid regurgitation (see Chapter 7). With RV failure, there may be an inspiratory increase in jugular venous pressure (Kussmaul's sign) and pulsus paradoxus.

Although the chest examination is abnormal with lung disease, a normal exam does not exclude cor pulmonale. Other causes such as sleep apnea, PPH, and recurrent pulmonary embolus may not affect the chest examination.

The chest x-ray findings of PPH and cor pulmonale are enlargement of the RV and central pulmonary arteries. Decreased vessel markings at the periphery in contrast to the large central vessels produce a pruned tree appearance.

The ECG is a nonspecific test. There may be RV hypertrophy and P pulmonale (Table 8.5, Figure 8.2), but their absence does not exclude cor pulmonale.

Table 8.5 Diagnosis of Right Ventricular Hypertrophy*	
Criteria	R/S in V_1 ≥1, *or* R in V_1 ≥7, *or* R in V_1 + S in V_5 or V_6 >10.5
Supportive findings	Right axis deviation >110 degrees Right atrial abnormality (inferior P waves >2.5 mm) ST depression + T wave inversion in V_1 or V_2 (RV strain)

*These findings are relatively nonspecific. For example right bundle branch block is a common ECG finding, and most patients with right bundle branch block do not have right ventricular hypertrophy; yet they have a tall R in V_1 and associated T inversion.

Low voltage is common with emphysema as is delay in R wave progression. Right bundle branch block (RBBB) or incomplete RBBB are nonspecific signs of RV overload, but they may also result from conduction system disease unrelated to the state of the RV.

The echocardiogram is the key test, detecting RV and possibly right atrial (RA) enlargement. RA measurement is not precise, but there may be a qualitative assessment. Both chambers are enlarged with cor pulmonale. RV wall thickness is difficult to measure, so the echo is not reliable for the diagnosis of RV hypertrophy. Most with pulmonary hypertension have mild tricuspid regurgitation (TR, often without a murmur), and the TR jet is used for Doppler estimation of PA pressure. The echocardiogram also excludes other causes of pulmonary hypertension such as occult mitral stenosis or left heart failure (systolic or diastolic). In many patients with advanced lung disease, the cushion of air between the echo transducer and the heart prevents good imaging. Transesophageal echocardiogram is an alternative, but slightly riskier in those with severe lung disease. The clinical diagnosis of cor pulmonale usually is sufficient, and a transesophageal echocardiogram is unnecessary.

An occasional patient has right heart catheterization. The major finding is elevated PA pressure. The pulmonary wedge pressure—e.g., left ventricular (LV) filling

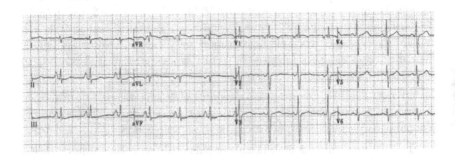

Figure 8.2 Right ventricular hypertrophy. The R wave is tall in V_1, and the S wave persists in V_{5-6}. There is right axis deviation, and a right atrial abnormality (P waves taller than 2.5 mm in inferior leads). (Reproduced by permission from Taylor GJ. The cardiology rotation. Malden, MA: Blackwell Science, 2001:282.)

pressure—is normal unless there is LV dysfunction. Normally the PA diastolic pressure is equal to the wedge pressure; during diastole the PA, pulmonary capillary bed, pulmonary veins, left atrium, and LV are in open communication. Pulmonary vascular resistance (PVR) is elevated with cor pulmonale. Thus, PA diastolic pressure is higher than a LA pressure (or pulmonary wedge pressure).

I indicated that cor pulmonale is pulmonary hypertension in the face of normal LV diastolic pressures; it is the lung disease and not left heart failure that causes right heart failure. Smokers get CAD and have MIs, so many with cor pulmonale have coexisting left heart disease. In such cases the pulmonary wedge pressure is high, but the PA diastolic pressure is even higher. This transpulmonary gradient defines elevated PVR and is a constant finding of cor pulmonale.

Other laboratory testing may be needed to determine the etiology. When there is no apparent lung disease, evaluate the patient for pulmonary embolus. A sleep study may be needed to diagnose sleep apnea. In such cases, bradyarrhythmias during sleep are common. Last month I consulted on a 70-year-old patient with edema who had 3.5-second sinus pauses on telemetry, while asleep. The QRS duration and PR intervals were normal. Rather than an urgent pacemaker, we documented sleep apnea and treated his arrhythmia and right heart failure with nocturnal positive-pressure ventilation.

Treatment—Improving oxygenation relieves pulmonary vasoconstriction. The usual indication for home oxygen is hypoxemia, but cor pulmonale is an additional indication in those with borderline oxygen saturation.[12] The goal is a PaO_2 greater than 60 mm Hg. Pulmonary hypertension may improve with part-time, overnight oxygen therapy. However, clinical trials have shown improved survival with continuous therapy for the general population needing oxygen for chronic lung disease, and those results would apply to patients with cor pulmonale. Supplemental oxygen must be used cautiously when there is chronic hypercarbia and respiratory acidosis. Vigorous treatment of the lung disease is critical.

Specific treatment of the heart failure is of limited benefit. Edema requires diuretic therapy. When there is splanchnic congestion, consider using the loop diuretics that are best absorbed (torsemide and bumetanide rather then furosemide; see Chapter 1). Vasodilator therapy has little effect on PVR when there is parenchymal lung disease, so afterload reduction therapy is not indicated, nor does beta blockade help.

Digoxin may be used for treatment of right heart failure, but it is less effective for controlling the ventricular rate when there are atrial tachyarrhythmias. Those with cor pulmonale are more susceptible to digitalis toxicity. Verapamil is a better choice for rate control. The successful treatment of atrial arrhythmias, like heart failure, requires control of the lung disease. Cardioversion may be considered for atrial flutter, but maintaining sinus rhythm is unlikely unless pulmonary function improves.

Primary pulmonary hypertension—This rare illness is marked by pulmonary vasoconstriction, intimal proliferation, and thrombosis in situ.[11] It is probably caused by endothelial dysfunction. Although more common in young women, others may be afflicted. They usually present with dyspnea, and other symptoms include chest pain, edema (right heart failure), light-headedness, and syncope. It is a fatal illness, with survival determined by the response to vasodilators.

All patients should receive anticoagulation therapy. Digoxin may relieve the symptoms of right heart failure.[11] Vasodilator therapy is critical. Calcium channel blockade is effective for some patients; in one study a favorable response led to a 94% 5-year survival, compared with 36% in those who did not respond.[11]

Prostacyclin is a vasodilator produced by the endothelium that is deficient in some patients with PPH. It has been shown to increase survival and relieve symptoms, even in those with advanced PPH (functional class 3-4). On average, patients have at least a 50% reduction in PVR, and the effect persists with chronic therapy. Epoprostenol (Flolan) is given by constant infusion through a permanent central catheter using an ambulatory pump.[11] A few patients have been on it 10 years. Oral and subcutaneous prostacyclins are being developed. More recently, bosentan, an endothelin receptor blocker, has been approved and as the first oral medicine available for PPH.[13] High dose sildenafil (Viagra) has been shown to improve exercise tolerance and other symptoms.[14]

Other Medical Conditions and their Cardiac Effects

A brief review text must focus on the big picture, and what is in that picture requires picking and choosing. To flesh out this overview—perhaps to jog your memory—Table 8.6 summarizes the cardiac effects of a number of medical illnesses that are not covered in detail.

Table 8.6 Cardiovascular Effects of Other Noncardiac Illnesses	
Condition	Cardiovascular Effects/Comment
Endocrine Disorders	
Cushing's syndrome	HBP in 80%. Diagnose with a dexamethasone suppression test.
Hyperaldosteronism (Conn's syndrome)	Expanded extracellular volume, moderate diastolic HBP, hypokalemia resistant to replacement therapy. Treat HBP with spironolactone (or resection of the adrenal adenoma).
Adrenocortical insufficiency	Chronic syndrome (Addison's disease): asthenia, fatigue, hypotension and a small heart on x-ray. Acute syndrome (Waterhouse-Friderichsen's syndrome with sepsis): shock
Hyperparathyroidism	Hypercalcemia and hyperphosphatemia. HBP common in elderly patients. Thiazides may aggravate the hypercalcemia.
Pheochromocytoma	HBP, sustained in 60% of cases, although labile. Half have paroxysms of flushing and HBP that can resemble anxiety attacks.

(Continued)

Table 8.6 (Continued)	
Condition	Cardiovascular Effects/Comment
Endocrine Disorders	
Chronic hypocalcemia (hypoparathyroidism)	Long QT interval.
Diabetes insipidus	Polyuria and polydipsia, an inability to concentrate the urine. If the patient cannot drink, volume depletion and hypotension soon develop.
Hyperthyroidism	Increased heart rate, decreased systemic vascular resistance, high systolic BP (and low diastolic BP with wide pulse pressure), atrial fibrillation (a common presenting sign in the elderly), high-output heart failure.
Hypothyroidism	Low heart rate, reduced LV contractility (though CHF is rare and function improves with treatment), increased diastolic BP in 20% but low systolic BP (a narrow pulse pressure), large and slowly accumulating pericardial effusion.
Connective Tissue Disease	
Systemic lupus erythematosus	Pericardial effusion (tamponade and constriction are possible). Atypical endocarditis (Libman-Sacks endocarditis, with valve nodules at autopsy that rarely cause valvular dysfunction). Cardiomyopathy and coronary artery lesions are possible, but rare.
Polyarteritis nodosa (PAN)	Segmental, necrotizing arteritis of small-medium vessels, including coronary arteries. MI and conduction system disease are possible but uncommon. Renal arteritis causes HBP and renal failure, leading to heart failure in 60%.
Rheumatoid arthritis (RA)	Fibrinous pericarditis occurs in 30% with RA. Usually clinically silent, but constriction is possible. Effusions can be large. Rheumatoid nodules can affect myocardium, valve or conduction system.
Ankylosing spondylitis	10% have aortic root inflammation, then sclerosis, then aortic regurgitation (usually with chronic disease). Conduction abnormalities possibilities.
Scleroderma (systemic sclerosis)	Raynaud's phenomenon is an early symptom (coronary spasm is possible). Fibrosis possible in heart, lungs and kidney. CHF, ventricular arrhythmia, or conduction disease occurs in one third of patients. Fibrosis can lead to pulmonary hypertension and cor pulmonale, or there may be primary pulmonary hypertension (vasospasm without lung fibrosis).
Polymyositis and Dermatomyositis	40% have cardiac involvement: conduction abnormalities, tachyarrhythmias, pericarditis with effusion, or dilated cardiomyopathy. Coronary arteritis is possible but rare.
Giant cell (temporal) arteritis	Aortitis may lead to chest pain, myocardial ischemia, aortic aneurysm, stroke, aortic regurgitation, or limb claudication.
Ehlers-Danlos syndrome	Multiple genotypes with variable cardiac involvement. MVP and aortic disease (rupture or dissection) the major problems.

(Continued)

Table 8.6 (Continued)

Condition	Cardiovascular Effects/Comment
Connective Tissue Disease	
Marfan's syndrome	Aortic root dilatation and dissection (beta blockade slows progression); mitral valve prolapse is common (Chapter 7).
Osteogenesis imperfecta	Fragile bones, blue sclera. AR and MR possible, plus large artery fragility.
Neoplastic Disease	
Metastatic tumors	30 × more common than primary tumors of the heart. Lung, breast, lymphoma, leukemia and melanoma most common. Most clinical disease is pericardial, with myocardial or intracavitary disease less common.
Atrial myxoma	Can mimic mitral valve disease. Thromboembolism (stroke) is common. Most have constitutional symptoms (fever, weight loss, fatigue) with an elevated sedimentation rate.
Rhabdomyoma	Benign tumor of myocardium in young children, often accompanies tuberous sclerosis. Surgically resectible. Rare.
Other benign myocardial tumors	Lipoma, papillary fibroelastoma, fibroma, hemangioma, mesothelioma involving mitral or tricuspid valves. Rare.
Angiosarcoma	Malignant, usually in the RA or pericardium. Right heart failure or pericardial pain. Death within a year. Rare.
Rhabdomyosarcoma	Malignant, in any cardiac chamber, and may alter valve function. Rare.
Complications of radiation	Pericarditis is the most common and may lead to constriction. Accelerated coronary atherosclerosis is possible. Radiation or surgery to the neck can cause carotid sinus syncope
Adriamycin	Cardiomyopathy may occur when the cumulative dose is >450 mg/m^2
5-Fluorouracil	Coronary artery spasm and angina.
Cyclophosphamide	At high doses (pre-bone marrow transplant), hemorrhagic myopericarditis is possible.
Neuromuscular and Neurologic Disease	
Duchenne muscular dystrophy	Cardiac involvement common: cardiomyopathy, conduction disorders, MVP (from papillary muscle disease), narrow and deep Q waves.
Myotonic dystrophy	80% have cardiac involvement, usually conduction disorders and other arrhythmias. Myocardial disease rare.
Friedreich's ataxia	Dilated cardiomyopathy (CHF is the most common cause of death). Degree of LV dysfunction does not parallel severity of the neuromuscular disorder.* There is an hypertrophic variant as well.

(Continued)

Table 8.6 (Continued)

Condition	Cardiovascular Effects/Comment
Neuromuscular and Neurologic Disease	
Stroke	Deep and symmetrical T wave inversion with troponin elevation (subendocardial myolysis); atrial and ventricular arrhythmias; hypertension in the initial stages, especially with hemorrhagic stroke (usually back to baseline in 10 days); noncardiac pulmonary edema (ARDS) is possible
End-stage Renal Disease (ESRD)	
Hypertension	HBP develops in most patients, regardless of the etiology of renal failure (see text)
Heart failure	Multiple complications of ESRD contribute: hypertension, hypervolemia, anemia, lipid abnormalities, disordered calcium metabolism, dialysis shunts, thiamine and other vitamin deficiencies.
Uremic pericarditis	Incidence is 20% with chronic hemodialysis. Tamponade is possible. More frequent dialysis is the treatment.
ASCVD	The process is accelerated, and MI is a common cause of death.
Nutritional Disorders	
Obesity	The metabolic syndrome, LVH plus dilatation (elevated preload and afterload, see Chapter 2), cardiomyopathy, obstructive sleep apnea, premature CAD, SCD.
Alcohol	HBP resistant to therapy, AF (holiday heart), cardiomyopathy (incidence in alcoholics is 10%–40%), favorable effect on CAD.
Thiamine deficiency (beriberi)	Vasodilatation, biventricular failure, edema. Common in alcoholics. It can be aggravated by diuretic therapy (increased excretion of thiamine parallels increased excretion of K and Mg). CHF may improve with replacement. (Consider this in a frail patient with CHF who is not eating well.)
Protein calorie malnutrition	A decrease in body weight is accompanied by smaller heart size, slower heart rate and QT interval prolongation. LVEF is normal. SCD possible with electrolyte disturbances.
Elevated homocysteine	Early ASCVD, increased risk of venous and arterial thrombosis (possibly through endothelial effects). Correct with folate and pyridoxine (see Chapter 3).
Selenium deficiency (Keshan's disease)	Cardiomyopathy (described in China)

BP, blood pressure; HBP, high BP; LV, left ventricle; LVEF, LV ejection fraction; CHF, congestive heart failure; CAD, coronary artery disease; AR, aortic regurgitation; MR, mitral regurgitation; ARDS, adult respiratory distress syndrome; SCD, sudden cardiac death (usually ventricular fibrillation); ASCVD, atherosclerotic cardiovascular disease

*This is true of most neuromuscular diseases that affect the myocardium.

References

1. Vasan RS, Beiser A, Seshadri S, et al. Residual lifetime risk for developing hypertension in middle-aged women and men: The Framingham Heart Study. JAMA 2002;287:1003–1010.

2. Chobanian AV, Bakris GL, Cushman WC, et al. The seventh report of the Joint National Committee on Prevention, Detection, Evaluation and Treatment of High Blood Pressure: the JNC 7 report. JAMA 2003;289:2560–2572.

3. Flack JM, Peters R, Mehra VC, Nasser SA. Hypertension in special populations. Cardiol Clin 2002;20:303–319.

4. Onusko E. Diagnosing secondary hypertension. Am Fam Physician 2003;67:67–74.

5. Aronow WS, Ahn C. Incidence of new coronary events in older persons with prior myocardial infarction and systemic hypertension treated with beta blockers, angiotensin-converting enzyme inhibitors, diuretics, calcium antagonists, and alpha blockers. Am J Cardiol 2002;89:1207–1209.

6. Ram CV, Fenves A. Clinical pharmacology of antihypertensive drugs. Cardiol Clin 2002;20:265–280.

7. Pearce WH. What's new in vascular surgery. J Am Coll Surg 2003;196:253-266.

8. Lederle FA, Wilson SE, Johnson GR, et al. Immediate repair compared with surveillance of small abdominal aortic aneurysms. N Engl J Med 2002;346:1437–1444.

9. United Kingdom Small Aneurysm Trail Participants. Long-term outcomes of immediate repair compared with surveillance of small abdominal aortic aneurysms. N Engl J Med 2002;346:1445–1452.

10. Khan IA, Nair CK. Clinical, diagnostic, and management perspectives of aortic dissection. Chest 2002;122:311-328. Also note, Januzzi JL, Isselbacher EM, Fattori R, et al. Characterization of the young patient with aortic disseciton: results from the International Registry of Aortic Dissection (IRAD). J Am Coll Cardiol 2004;43:665–669.

11. McLaughlin VV, Rich S. Severe pulmonary hypertension: critical care clinics. Crit Care Clin 2001;17:453–467.

12. Crockett AJ, Cranston JM, Moss JR, Alpers JH. A review of long-term oxygen therapy for chronic obstructive pulmonary disease. Respir Med 2001;95:437–443.

13. Lehrman S, Romano P, Frishman W, et al. Primary pulmonary hypertension and cor pulmonale. Cardiol Rev 2002:10:265–278.

14. Sastry BKS, Narasimhan DM, Reddy NK, Raju BS. Clinical efficacy of sildenafil in primary pulmonary hypertension: a randomized, placebo-controlled, double-blind, crossover study. J Am Coll Cardiol 2004;43:1149–1153.

Additional Reading

Medalion B, Katz MG, Cohen AJ, et al. Long-term beneficial effect of coronary artery bypass grafting in patients with COPD. Chest 2004;125:56–62. (*While not discussed in this chapter, many of our patients with heart disease also have chronic lung disease—without cor pulmonale. This study found that the 9-year survival after CABS was 62% for those with COPD vs. 95% for a control group without lung disease. Nevertheless, the authors claim a survival benefit for CABS when compared to medical therapy.*)

CHAPTER 9

CARDIOLOGY CONSULTS

Abbreviations

ACC	American College of Cardiology	LV	left ventricle (ventricular)
		LVEF	LV ejection fraction
AHA	American Heart Association	MI	myocardial infarction
ASD	atrial septal defect	PA	pulmonary artery
CAD	coronary artery disease	PDA	patent ductus arteriosus
CHF	congestive heart failure	PFO	patent foramen ovale
DC	direct current	RA	right atrium
ECG	electrocardiogram	RV	right ventricle
LA	left atrium	VSD	ventricular septal defect

Preoperative Care of the Patient Having Noncardiac Surgery

The Screening Protocol

Coronary artery disease (CAD) is ubiquitous, and myocardial ischemia is a common cardiac problem during anesthesia and surgery. Primary care doctors and cardiologists are asked to assess cardiac risk, and to clear the patient for surgery.

Identification of high- or low-risk patients is now evidence-based.[1] Prospective studies gathered clinical data before surgery, monitored patients for cardiac complications during and after the operation, and identified risk factors for perioperative myocardial infarction (MI). These studies are the basis of the risk assessment protocol offered by the American College of Cardiology (ACC) and American Heart Association (AHA).[1] The preoperative screening process is outlined in Figures 9.1 to 9.3.

As a rule, I dislike algorithms; they seem to complicate a straightforward problem. But in this case the algorithm works well and clearly defines the standard of care. Without it you will err. Make a copy for your clinic bulletin board, and refer to it whenever you see a preoperative consult—after a couple uses, the process will become clear.

Most of the data used to define the patient's risk come from the history and physical examination. There are three stages of screening.

Stage-1 screen (Figure 9.1)—A patient needing emergency, life-saving surgery requires no special cardiac testing. In such cases, your assessment of cardiac risk is

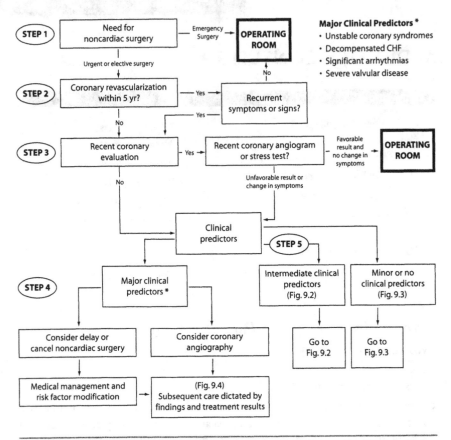

Figure 9.1 Stage 1: Initial screening based upon history and physical exam, identifying the highest risk patients. (Modified with permission from Eagle KA, Berger PB, Calkins H, et al. ACC/AHA guideline update for perioperative cardiovascular evaluation for noncardiac surgery—executive summary. J Am Coll Cardiol 2002;39: 542–553. Copyright © 2002, American College of Cardiology Foundation.)

based on the history and physical exam; the patient and family should have a clear understanding of risk, especially when it is high.

An *asymptomatic* patient who has had coronary revascularization *within 5 years* does not need a stress test or noninvasive imaging study.

In general, a patient who has had an angiogram or imaging study within 2 years does not require repeat evaluation as long as symptoms are stable. This is especially true if the study showed low-risk disease. If the earlier study indicated high-risk disease (e.g., diffuse or anterior wall ischemia), but revascularization was not possible because of comorbidities or coronary arteries that were unsuitable for revascularization, repeating that work-up is not indicated unless there has been a change in symptoms. A high-risk patient usually remains high risk, and more study will not change that.

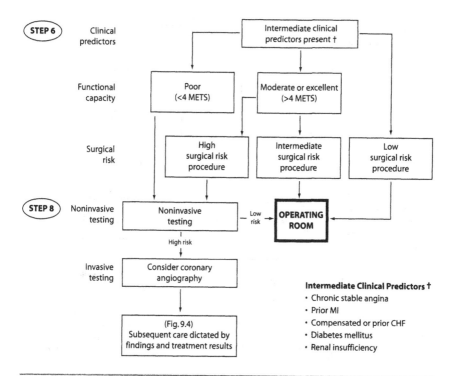

Figure 9.2 Stage 2: Further screening of the intermediate risk patient to determine who needs noninvasive testing (stress ECG, perfusion scanning, etc.). (Modified with permission from Eagle KA, Berger PB, Calkins H, et al. ACC/AHA guideline update for perioperative cardiovascular evaluation for noncardiac surgery—executive summary. J Am Coll Cardiol 2002;39:542–553. Copyright © 2002, American College of Cardiology Foundation.)

The presence of a major clinical predictor indicates that the surgery has a high risk of cardiac complications, greater than 15%. As high risk is identified, the guidelines call for additional work-up only if the cardiac condition requires it. For example, a patient with an unstable coronary syndrome or with symptomatic valvular heart disease should have the heart disease addressed before an elective operation. That is another way of saying that any patient with heart disease should be optimally tuned before surgery.

No surgeon would consider fixing the hernia of a patient with unstable angina. But the fact is that a subtle change in cardiac symptoms may be unrecognized by the doctor who is concentrating on the surgical condition, and it may not be uppermost in the patient's mind, either. That is a good reason for preoperation evaluation by the primary care physician.

Unstable coronary disease includes MI within the last 6 months. The highest risk would be with large infarction, substantial LV injury, and heart failure. A patient with recent incomplete infarction who might have recurrent ischemia is also high risk, and if possible should have revascularization before noncardiac

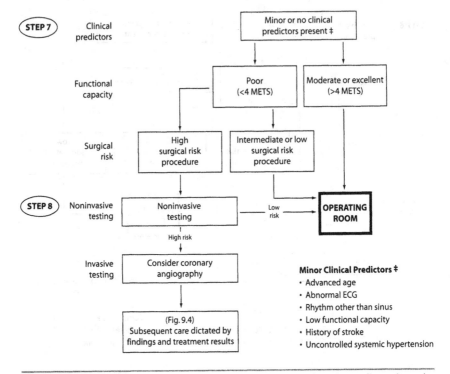

Figure 9.3 Stage 3: Final screening of lowest risk patients to select the small number who need preoperative testing (e.g. those with poor exercise tolerance having high risk surgery). (Modified with permission from Eagle KA, Berger PB, Calkins H, et al. ACC/AHA guideline update for perioperative cardiovascular evaluation for noncardiac surgery—executive summary. J Am Coll Cardiol 2002;39: 542–553. Copyright © 2002, American College of Cardiology Foundation.)

surgery is considered (see Chapter 5). This often means delaying an elective operation, because coronary intervention may necessitate aggressive antiplatelet therapy for a month.

A high-risk patient with heart disease that cannot be corrected must either accept the risk of noncardiac surgery and proceed or pursue an alternative therapy. When describing high risk to the patient and family my message is this: "You know that you have this heart condition, and it will come as no surprise that the chance of a heart complication during any operation is higher for you than it would be for another person your age who does not have heart disease. That does not mean you cannot have the operation, just that the risk is higher. You, your family and the surgeon must go into this with your eyes open." It makes sense, and most patients are nodding halfway through this speech (and not nodding off).

Stage-2 screen (Figure 9.2)—Patients without major clinical predictors are screened a second time using intermediate clinical predictors. Prior MI is based on history or the presence of Q waves on the ECG.

Table 9.1 The Cardiac Risks of Non-cardiac Operations	
High risk (>5% chance of cardiac complications*)	Emergent major operations, particularly in the elderly Aortic or other major vascular surgery Peripheral vascular surgery Long operations with large fluid shifts or blood loss
Intermediate risk (1–5%)	Carotid endarterectomy Head and neck surgery Intraperitoneal and intrathoracic surgery Orthopedic surgery Prostate surgery
Low risk (<1%)[†]	Endoscopic procedures Superficial procedures Cataract surgery Breast surgery

*Combined incidence of cardiac death, and nonfatal myocardial infarction.
[†]Do not generally require further preoperative cardiac testing.

Reproduced by permission from Eagle KA, Berger PB, Calkins H, et al. ACC/AHA guideline update for perioperative cardiovascular evaluation for noncardiac surgery—executive summary. J Am Coll Cardiol 2002;39:542–553. Copyright © 2002, American College of Cardiology Foundation.

At this stage, the nature of the operation and the patient's functional capacity come into play. The major difference between earlier guidelines and the present edition is the emphasis on the patient's exercise tolerance. Table 9.1 summarizes the cardiac risk of surgical procedures, and Table 9.2 describes the energy requirements for common activities. Thus, a middle-aged patient with no prior heart disease and normal exercise tolerance does not need a stress perfusion scan before hernia repair, knee surgery, or prostatectomy (low- or intermediate-risk procedures). Even one

Table 9.2 Estimated Energy Requirements for Common Activities	
1–4 METs*	Dress and use the toilet Walk a block slowly on level ground Do light housework
4–10 METs[†]	Climb a flight of stairs Run a short distance Do heavy housework (scrubbing floors, moving heavy furniture) Participate in light recreational activities (bowling, golf, doubles tennis, dancing)
10+ METS	Participate in strenuous sports (swimming, running, skiing, singles tennis)

*MET, metabolic equivalent, roughly the energy that is expended (or the oxygen consumed) sitting in a chair at rest.
[†]The cut-off for higher surgical risk is an inability to exercise at the 4 MET level (e.g., the patient hesitates to walk up a flight of stairs as a normal daily activity, or is unable to walk a block at a moderate pace).

Modified with permission from Eagle KA, Berger PB, Calkins H, et al. ACC/AHA guideline update for perioperative cardiovascular evaluation for noncardiac surgery—executive summary. J Am Coll Cardiol 2002;39:542–553. Copyright © 2002, American College of Cardiology Foundation.

with diabetes or prior MI would not require testing as long as exercise tolerance is good. Stress testing is needed for all with poor exercise tolerance and for those having high risk surgery (Table 9.1).

Stage-3 screen (Figure 9.3)—Those who have passed the stage 1 and 2 screens have a final screen using minor clinical predictors. If present, no preoperative testing is needed if exercise tolerance is good. If it is not, screening is needed before high-risk surgery. Note that poor exercise tolerance is a minor clinical predictor; the guidelines call for noninvasive testing if exercise tolerance is poor and the proposed surgery is high risk.

It is helpful to understand what low risk means in this context. After going through the screening process, the low risk patient's chance of a cardiac complication is less than 3%. At this low level of risk, noninvasive testing does not allow further risk stratification. A perfusion scan does not reliably differentiate between 1% and 3% risk. For that matter, nor would coronary angiography.

Low risk does not mean zero risk. Every patient takes a chance when having anesthesia or surgery and should understand that. On the consult—and to the patient—I state that "the risk of surgery and anesthesia is average for the patient's age, and no further cardiac testing is indicated."

High risk means that the chance of a cardiac complication with surgery is greater than 15%. Much of the screening process involves sorting out the group with *intermediate risk*, whose chance of a complication is between 3% and 15%. That is the role of noninvasive testing. If positive the cardiac risk is closer to 15%, and if negative it is closer to 3% (or lower—but never zero!).

The intermediate risk group is a large number of patients, and deciding which of them requires preoperative testing is the essential task of the preoperative medicine consultation.

Laboratory Testing

The AHA/ACC practice guidelines indicate that the stress ECG is "the test of choice" for ambulatory patients, and a negative study with good exercise tolerance indicates low risk.[1] However, many are unable to accomplish a diagnostic stress ECG, or have conditions that preclude treadmill testing. Our older patients who need screening usually require a cardiac imaging study.

Imaging studies are expensive. The retail cost of a stress thallium study in our hospital is $3500. The screening protocol also identifies the patient who does not require testing. The guidelines recommend "a conservative approach to the use of expensive tests."[1] This makes medical as well as economic sense. Laboratory testing without a clinical indication seldom improves outcomes, and that is certainly the case with preoperative screening.

Pharmacologic stress imaging has the largest and best record of performance, and dipyridamole perfusion scanning, and dobutamine stress echocardiography are both effective (see Chapter 4). One study of intermediate risk patients found a 1% incidence of MI or cardiac death with a negative perfusion scan, compared with a

23% risk when the scan showed reversible ischemia.[2] When the imaging study shows no active ischemia, further cardiac evaluation is not indicated.

A person with previous MI may have a fixed perfusion abnormality, a scar but no reversible ischemia; this is not active ischemia and further testing is not required. An occasional scan shows scar with peri-infarct ischemia. If other vascular regions are normal and symptoms are stable, angiography is not required.

Measurement of LVEF is not part of routine screening protocols. It may be helpful in sorting out dyspnea of uncertain cause, or to support a diagnosis of heart failure.

Management of the High-Risk Patient

The indication for revascularization or another cardiac procedure is based on the patient's heart disease and not on the need for noncardiac surgery. Do not recommend intervention to lower the risk of surgery, to "get the patient through" a proposed operation (Figure 9.4).[1] A decision to perform angiography is made using the usual indications (see Chapter 4), irrespective of the need for surgery.

An apparent exception to this would be a screening study that suggests unusually high-risk disease such as left main coronary artery stenosis (Figure 9.4). But it is not really an exception, as left main disease is itself an indication for surgery, regardless of symptoms. Finding it requires fixing it, barring contraindications.

What this means in practice is that we often complete the screening process, identify risk, and then recommend no further action before surgery. If we are not going to do anything about it, why go through the process? The simple answer is that defining risk and prognosis is useful, and it may influence the surgeon's approach. For example, a patient with diabetes and silent myocardial ischemia may fare better with amputation of toes rather than a long vascular operation.

Perioperative Therapy

Beta blockade—There have been multiple studies showing a protective effect. The Multicenter Study of Perioperative Ischemia Research found that atenolol given throughout hospitalization lowered the risk of cardiac events by 15% and mortality by 8%.[3] Patient selection for this treatment included known CAD or two risk factors for CAD (in this study, age 65 years or older, current smoking, hypertension, diabetes or cholesterol 240 mg/dL or greater), and no contraindications to beta blockade. Those with heart rate below 55 beats per minute were excluded.

The protocol prescribed atenolol 5 mg intravenously 30 minutes before surgery and again just after surgery, then atenolol 50–100 mg orally each day depending on baseline heart rate. Those unable to take oral medications were given 5–10 mg atenolol intravenously at 12-hour intervals. The present guidelines suggest starting beta-blockers days or weeks before elective surgery, and adjusting the dose to bring the heart rate to 50 to 60 beats per minute.

This and similar studies included few patients with congestive heart failure (CHF). Starting beta-lockers shortly before surgery in a marginally compensated

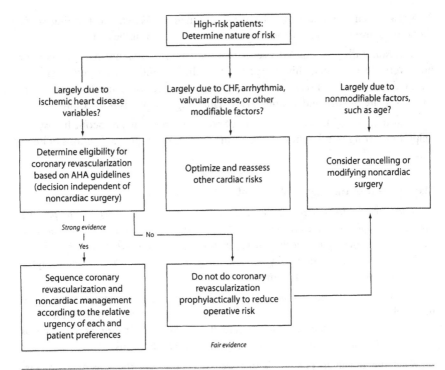

Figure 9.4 An algorithm for the management of patients at high risk for perioperative cardiac complications. Boxed phrases indicate recommended actions, and italicized words below the boxes indicate the level of evidence supporting the recommendation. If no italicized word is present, no evidence exists for or against use. AHA, American Heart Association; CHF, congestive heart failure. (Reproduced by permission from American College of Physicians. Guidelines for assessing and managing the perioperative risk from coronary artery disease associated with major noncardiac surgery. Ann Intern Med 1997;127:309.)

patient with heart failure is thus untested, and should be undertaken with caution (if at all).

Other therapies—There is no single anesthetic technique or drug that provides the best cardiac protection. Spinal anesthesia is not necessarily safer for the heart. There may be less myocardial depression, but spinal anesthesia can block the sympathetic nervous system and cause hypotension. A drop in blood pressure may lower coronary or carotid perfusion pressure.

Intravenous nitroglycerin has not been proven as prophylactic therapy, but is often added during surgery for control of blood pressure or ischemia (i.e., new ST segment changes). Most anesthesiologists do not want cutaneous delivery systems in place during surgery. There may be variation in cutaneous blood flow, and the delivery of nitroglycerin, or any medicine delivered by patch, is unpredictable.

Adequate perioperative pain control prevents sudden increases in sympathetic tone, preventing ischemia. It may also limit the hypercoagulability that is common after surgery.

Other Cardiac Illnesses

Valvular heart disease—Critical aortic stenosis should be repaired before elective noncardiac surgery. Endocarditis prophylaxis is a consideration for all with valvular or congenital disease. In general, antibiotic coverage is indicated for drainage of an infected site, or for oral, lower gastrointestinal, gallbladder, and genitourinary procedures (see Chapter 7). The management of anticoagulation for those with a valve prosthesis is reviewed in Chapter 7.

Congestive heart failure—CHF is a big problem, and there has been little progress with its perioperative management. CHF increases the mortality of noncardiac surgery, and it is associated with longer hospitalization. The rate of readmission to hospital during the month after surgery is much higher. Experience suggests this often is because the patient is managed by the surgeon after the operation, and is discharged without his heart failure medicines. A patient with CHF might do better if an internist was actively involved, but that is not the usual pattern of practice in most hospitals (nor will Medicare pay for the service).

A patient with CHF should be at dry weight and well compensated at the time of surgery. Careful monitoring of fluid status and electrolytes is needed after surgery, and fluid overload avoided. That is the essence of perioperative management. Remember that low magnesium as well as potassium increases the risk of atrial and ventricular tachyarrhythmias after surgery (see Chapter 6). Magnesium often falls after large operations (the reason is uncertain, and I wonder if freshly cut tissue soaks up magnesium), and this may be aggravated by diuretic therapy.

There has been controversy about the use of pulmonary artery (PA) pressure monitoring in general, and none of the available trials has documented any benefit in the perioperative setting. On the contrary, patients having right heart catheterization fare slightly worse than those managed using clinical parameters (patient selection issues make this hard to sort out, but at least there is no clear benefit). The practice guidelines allow their perioperative use in high-risk patients, but do not require it.[1] Our heart failure team often uses hemodynamic monitoring and tailored therapy to tune a patient with decompensated CHF before noncardiac surgery. This includes aggressive treatment with vasodilators, inotropes, and diuretics, and, rarely, intra-aortic balloon pumping.

Isolated Right Heart Failure

Left Heart Failure

It is a conundrum—the patient with systemic congestion and altered left ventricular (LV) function who has never had pulmonary congestion. How can the cause of right heart failure be left heart failure if (clinically) there is no left heart failure? But it can occur in patients with a variety of left heart disorders, including low LVEF, LV diastolic dysfunction, or mitral stenosis.

The probable explanation is that there is a percentage of the population with hyperreactive pulmonary vasculature. When stressed with hypoxia or hemodynamic

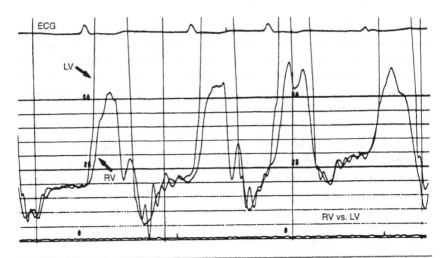

Figure 9.5 Simultaneous left and right ventricular (LV and RV) pressures in a patient with constrictive pericarditis. Normally, the left ventricular pressure is much higher than the right ventricular pressure during diastole, and identical pressure during diastole is a hallmark of both constriction and pericardial tamponade. In addition, this patient has the elderly diastolic pressure dip and then plateau that is typical of constriction (best seen in the first and last beats). (Reproduced by permission from Kern MJ. The Cardiac Catheterization Handbook. St. Louis: Mosby, 1999:203.)

overload these patients develop pulmonary hypertension. Because the PA clamps down, the pulmonary capillary bed is protected, and congestion develops proximal to it, but not in the lungs. The clinical picture is isolated right heart CHF.

Cor Pulmonale

While thinking of reactive pulmonary hypertension, we should revisit cor pulmonale (see Chapter 8). Not everyone with chronic lung disease gets it, and developing it requires lung disease plus susceptibility—probably a touchy pulmonary vasculature. The extreme example of this is primary pulmonary hypertension, a vasospastic disorder probably caused by endothelial dysfunction (see Chapter 8).

Pericardial Disease

Both pericardial tamponade and constriction limit cardiac filling. Consider them external causes of right heart failure. The right atrium (RA) and ventricle (RV) are compressed, and just cannot accommodate normal volume. This inadequate preload (as that is what it is) results in reduced stroke volume (see Chapter 2).

Clinically, acute tamponade causes a precipitous fall in blood pressure.[4] An example is cardiac rupture after MI (see Chapter 5). Subacute pericardial tamponade presents with symptoms of low cardiac output such as fatigue or weakness, and with systemic congestion.[5,6] On the other hand, when the pericardial effusion develops slowly the pericardium has time to stretch, and there may be no compression of the heart. That is often the case with the pericardial effusion of hypothyroidism, which can be massive. Constrictive pericarditis (Figure 9.5) usually develops slowly, with symptoms of low cardiac output and right heart failure.[7] We see one or two cases of cryptogenic cirrhosis and massive ascites a year on the liver transplant service that turn out to have constriction. Stripping the pericardium cures the liver disease.

A discussion of pericardial effusion and constriction is in Chapter 2.

Congenital Heart Disease Seen in Adults

We will review three topics: Eisenmenger's syndrome, because management can be tricky and primary care practitioners often follow patients with this condition; atrial septal defect (ASD), because it is common, easily missed and often encountered on board exams; and patent foramen ovale (PFO), as there has been renewed interest in it as a cause of peripheral embolism.[8,9]

Eisenmenger's Syndrome

Adults who are cyanotic and have congenital heart disease have Eisenmenger's syndrome, with pulmonary hypertension and possibly right heart failure.[10,11] The most common causes are ventricular septal defect (VSD), patent ductus arteriosus (PDA), transposition of the great vessels, and rarely, ASD. The size of the shunt is the key factor in developing pulmonary hypertension. About half of those with large VSD or PDA develop Eisenmenger's syndrome.

Lesions that transmit both high pressure and volume to the PA tend to provoke pulmonary hypertension, explaining why VSD and PDA are common causes. With these high-pressure lesions, pulmonary hypertension becomes fixed in infancy. ASD, which delivers high volume but not pressure to the PA, may rarely cause Eisenmenger's syndrome. In such cases, it develops later in life. As with other causes of isolated right heart failure, a susceptible pulmonary vasculature may be a requirement.

High pulmonary blood pressure leads to irreversible microvascular changes. Endothelial dysfunction, growth factors and platelet aggregation appear to contribute to intimal proliferation and progressive occlusion of small arterioles. Once these anatomic changes are present, high pulmonary vascular resistance is irreversible.

Eventually pulmonary resistance exceeds systemic resistance. The direction of shunting reverses, becoming right to left. Desaturated blood reaches the left heart, and the resulting arterial hypoxemia stimulates erythrocytosis.

Clinical presentation and management—Most patients have symptoms of low cardiac output, including fatigue and poor exercise tolerance. Right heart failure is common, and there may be an element of left heart congestion as well. The patient's appearance is striking, with central cyanosis and clubbed fingers. The cardiac exam reflects the underlying condition.

Erythrocytosis causing hyperviscosity is the major day-to-day management issue. Formerly we used frequent phlebotomy to keep the hematocrit under 65%. Targeting the hematocrit is not the current practice. Rather, the indication for phlebotomy is symptoms of hyperviscosity, including headache, irritability, lethargy, fatigue, dizziness, and visual disturbances. Most develop symptoms when the hematocrit approaches 70%, and the goal of phlebotomy is to reduce it below 65%. Simultaneous volume replacement with saline is needed.

Iron deficiency and microcytosis are common, especially with recurrent phlebotomy. The small red blood cells are rigid, do not deform normally, and thus do not pass through capillaries as easily. This contributes to sludging. When red cell indices indicate microcytosis, or there is low serum iron, iron therapy is needed (an apparent paradox in a patient with an elevated hematocrit).

There are a number of other complications of Eisenmenger's syndrome. With right-left shunting, paradoxical embolus is a possible cause of stroke. For the same reason, brain abscess may be a consequence of transient bacteremia. Stress is poorly tolerated. With pregnancy, maternal mortality is about 50%, and pregnancy is inadvisable. The perioperative mortality is high with noncardiac surgery. High altitude travel should be avoided, and commercial air transportation is best tolerated with the patient on supplemental oxygen. Although pressurized, airplane cabins do not have sea level pressures; there is an altitude effect.

Clinical course—The prognosis with Eisenmenger's syndrome is better than it is with other causes of pulmonary hypertension. Survival is 80% at 10 years, 77% at 15 years, and 42% at 25 years. Predictors of early mortality include syncope, elevated RV filling pressure and right heart failure, and more severe hypoxemia (an oxygen saturation less than 85% at rest). The location of the right-to-left shunt does not affect prognosis. Causes of death include ventricular fibrillation, heart failure, hemoptysis, stroke, brain abscess, thromboembolism, and complications of surgery or pregnancy.

Atrial Septal Defect

There are three possible sites of communication between the right and left atria. The most common defect (more than 80% of cases) is the ostium secundum ASD, located in the mid-septum, well above the atrioventricular valves.

The ostium primum defect (15% of cases) originates in the endocardial cushion, a structure in the center of the fetal heart that also contributes to the formation of the mitral and tricuspid valves and the upper part of the interventricular septum. The most extreme form of endocardial cushion defect is the absence of these structures, resulting in a single-chambered heart. With primum ASD, there may be cleft mitral or tricuspid leaflets and regurgitation. The interventricular conduction system also is affected, and left axis deviation (usually left anterior fascicular block) is a marker of primum ASD.

The sinus venosus defect is the least common ASD, occurring at the junction of either the superior or the inferior vena cava and right atrium.

The usual ASD is large, often 2 cm in diameter. Because of its size, there is no jet effect and little turbulence. Thus, the ASD itself does not generate a murmur. The large defect also means that pressures in the two atria are equal. Blood flows toward the RA because the RV is more compliant than the LV during diastole.

The major hemodynamic effects are RA, RV, and PA volume overload. When the catheterization report indicates a 2:1 shunt, it means that the pulmonary blood flow is twice the systemic blood flow, and that the RV is handling twice as much volume as the LV.

Increased pulmonary blood flow may provoke a rise in PA pressure, and a form of Eisenmenger's syndrome occurs in about 10% of patients, usually appearing in adolescence. The incidence of Eisenmenger's reaction with VSD or PDA is higher and the onset is younger. These conditions increase flow to the PA, but they also transmit systemic pressure (either LV or aortic systolic pressure) to the PA. The combination of high pressure and high flow is a stronger stimulus of pulmonary vascular reactivity.

Clinical presentation, laboratory evaluation, and treatment—ASD is often diagnosed late in life. Young adults are rarely symptomatic; the diagnosis may be made with routine physical examination or chest x-ray. Middle-aged patients usually present with atrial arrhythmias. Heart failure may develop as the initial symptom in older people. It would seem that the LV would be protected, but a common pattern is biventricular failure and not isolated RV failure.

This probably has to do with how the interventricular septum works. It has to choose sides, to work as a part of either the LV or RV. It chooses the side with the greater workload, normally the LV. With chronic RV overload, it works instead with the RV, moving away from the lateral wall of the LV rather than toward it during systole. This is the so-called *paradoxical septal motion* seen on the echocardiogram when there is RV overload. Loss of septal function may contribute to the eventual failure of the LV when there is chronic RV overload. In this case, chronic may mean five or six decades of abnormal cardiac loading before symptoms develop.

The physical findings of ASD are not subtle. S_2 is widely split, with no respiratory variation. Because of volume overload, emptying of the RV is delayed, and P_2 is late. The large ASD distributes the increased venous return to the heart during inspiration equally to both atria. Fixed splitting of S_2 is a reliable finding, and its absence excludes ASD.

There is usually a systolic murmur at the left base. This is not caused by flow across the ASD, but rather by high flow across the normal pulmonic valve (with a 2:1 shunt, the pulmonic valve has twice the normal flow). With a primum defect, a cleft mitral or tricuspid leaflet causes the typical regurgitant murmur.

The typical pattern of RV volume overload on the ECG is incomplete right bundle branch block, a usual finding with ASD. The primum defect causes left anterior fascicular block, and checking the QRS axis in a patient with ASD is a mark of clinical sophistication. Pulmonary plethora on the chest x-ray is always present, and experienced radiologists claim that it is not subtle (although I have a hard time seeing it). *A normal chest x-ray and ECG exclude significant right-left shunting and ASD.* (It is surprising how many doctors assume that the echocardiogram is needed to diagnose or exclude all structural heart disease.)

The echocardiogram confirms RV enlargement and paradoxical septal motion. The ASD is easily visualized, and flow across the defect may be documented with echocardiographic contrast agents and Doppler. In addition, the echo-Doppler study allows estimation of PA pressure.

Surgical repair of ASD is recommended when the pulmonary to systemic blood flow is above 1.5:1, especially when the RV size is increased. Surgery is not done to prevent pulmonary hypertension, a rare complication that develops before age 30 when it does occur. In middle age, repair is done to prevent atrial arrhythmias and eventual heart failure. There is a survival benefit with surgery even for patients older than 50 years, most of whom are symptomatic.

Since there is no jet effect, endocarditis prophylaxis is not indicated for ASD. A patient with primum ASD and mitral regurgitation needs antibiotic prophylaxis because of the valve lesion.

Patent Foramen Ovale and Embolic Stroke

Most *arterial emboli* originate from the left heart (atrial fibrillation or flutter, mitral stenosis, valve vegetations, dilated cardiomyopathy, atrial myxoma), or from aortic or large artery atheroma. With the Eisenmenger syndrome and right to left shunting across a cardiac lesion (i.e., VSD, PDA, or ASD), clot from leg veins may cross to the arterial circulation—so-called paradoxical embolization. One of the worst complications of Eisenmenger's is the passage of infected material from the venous circulation leading to brain abscess.

About 25% of us have incomplete closure of the foramen ovale at birth.[12] This communication between RA and LA is small and functionally insignificant. Higher pressure in the LA should cause any shunting to be left-to-right. The PFO can be an exception to this. Those of us who worked in the catheterization laboratory in the 1970s used green dye to test for shunts. With PFO, injection of the dye into a femoral vein results in the early appearance of a small amount of the dye in the arterial circulation (right-to-left shunting). Dye injected from the arm vein does not cross from right to left. The PFO seems to work as a baffle, shunting a tiny amount of the return from the inferior vena cava, from the RA to the LA (but it does not catch blood from the superior vena cava). It is possible for this baffle to catch small venous emboli, sending them to the arterial circulation.

Case-controlled studies have shown that the incidence of PFO is somewhat higher than usual in young patients who have had *cryptogenic stroke*, that is, stroke despite normal carotid arteries. The highest risk anatomy is PFO plus an associated atrial septum aneurysm. The aneurysm either increases the chance of interatrial shunting or provides a locus for thrombus formation. In a European study of patients who had cryptogenic stroke, those with PFO plus aneurysm had an almost fourfold increase in recurrent stroke during follow-up.[12]

The other element of the equation is a source of embolus. The diagnosis of paradoxical embolus is more believable if venous stasis or a hypercoagulable state is demonstrated.

Medical therapy for paradoxical embolism is anticoagulation with warfarin. Thus, it is treated like other illnesses where embolus originates from the heart, including atrial fibrillation and LV mural thrombus. (One exception to this is bacterial endocarditis; anticoagulation does not seem to prevent thromboembolism.)

An inability to take warfarin is an indication for surgical or catheter repair of the PFO.[12] Many advocate PFO closure for all patients, arguing that the catheter-based repair of PFO is safer than lifelong anticoagulation. New closure devices delivered by catheter are highly effective, but there are no data to support their use for all patients with stroke, PFO, normal carotid arteries, and no other apparent source of embolus. A randomized trial is in progress comparing anticoagulation and PFO closure in such patients with cryptogenic stroke.

Pregnancy and Heart Disease

Normal pregnancy leads to hemodynamic changes that increase the workload of the heart.[13] There is a 40% increase in maternal blood volume and cardiac output. Vasodilatation leads to a decline in both systemic vascular resistance and diastolic blood pressure. Pulse pressure and heart rate increase. These changes peak in the second trimester.

The cardiovascular system is thus hyperdynamic. With volume overload and increased rapid filling of the LV in early diastole, there may be an S_3 gallop. A heart murmur is common. Most patients have no structural abnormality; the murmur is the result of high flow across the pulmonic valve. Or what you think is a murmur may be a bruit from the breast. One of my teachers commented that the cardiac examination in a normal pregnant woman can sound like a washing machine. Murmurs with valve stenosis become louder with increased flow. On the other hand, the physical findings of mitral valve prolapse or hypertrophic subaortic stenosis may disappear with increased LV volume.

There are a number of cardiac illnesses that increase *maternal mortality* (Table 9.3). The risk increases with worsening functional class.[13] The highest risk conditions are considered contraindications to pregnancy. The usual medical indications for terminating pregnancy are pulmonary hypertension (PA pressure >50 mm Hg, either primary pulmonary hypertension or Eisenmenger's syndrome), dilated cardiomyopathy, Marfan's syndrome with marked aortic root dilatation, pulmonary arteriovenous fistulae, and any uncorrectable cardiac disease with class 3 or 4 symptoms that are refractory to medical therapy.[13]

There is concern about inheritance. The risk of transmitting Marfan's syndrome to the child is about 50% (it is autosomal dominant), and that is the case with familial hypertrophic cardiomyopathy as well (although the familial form is uncommon). For other congenital heart diseases with polygenic inheritance, the chance of a fetal abnormality is about 13%, roughly 12 times the risk in the

Table 9.3 Mortality Risk Associated with Heart Disease in Pregnancy	
Low risk (<1%)	Septal defects Patent ductus arteriosus Pulmonic, tricuspid valve lesions NYHA classes I and II
Moderate risk (5–15%)	NYHA class III or IV mitral stenosis Aortic stenosis Marfan's syndrome with a normal aortic root Uncomplicated coarctation of the aorta Prior myocardial infarction
High risk (25–50%)	Eisenmenger's syndrome Pulmonary hypertension Marfan's syndrome with a dilated aortic root History of peripartum cardiomyopathy

normal population.[13] This estimate is higher than the 5% that we quoted a decade ago, and it varies with different conditions. There are about 200 inherited conditions with associated heart disease, and 85 of them allow survival to the reproductive age. Genetic counseling is important when considering pregnancy.

Management

Arrhythmias may develop or worsen during pregnancy. However, most with preexisting arrhythmias tolerate pregnancy well. The first step in management is exclusion of correctible causes: electrolyte abnormalities, thyroid disease, alcohol, other drugs, caffeine, and smoking. Try to avoid drug therapy unless the arrhythmia is symptomatic, hemodynamically important or life-threatening. Digoxin, metoprolol, diltiazem, and quinidine may be used during pregnancy. Amiodarone is not safe (intrauterine growth retardation, thyroid dysfunction, fetal distress). Animal studies with high drug doses have raised concerns about most other available drugs. I am reluctant to begin antiarrhythmic therapy in the first trimester unless it is absolutely necessary. Low-moderate dose DC cardioversion is relatively safe for the fetus.

The usual indications for *anticoagulation* apply for those with atrial fibrillation and *valve prostheses.* Heparin is safer for the baby while warfarin is safer for the mother. Warfarin crosses the placenta and may cause a variety of defects, including cerebral hemorrhage, fetal wasting, optic atrophy, mental retardation, etc. The highest risk is from conception to the 14th week, and risk increases with the dose of warfarin.[13] There are no clear guidelines for management, and some recommend subcutaneous heparin during the first trimester, then switching to warfarin. Unfortunately, unfractionated heparin twice daily does not provide full anticoagulation, and has been associated with embolism from valve prostheses. There is little experience with low-molecular-weight heparin, and teratogenic effects are possible.[14] One small trial was complicated by thrombosis of a valve prosthesis, but the dose of LMW heparin was not increased as the mother's weight increased. The role of this therapy is uncertain.

Severe LV dysfunction is a contraindication to pregnancy. Those with advanced heart failure—functional class 3 or 4—have a significant mortality risk, and termination of pregnancy should be considered.[13,15] The usual treatment principles for heart failure apply. The one exception is angiotensin-converting enzyme (ACE) inhibitors (and probably receptor blockers); fetal renal dysfunction is common. In fact, ACE inhibitor therapy during early pregnancy may be an indication for therapeutic abortion. Calcium channel blockers and/or hydralazine are preferred for afterload reduction.

Endocarditis prophylaxis is suggested as an option during vaginal delivery for highest risk patients, although most prescribe it for these conditions: complex congenital disease, a prosthetic valve, previous endocarditis, a surgically created arteriovenous shunt, valve disease including mitral valve prolapse with regurgitation and/or thickened leaflets.[4] It is not required for ASD, previously repaired VSD, PDA or a functional heart murmur (with a no apparent structural abnormality on the echocardiogram).

For most patients, vaginal delivery at the 38th week is safer than cesarean section. The one exception may be Marfan's syndrome. Immediately after delivery, pressure on the inferior vena cava is relieved increasing venous return to the heart. This auto-transfusion effect may aggravate cardiac symptoms. Cardiac output may remain above pre-pregnancy levels for weeks, especially if the mother is breast-feeding.

Peripartum Cardiomyopathy

This form of dilated cardiomyopathy affects women with no previous heart disease.[16] It may occur in the last month of pregnancy or during the first 6 months postpartum; peak incidence is 1 to 2 months postpartum.

The cause is unknown. It is more common in black women, and the highest incidence is in Africa. Other risk factors for developing cardiomyopathy are maternal age older than 30 years, multiparity, twin pregnancy, malnutrition, hypertension, or toxemia of pregnancy. It recurs in 50% with subsequent pregnancies, even when LV function has returned to normal. A second episode often is worse than the first, and possibly fatal, especially for those who do not have complete recovery of LVEF.[17] Most consider postpartum cardiomyopathy a reason to avoid future pregnancy.

The treatment includes standard therapy for heart failure (see Chapter 1). An exception is ACE inhibitors and angiotensin receptor blockers, which affect the fetal kidneys and should be avoided during pregnancy. Hydralazine and/or calcium channel blockers are safer prepartum afterload reducers.

More than half of the patients recover. The prognosis is good for those with normalization of LV size and ejection fraction within 6 months. Clinical features indicating a worse prognosis are onset of symptoms late after delivery, severe depression of LVEF, marked LV enlargement, and new left bundle branch block.

End-of-Life Decisions and Palliative Care for Patients with Heart Disease

You will observe a general reluctance to give up on the patient with heart disease. There is always the possibility of one more interventional procedure. Scientific medicine's central ethic is prolongation of life, and aggressive therapy often is life-saving. But there is a dilemma when life-prolonging surgery seems too aggressive for an elderly or severely disabled person. This is especially true for the patient who has had multiple cardiac procedures in the past.

The first step in resolving the dilemma is considering the patient's wishes. The new medical ethics, which has evolved in recent decades, is based on patient autonomy. As doctors we do not have unquestioned control over what happens to patients. Instead, our responsibility is to inform, recommend alternatives, and then to respect and support the patient's decision. This means that when we are old and sick no one can make us do something we do not want. It is what we want for ourselves, and it should be what we want for our patients.

Even so, surveys of elderly patients and their families document concern about inappropriate and aggressive care at the end of life. Old people often feel that they are convinced to have procedures they do not want.

Peaceful Death, Another Goal of Medicine

In addition to prolonging life and relieving suffering, at some stage of our lives the goal of medical care is a peaceful death. We wince at the spectacle of the hopelessly ill old person subjected to the savagery of a prolonged intensive care unit death.

The trend in scientific medicine has been the elimination of illnesses that are rapidly fatal. What remains are conditions like dementia, stroke, and heart failure. I occasionally encounter a chronically ill, elderly person who has decided to reclaim the traditional old man's friends by declining curative treatment for acute illnesses such as pneumonia, heart attack, or urosepsis. This usually meets resistance from the doctor. However, an autonomous person has the right to refuse any treatment, whether it is antibiotics for pneumonia or chemotherapy for advanced cancer.

This is not an argument against life-prolonging therapy for old people. Indeed, treatment known to prolong life should be applied irrespective of age, *if that is what the patient wants*. Instead, you should support your patient who has decided to avoid possibly life-prolonging but *unwanted* therapy. (That would include surgical correction of aortic stenosis, an implanted defibrillator after MI or any cardiac intervention.)

If you do not convince your patient to accept a cure, are you are in some way responsible for the resulting death? If you believe that you are, you have fallen prey to the doctor's delusion of control over life and death. In matter of fact, a terminally ill patient dies of a disease. Our intervention affects only the timing and the amount of suffering. By avoiding life-prolonging therapy at the patient's direction, the doctor is not responsible for death, nor is the patient. Daniel Callahan develops this line of reasoning in *The Troubled Dream of Life*, and I recommend it to you and your patients.[18]

Palliative Care

Those with terminal heart failure or CAD should have aggressive medical therapy, as it relieves symptoms. When usual drug therapies become ineffective, it helps to involve hospice.[19]

Current federal regulations provide for hospice care if survival is estimated to be less than 6 months, and patients with advanced heart disease meet this criterion. Hospice nurses are good at regulating heart failure therapy. Their day-to-day adjustment of diuretics and other medicines may allow the patient to remain at home, out of the hospital. For those with heart disease, hospice care often leads to dramatic improvement of symptoms, so much so that it is possible to discontinue hospice (at least for awhile). This has been observed for those with advanced lung disease as well.

Morphine—Morphine is the key addition to end-stage care when standard therapy no longer controls cardiac symptoms. As a venodilator, it reduces blood return to the heart and relieves pulmonary congestion. In addition, it blunts the anxiety that comes with severe dyspnea.

There is concern that morphine may depress respiration. In practice, with all but extreme doses, this is rare for patients with pulmonary edema (or with severe dyspnea in advanced lung disease).

Oral morphine (Roxanol) may control symptoms, and it can be supplemented with a nebulized preparation. Parenteral morphine is more difficult to administer in the outpatient setting. Hospice nurses have experience with the opioids—more than most physicians—and can competently regulate even parenteral use for patients with heart failure or intractable angina. A brief inpatient stay may help with determining the effective dose.

Rest therapy—Another option for those with uncontrolled angina or advanced heart failure is reduced activity, a bed-to-chair lifestyle. This was a common approach before the 1960s. I was introduced to it by a master clinician of that era, Dr. Julian Beckwith. At times it is still appropriate. Don't get me wrong; I am convinced of the value of exercise therapy for CAD and CHF. But there comes a time when it may not work, and reduced activity offers palliation. Some elderly patients prefer this alternative to open heart surgery.

Extreme symptoms in the terminal patient—What can we do for a patient with end-stage disease who comes to the emergency department with extreme symptoms? A common issue is pulmonary edema unresponsive to intravenous diuretics. It is unfortunate when the doctor offers (or demands) intubation and mechanical ventilation to control congestion. Despite a previous decision to avoid ventilator therapy, a desperate patient and family may have a change of mind when this seems the only chance for relief.

An effective alternative is higher dose morphine, titrated to relieve dyspnea. There may be depression of respiration with a dose sufficient to relieve symptoms. In this case the moral imperative is to provide relief of suffering for the dying patient, even if high-dose opiates contribute to more rapid death. There is no culpability. This is not assisted suicide or euthanasia, but rather necessary therapy for extreme symptoms.[19,20]

References

1. Eagle KA, Berger PB, Calkins H, et al. AC C/AHA guideline update for perioperative cardiovascular evaluation for noncardiac surgery—executive summary. J Am Coll Cardiol 2002;39:542–553.

2. Eagle KA, Coley CM, Newell JB, et al. Combining clinical and thallium data optimizes preoperative assessment of cardiac risk before major vascular surgery. Ann Intern Med 1989;110:859–866.

3. Mangano DT, Layug EL, Wallace A, Tateo I. Effects of atenolol on mortality and cardiovascular morbidity after noncardiac surgery. Multicenter Study of Perioperative Ischemia Research Group. N Engl J Med 1996;335:1713–1720.

4. Spodick DH. Acute cardiac tamponade. N Engl J Med 2003;349:684–690.

5. Myers RB, Spodick DH. Constrictive pericarditis: clinical and pathophysiologic characteristics. Am Heart J 1999;138:219–232.

6. Swami A, Spodick DH. Pulsus paradoxus in cardiac tamponade: a pathophysiologic continuum. Clin Cardiol 2003;26:215–217.

7. Garcia MJ. Constriction vs. restriction: how to evaluate. ACC Curr J Rev 2003;12:49–52.

8. Deanfield J, Thaulow E, Warnes C, et al. Management of grown up congenital heart disease. Eur Heart J 2003;24:1035–1084.

9. Therrien J, Webb G. Clinical update on adults with congenital heart disease. Lancet 2003;362:1305–1313.

10. Perloff JK, Warnes CA. Challenges posed by adults with repaired congenital heart disease. Circulation 2001;103:2637–2643.

11. Vongpatanasin W, Brickner ME, Hillis LD, Lange RA. The Eisenmenger syndrome in adults. Ann Intern Med 1998;128:745–755.

12. Castello R, Brott TG. Patent foramen ovale: friend or foe? J Am Coll Cardiol 2003;42:1073–1075.

13. Gei, AF, Hankins GD. Cardiac disease and pregnancy. Obstet Gynecol Clin North Am 2001;28:465–512.

14. Hung L, Rahimtoola SH. Prosthetic heart valves and pregnancy. Circulation 2003;107:1240–1246.

15. Avila WS, Rossi EG, Ramires JA, et al. Pregnancy in patients with heart disease: experience with 1,000 cases. Clin Cardiol 2003;26:135–142.

16. de Beus E, van Mook WN, Ramsay G, et al. Peripartum cardiomyopathy: a condition intensivists should be aware of. Intensive Care Med 2003;29:167–174.

17. Elkayam U, Tummala PP, Rao K, et al. Maternal and fetal outcomes of subsequent pregnancies in women with peripartum cardiomyopathy. N Engl J Med 2001;344:1567–1571.

18. Callahan D. The Troubled Dream of Life. New York: Simon and Schuster, 1993.

19. Taylor GJ, Kurent JE. A Clinician's Guide to Palliative Care. Malden: Blackwell Publishing, 2003.

20. Johnson-Neely K, Crammer LM. End-of-life care: palliative strategies for vomiting and dyspnea. Fam Prac Recert 1998;20:13–22.

INDEX

Note: Page numbers followed by *f* refer to figures; page number followed by *t* refer to tables; page numbers followed by *b* refers to boxes.